Meditation in Psychiatry and General Medicine

Jeong-Ho Chae • Hwa-Young Lee
Editors

Meditation in Psychiatry and General Medicine

Springer

Editors
Jeong-Ho Chae
Department of Psychiatry
The Catholic University of Korea
Seoul, Korea (Republic of)

Hwa-Young Lee
Department of Psychiatry
Soonchunhyang University
Cheonan, Korea (Republic of)

ISBN 978-981-95-7146-8 ISBN 978-981-95-7147-5 (eBook)
https://doi.org/10.1007/978-981-95-7147-5

This Springer imprint is published by the registered company Springer Nature Singapore Pte Ltd.
The registered company address is: 152 Beach Road, #21-01/04 Gateway East, Singapore 189721, Singapore

Preface

In a world where the pace of life seems to accelerate endlessly and the pressures of modern living take their toll on our health and happiness, it's more crucial than ever to explore the synergies between traditional medicine and ancient contemplative practices.

In recent years, there has been a surge of interest in meditation as a panacea for all manner of health woes. From stress and anxiety to chronic pain and insomnia, proponents of meditation tout its myriad benefits, often presenting it as a cure-all for the ailments of modern life. Yet, as we delve deeper into this trend, it becomes increasingly apparent that the reality is far more nuanced.

As practitioners deeply rooted in both the spiritual and scientific realms, we have observed with both fascination and concern the growing popularity of meditation as a catch-all solution for health promotion. While we hold a profound reverence for the spiritual heritage of meditation and acknowledge its potential to enhance well-being, we are also acutely aware of the limitations and complexities that arise when attempting to apply ancient practices to modern healthcare.

This book represents an exploration into the harmonious relationship between two seemingly disparate realms: the art and science of medicine and the profound practice of meditation.

As physicians with a deep appreciation for the complexities of the human body and mind, we have witnessed firsthand the incredible advancements in medical science that have revolutionized the way we diagnose, treat, and prevent disease. However, we have also come to recognize the limitations of a purely mechanistic approach to health—one that often overlooks the interconnectedness of mind, body, and spirit. Conversely, as practitioners of meditation, we have experienced the transformative power of these ancient practices to cultivate inner peace, resilience, and compassion. Through meditation, we can tap into a wellspring of wisdom and healing that lies dormant within each of us, transcending the boundaries of our physical bodies to connect with something greater than ourselves.

Medicine and meditation are two distinct approaches to health and well-being, each with its own principles, methods, and benefits. Medicine refers to the practice of diagnosing, treating, and preventing diseases and injuries using pharmaceuticals, medical procedures, and other interventions. It is based on scientific research, clinical trials, and evidence-based practices. Modern medicine encompasses various fields such as allopathic, alternative medicine, and integrative medicine, which combines conventional and complementary approaches. On the other hand, meditation is a mind-body practice that involves training the mind to focus, cultivate awareness, and achieve a state of mental clarity, relaxation, and inner peace. It has been practiced for thousands of years in various cultures and spiritual traditions. While medicine primarily targets physical symptoms and illnesses, meditation addresses the mental, emotional, and spiritual aspects of health. However, there is growing evidence that meditation can also have physiological benefits, such as reducing stress, lowering blood pressure, improving immune function, and promoting overall well-being. In some cases, medicine and meditation can complement each other. Several integrative meditation techniques with conventional medical treatment help manage chronic pain, anxiety, depression, and other health conditions. Similarly, some hospitals and healthcare providers offer integrative medicine programs that combine conventional treatments with meditation to support patients' holistic health.

Especially, in the field of psychiatry, we confront the complexities of the human mind—the intricate interplay of thoughts, emotions, behaviors, and experiences. As psychiatrists, therapists, and mental health professionals, we are tasked with understanding and alleviating the suffering that arises from mental illness and emotional distress. In recent years, there has been a growing recognition of the role that contemplative practices, particularly mindfulness meditation, can play in promoting mental health and well-being. Meditation offers a unique pathway to healing—one that goes beyond the traditional approaches of pharmacotherapy and psychotherapy to address the underlying roots of suffering at their core.

Drawing on insights from neuroscience, psychology, and contemplative traditions, the concept of "mindful healing" in this book explores the integration of meditation into psychiatric practice. Unfortunately, while we don't have enough rigorous scientific and empirical evidence yet, this book may offer a comprehensive framework for understanding how meditation can complement existing psychiatric treatments and enhance therapeutic outcomes. We hope this book provides a roadmap for harnessing the power of meditation to promote healing and transformation.

While this is a new challenge for our current understanding, there will be future work to reinforce the following more important factors. Despite the widespread enthusiasm for meditation as a therapeutic intervention, the empirical evidence supporting its efficacy for various health conditions remains limited and often inconclusive. We will explore the gaps in our understanding of how meditation works, who it benefits most, and its potential risks and limitations. Health problems are rarely isolated phenomena but rather multifaceted manifestations of biological, psychological, social, and environmental factors. We will examine the limitations of a reductionist approach that attempts to address complex health issues solely through meditation, overlooking the broader context of modern healthcare. As meditation has gained mainstream popularity, it has also become increasingly commodified, marketed as a consumer product promising instant relief from life's challenges. We will interrogate the commercial forces driving the meditation industry and the implications for individual well-being and societal values.

Meditation practices are deeply embedded within cultural, religious, and philosophical traditions, each with its own unique worldview and ethical framework. We will explore the dangers of decontextualizing meditation from its spiritual roots and appropriating it for secular, therapeutic purposes without regard for its broader implications. While acknowledging the potential benefits of meditation in promoting health and well-being, we will advocate for a more nuanced and balanced approach—one that integrates meditation into a broader toolkit of evidence-based interventions, respects individual differences and preferences, and acknowledges the inherent complexities of human health and healing.

Even with these unresolved issues, in "Meditation and Medicine" we invite you on a journey of exploration and discovery—one that bridges the gap between the tangible world of medicine and the intangible realm of meditation. Drawing on the latest scientific research, as well as timeless wisdom from contemplative traditions around the globe, this book offers practical insights and tools for integrating meditation into your healthcare routine. Whether you're a healthcare professional seeking to enhance your patient care practices, a patient looking for holistic approaches to healing, or simply a curious seeker on the path to greater well-being, this book is intended to be a guide and companion on your journey. Through its pages, may you find inspiration, guidance, and the wisdom to cultivate harmony and balance in your life.

The fact that this book was written by authors trained in Western-derived medicine in Korea, a country with a long tradition of Eastern meditation, is particularly encouraging in terms of integrating the East and West, past and present. As we embark on this journey together, our hope is that this book will serve as a catalyst for critical reflection and dialogue, challenging prevailing narratives and inviting readers to explore the intersection of spirituality and science with open minds and discerning hearts.

With humility, curiosity, and a commitment to truth-seeking, on behalf of all the authors who contributed to this book.

Seoul, Republic of Korea — Jeong-Ho Chae
Cheonan, Republic of Korea — Hwa-Young Lee

About the Translator

Hanul Jun graduated with a Master of Arts in Asian Languages and Cultures from the University of Michigan in 2017, where his primary focus was on Buddhist meditation practice. During his undergraduate studies, he initially pursued a major in psychology before switching to Buddhist studies.

He has worked on several translation projects, including *Samatha, Jhana, and Vipassana Practice at the Pa-Auk Monastery: A Meditator's Experience*, published by Wisdom Publications in 2018, and *Buddhist Psychotherapy: Wisdom from Early Buddhist Teaching*, published by Springer in 2021. He is also a contributing author for *Hyecho's Journey: The World of Buddhism,* originally published by the University of Chicago Press in 2017.

He has been practicing mindfulness meditation for over 20 years, having been ordained as a novice monk in Myanmar for 3 months in 2002, and as a fully ordained bhikkhu for 3 months in 2013. Throughout the years, he has traveled to many countries to learn about different traditions of Buddhist meditation, including Korean Seon meditation (Zen), Tibetan meditation, and Theravada Vipassanā meditation. He has taught meditation at various youth camps in both the United States and Korea.

Currently, he is a Program Manager at Google in Seattle, Washington, where he continues to lead bi-weekly guided mindfulness meditation sessions. He is also an active member in various Buddhist and meditation communities in the area, including the Seattle Insight Meditation Society (SIMS) and Clear Mountain Monastery.

Contents

1 Introduction

Hoon-dong Choe

Meditation is a mental health therapy that has its origins in the East since ancient times, while psychotherapy is a mental health therapy from the West. Meditation is the practice of objectively observing changes that arise inside oneself, and the key to the practice is seeing things as they are without assigning any meaning, interpretation, or judgment. When you first start paying attention to breathing, it is difficult to maintain focus on the breath as it is difficult to concentrate in the beginning. You focus on each movement of the body as it occurs, and when thoughts arise, you recognize clearly that they have arisen. You observe how thoughts arise and pass away, and how sensations arise and pass away. You become free from all attachments when practicing meditation in this way, and your mind becomes calm when you are liberated from anxiety, anger, and sensual desire. Once you reach a state where you are one with the object and then recognize that you are connected with everything, you become compassionate and wise.

What meditation and psychotherapy share in common is introspection. Meditation involves turning your attention to focus on what is happening inside rather than what is 'out there.' When facing discomfort, people usually exert their energy to resist, criticize, correct, or avoid it. Suffering arises not from the things that happen in one's life, but due to the belief in the stories that one creates based on the things that occur in one's life. The people who maintain their inner strength even after going through tremendous suffering are those who recognize they are nervous and are aware of the stories instead of creating them. Looking into yourself, paying attention to your inner monologues, and recognizing your suffering lead to a healing effect. Both mediation and psychotherapy allow you to see a distorted reality as it is, which makes your mind free and peaceful.

What all spiritual traditions of the East and West have in common is the practice of meditation. Here, spirituality refers to progressing towards a transcendent consciousness by looking into oneself, particularly one's unconscious, and finding happiness not from the outside but from within. There is no difference between how people in ancient and modern times deal with mental pain. Meditation has been critical to resolving pain within one's mind, passed down from ancient shamans to priests, monks, all the way to modern psychotherapists. Meditation finds its solution from within, not from the outside. It is also not exclusive to monks or yogis. Even the Desert Fathers or Sufi Sheikhs practiced meditation. Meditation is not a method of a particular religion, but can be considered as the essence and path to pursuing spirituality for all religions.

H.-d. Choe (✉)
Korean Academy of Meditational Medicine,
Seoul, Republic of Korea

J.-H. Chae, H.-Y. Lee (eds.), *Meditation in Psychiatry and General Medicine*,
https://doi.org/10.1007/978-981-95-7147-5_1

The pure lotus in a dirty pond symbolizes religious transcendence where one reaches purity and salvation in one's life without leaving the secular world. Within the awakening through meditation is unconditional purity and salvation. Being awake at this very moment, it is a salvation described as 'already arrived' or 'already at home'. It is dwelling in a world of light by being fully awake in this moment rather than being saved at some point in the far future. On the other hand, not being awake in this moment is being shrouded in darkness and drowned in the impulses of the unconscious. If you act unconsciously and live by impulse, your life will become difficult as if you are wandering around in the dark, constantly bumping into things. If you are always awake in observing each of your actions, and you reflect on and carefully watch over your intentions and their context, the darkness will turn into light and you will become happy. When we breathe fully awake, we feel the nature that surrounds us and the stars in the night sky become one with us. In addition, all of humanity with whom we share blood throughout the countless ages becomes one family and one body. Just as we are not separate from our food or the air that we breathe in and out, we are not separate from the water, rivers, clouds, mountains, winds, and flowers.

The barbarism of a body that bites and rips at itself is darkness, whereas sharing love and compassion even with complete strangers is light. The core of meditation and training the mind is to turn impulsive barbarism to controlled maturity, stiffness into softness. Taming the mind like that of a wild bronco cannot occur on its own without making an effort to train the mind. The transition from darkness to light is the nature of all salvation and is spirituality itself. It signifies the transition from despair to hope, from ignorance to enlightenment, from conflict to tranquility, from suffering to happiness. This major transformation is only possible through self-reflection. Salvation is not granted from the outside, but must be obtained by oneself, and true salvation is not the resurrection of one's body, but the rebirth and spiritual purification of one's mind. Once spirituality is attained, it transcends language, and even the differences between religions lose their meaning in the face of spirituality. Once we understand that separating religions into 'my religion' and 'your religion' is akin to children fighting with one another, arguing about dogma or the superiority of religion becomes very childish, and the only important problem that remains is the inability for us to love and understand each other.

When asking what the purpose of meditation is, one must first ask whether one's mind is peaceful and happy. Proper meditation is a journey that takes you to a place free from pain, so if pain returns, it is not true meditation. It is like muddy water, which appears clear when the mud sinks and settles, but becomes murky again when it is shaken up. If concentration meditation (samathā) is calmly settling the mind down, then insight meditation (vipassanā) is completely burning all of its scraps on the bottom until there is nothing left. In meditation, one sees calm within movement and movement within calm. It includes both macroscopic and microscopic observation and involves contemplating and reflecting on the full context.

Meditation dismantles concepts so that one can experience reality as it is. The essence of meditation is emptying out any learned knowledge or belief. It is completely empty and quiet, yet it conceives all things. The silence of calmness is immovable and unshakeable. However, it is a calmness that is extremely bright and limitless. So long as we are armed with the clouds of faith, what we cannot encounter is like the reason why we cannot see the sky through the clouds. A world that is perceived and understood through concepts is different from reality. The state of pure consciousness before perception is a place of unconditional love and compassion. The aim of meditation is ultimate peace and happiness. Therefore, the main method of meditation is a deep introspection and reflection on suffering. It is difficult to arrive at an understanding of the hidden aspects of suffering simply through concentration and observation. To do this, one must reflect on it and look into it deeply by shining the light of wisdom onto it. The destination of meditation points to a place beyond language and thought. However, one can only enter this place through meditative contemplation.

Once you realize through contemplation and insight that your belief in 'self' consists of an interaction of various processes that occur every moment in the body and mind, you come to understand that there is no self to cling onto. If we take the act of walking as an example, it occurs through a symbiotic interaction of the body and mind. To walk, there is first the intention to take a step. Then there is the knowledge of lifting your foot, pushing it forward, setting it back down, and then lifting the other foot. Walking stops when there is an intention to stop. Thinking of this as 'I walked' or 'I took a step' is simply just a concept. Strictly speaking, there is no separation between an action and the person performing the action. The mind is the cause of bodily motions, and bodily sensations give rise to desire in the mind and serve as the cause of our intentions. The concept of 'self' is the most deeply rooted concept. We come to believe that the conceptual self is real under the idea that it is something eternal and the essence of our being. Through this, we believe there is such a thing as 'mine' or 'myself' and identify the various functions of the body and mind as 'me.' We exert a lot of energy defending and protecting an imaginary self and devote our efforts to satisfy this self physically and mentally. Meditation helps us realize that this imaginary self does not actually exist. It helps us see clearly that this 'self' is just a concept, a shadow, and that all we are doing is identifying the various phenomena that arise moment to moment as 'self'.

In this way, meditation is awakening from the cocoon that we call 'self,' much like a caterpillar transforms into a butterfly. There is no psychological awakening without the awakening of wisdom. True awakening goes beyond thought and contemplation and is attained through contextual thinking and insight of 'cause followed by cause.' This contemplative meditation is what is known as the Buddha's theory of dependent origination (paṭiccasamuppāda, 緣起觀). By taking suffering as your teacher, you become awakened, and suffering becomes a blessing. If your enemy becomes your benefactor, you will have no choice but to love them. This is spiritual transformation. Through meditation, one breaks through the ontological perspective that treats the constantly dynamic and changing phenomena in life as fixed entities. The dismantling of concept is the dismantling of existence, and it connects one to experience, joy, and life itself. Rather than struggling with the ebbs and flows of life, you enjoy riding its waves. Rather than trying to remove or change one's body and mind, you take care of and respect them.

The peak of meditation is pure concentration and gentle insight. Concentration and insight, the two wings of meditation, combined with wisdom, the body, rise up as the ultimate solution to suffering. Through concentration one attains peace and calmness of the mind, and through insight one becomes connected with wisdom, leading to clear enlightenment. When the practice involving quiet thought and deep introspection emphasizes thoughtlessness (無念無想) partially, it is called concentration meditation (samathā), and when it involves dynamically contemplating all of the processes of the body and mind, it is called insight meditation (vipassanā). When the practice involves reaching enlightenment by deeply contemplating oneself, it is called wisdom meditation or contemplative meditation. Just as a blind person describes an elephant by touching each part of its body, emphasizing one external form of mediation becomes various forms of meditation.

On the basis of unconditional love and compassion towards the world, meditation is quite in line with the humanistic approach to medicine. While being central to all religions, meditation is at the same time both scientific in that it transcends religion by being neutral to all beliefs, and medical in that it treats the body and mind. Meditation helps cultivate a nondiscriminatory respect and compassion for life, which are qualities that a medical professional should possess. While based on the principle of reciprocity between body and mind, where one treats the mind with the body and treats the body with the mind, meditation at the same time also transcends the structure of the body and mind. Already proven through experiments in quantum mechanics, the infinite and shining transcendent consciousness goes beyond the duality of matter and mind. Consciousness is the foundation of all existence (the universe). When Heisenberg observed the inside of an atom in 1920, he discovered that it is impossible to completely separate the observer from the object of observation. What he found is that objects that appear to be distinct (such as a desk, chair, a person, or a star) are all closely connected with each other at the atomic level. The feeling that things are separate is just an illusion. No reality can be explained while excluding consciousness. We are all connected to each other within the larger universe. Within the core of existence is consciousness. Neither particle science nor brain science can completely explain a consciousness that is outside of the body, brain, or mind. Meditation will become the protector of the humanistic foundations of medicine within modern society that has become dehumanized under the influence of materialistic and scientific trends and within medical science that is being replaced by artificial intelligence.

Meditation speaks of healing while medicine speaks of curing. Meditation calls for inaction and follows the flow of nature. Medicine often goes against nature and boasts of the superiority of artificial manipulation. This is similar to the way that humans have harmed nature. The key to healing is the inherent inner power of life, while the key to curing is a person prescribing a cure or a method of treatment. Healing cannot arise without the function of life's energy even through medicine or (either physical or mental) procedures. The source of life is love. As Laozi (老子) once said, meditation follows the principles of 'creating but not possessing' (生而不有) and 'cultivating but not controlling' (長而不宰). Rather than exerting energy to try and manipulate or fix things, one acknowledges, accepts, and embraces things as they are. One does not stay or cling to things, but lets them go so they can flow. Rather than judging, evaluating, or reacting with attachment or aversion, one observes what is happening with compassion. The source of healing is unlimited love. The universe is full of the energy of love. Death and destruction are the results of artificial manipulation and the obsession with possession.

That meditation reminds us of Buddhism shows how important it is to Buddhism. In fact, this is because the Buddha, who criticized the religious and ceremonial behavior of the Brahmans that preceded Buddhism by saying they 'bathe without water,' emphasized the importance of studying the mind. Therefore, Buddhism cast aside all hints of religion from the very beginning and emphasized the cultivation of one's mind, which also facilitated the systematization of yogic meditation and contributed to the establishment of Hinduism. The meditation that was introduced to the West was developed in a scientific framework, and it is currently actively being introduced to Korea. It is thanks in large part to the rational approach of the West that meditation has become popular amongst the masses and is considered as something that can be practiced by any ordinary person rather than being some mystical practice of ascetics. However, in order to preserve the tradition of the East, the original form of meditation must be preserved and passed on.

In this book, the authors attempt to cover not only the history of meditation and its various forms, but also its anthropological considerations and the achievements of psychiatry brought about through modern brain research. While the mental aspect of the body has been explained thoroughly through brain research, this book attempts to present that the spiritual dimension is inherent to the human consciousness through more nature (mind-based) or psychological research. Through the emergence of psychoanalysis, analytical psychology, and transpersonal psychiatry (psychology) that accepts meditation, it was possible to establish a relationship between psychology and meditation, and furthermore, a relationship between meditation and spirituality. At the apex of the human mind is a level of consciousness where all borders and conceptual limitations disappear and individual consciousness is transcended, just as spirituality is both the pursuit of religious nature and that which transcends it, and meditation, which is both a religious tradition and a secular practice. Christian practices of contemplation and physiognomy should also be considered carefully. Additionally, Xinxue (心學) of Confucianism that appears in "The Great Learning (大學)" and "The Doctrine of the Middle Way (中庸)" as well as inaction (doing nothing) of Laozi (老子) and Zhuangzi (莊子) are based on meditation and are therefore the subjects of future research. Although the book attempts to cover the entire relationship between meditation and psychiatry as well as psychology and religion, admittedly the authors who have all majored in medicine are unable to fully experience the essence of the East. However, we hope that this book will become a useful guide to anyone who wishes to pursue meditation-based medicine by shedding light on meditation from a variety of unbiased perspectives and by allowing the reader to see modern academic accomplishments at a glance. Based on this, we hope that more extensive and deeper medical research will continue to be conducted, and that more refined textbooks on meditation-based medicine will continue to be published.

2 The History of Meditation

Sungwon Jung

'Through meditation, one obtains wisdom, otherwise one will remain ignorant. One should clearly know what leads them forward and what holds them back.'

—Sakyamuni

Meditation is a method of self-reflection where one observes objectively, taking oneself out of subjective perspectives and immersing oneself in their inner self. Meditation is used to purify the mind, reduce stress, promote rest, and train the mind. Meditation techniques include repeating mantras in a quiet environment or observing one's breath. It is said to have been practiced for about 5000 years. Initially, it mainly referred to the practices of Hinduism or Buddhism that originated in India, but as time passed, its meaning gradually expanded to encompass the specialized spiritual practices of various religions. Following the nineteenth century and with the rise of counter-cultural and New Age movements due to events such as the World Wars, Westerners began to take an interest in Eastern philosophy. As a result, meditation gradually became popularized and spread from Asia to Western cultures.

The History of the Word Meditation

Meditation means to calmly close one's eyes and think deeply. In English, it carries meanings such as 'to think deeply' or 'to plan.' In Chinese, the term 'meditation' is written as '瞑想' (míngxiǎng) or 冥想 (míngxiǎng). Meditation can be used to mean 'to close one's eyes (瞑) and think calmly (想),' and 'to quiet (冥) one's mind(想).' In Eastern Philosophy, the meaning 'to still one's thoughts' may be more appropriate, but in reality, both meanings are achieved within the same context. After one concentrates the mind and arrives at a state where they can think deeply and calmly, they can even reach the point where their thoughts cease entirely. The Eastern concept of meditation can be seen as primarily a static concept that puts emphasis on calming one's thoughts, while the Western concept includes a more dynamic concept of thinking. The concept of meditation originates from ancient India, and was derived from the Aryans who resided in the upper reaches of the Ganges River. Meditation is thought to have originated from the meaning of 'dhyāna' (a state of being fully immersed in an object without any distractions) that the Aryans strived to attain. As this concept of meditation crossed over into China, it was translated both phonetically and semantically. In the case of its phonetic translation, the sound of the Sanskrit word 'dhyāna' was translated as 'chánnà' (禪那), which was then abbreviated as 'chán' or Zen (禪). In the case of its semantic translation based on meaning of the word 'dhyāna,' it was translated into Chinese as 'dìng' (定), and also as 'jìnglǜ' (靜慮), 'sīwéixiū' (思惟修) 'qì è' (棄惡), and 'gōngdélín' (功德林). Here 'jìnglǜ' (靜慮) means to contemplate

S. Jung (✉)
Department of Psychiatry, Keimyung University School of Medicine, Daegu, Republic of Korea

J.-H. Chae, H.-Y. Lee (eds.), *Meditation in Psychiatry and General Medicine*,
https://doi.org/10.1007/978-981-95-7147-5_2

the true nature of reality and to think calmly to keep the mind from being disturbed, 'sīwéixiū' (思惟修) means to cultivate oneself through thought and contemplation, 'qì è' (棄惡) means to abandon that which is evil, and 'gōngdélín' (功德林) means to accumulate many wholesome virtues. As this culture of 'jìnglǜ' (靜慮) or 'chán' (禪) entered Europe and the United States, it was translated as 'meditation.' The etymology of the English word 'meditation' itself is derived from the two Latin words 'meditārī' and 'medērī,' of which the former means 'to think deeply, to think carefully, or to examine the mind,' and the latter means 'to heal, or to cure.' It is also used in religious contexts to mean 'contemplation' or 'mòxiǎng' (默想). Later, when Japan readopted this culture, 'meditation' was translated back into Chinese characters as 'míngxiǎng' (瞑想/冥想), and both forms are currently written and used.

How Long Has Meditation Existed?

The Beginning of Human Existence on Earth

When looking at meditation through its general meaning of 'closing one's eyes and thinking,' it can be said that even the Neanderthals, who are even older than our human ancestors, the Homo sapiens, possessed the potential capacity for meditation. The Neanderthals had an interest in the afterlife and had customs for burying the dead.

The Indus, Ganges Civilization

Meditation, in a narrower sense as a form of self-reflection involving immersion in one's inner being to transcend subjectivity and observe objectively—rather than simply thinking—can be traced back to the ancient ruins of 'Mohenjo Daro' and 'Harappa' in the Indus Valley Civilization of India, one of the cradles of the four great civilizations. From this, it can be inferred that the history of meditation spans at least 5000 years.

The Vedic Period of Hinduism

During this period, Indian society was dominated by Brahmanism, a religion founded upon the teachings of the 'Vedas' and 'Upaniṣads.' Within Brahmanism, the central philosophy of 'Brahma-ātman-aikyam' held that the ultimate origin of the universe, 'Brahman,' and the inner principle within each individual, the 'Ātman,' are one and the same. Brahmanism also embraced the doctrines of karma and rebirth (saṃsāra), teaching that a person's present life is determined by the actions of past lives, and that present actions shape future existences. Philosophers and spiritual leaders of the time asserted that liberation from the endless cycle of rebirth could be achieved through both theoretical understanding and the practical application of meditation.

The earliest comprehensive records of meditation are found in the 'Upaniṣads,' the sacred texts of Brahmanism and the precursors to Hinduism, written between the fifth and sixth centuries BCE. The 'Upaniṣads' teach that to escape the suffering of saṃsāra, one must seek the true self, or 'Ātman', and that this realization is attained through meditation —a process of deep introspection into one's inner being.

The Foundation of Buddhism and Meditation

At around the same time as Brahmanism, Buddhism was founded, after which the system of mediation became more established. Gautama Siddhartha developed a method called 'vipassanā,' which can be described as the essence of mindfulness. Before attaining what is known in Buddhism as peerless and perfect enlightenment (anuttarā-samyak-saṃbodhi), Siddhartha also followed the practices of the Brahmanical tradition of the prevailing religious culture. After renouncing the world at the age of 29, Siddthartha chose to practice asceticism (samathā, Chinese: 禪定) and austerity (duḥkha-cāritā, Chinese: 苦行), which were the popular methods of meditation at that time. Siddhartha initially practiced under the guidance of the teachers Āḷāra Kālāma and Uddaka Rāmaputta. However, unsatisfied with their teachings, he left them and embarked on a 6-year-long practice of austerity along with five other ascetics. However, Siddhartha was unable to attain enlightenment even after 6 years of practicing austerity, and so he abandoned the practice and chose the Middle Way (Pāli: Majjhimāpaṭipadā). Eventually, at the age of 35, Siddhartha achieved enlightenment under a Bodhi tree and embodied the world of Nirvana (Pāli: Nibbāna), extinguishing the cause for birth, old age, sickness, death and rebirth in saṃsāra.

It can be said that the core doctrine of Buddhism is the system of meditation itself. The goal of Buddhism is for one to attain liberation by personally realizing the truth through meditation. The meditation methods of Early Buddhism, or in other words those that the Buddha taught to his disciples can be found in the Sanskrit 'Āgamas' or the Pali 'Nikāyas.' According to the 'Noble Eightfold Path' (Pāli: ariya-aṭṭhāṅgika-magga), the Buddhist practice of meditation is as follows. First, practitioners train themselves to refrain from speech or action that is harmful to themselves and others. Once this is achieved to a certain extent, one goes beyond speech and action to practice temporarily calming the unwholesome mind. Among the most famous of these practices is singularly focusing the mind on the breath or on a particular image to calm the unwholesome mind and create a peaceful and purified state of mind. There are also various other methods, including observing the body or diligently cultivating loving-kindness and compassion in the mind. It is said that choosing a method of practice that suits one's temperament leads to faster progress. Afterwards, using the purified and concentrated mind that has become very powerful, one cultivates wisdom to see one's own existence and the world as they really are. As this wisdom deepens through practice, there comes a time when all ignorance disappears and all attachment towards existence and the world is forever severed, at which point one achieves liberation. Typically, the type of meditation where one develops a calm and concentrated mind by focusing on a single point, often the breath or a specific image, is called 'Samathā' meditation, whereas the type of meditation that cultivates insight into the nature of existence and the world is called 'Vipassanā' meditation. These two types of meditation are not clearly distinguished in the Noble Eightfold Path. Disciplining one's speech and behavior is known as keeping the precepts, and although it is not usually directly included in teachings on meditation, it becomes an important foundation for the practice. Another important foundation to meditation is learning and familiarizing oneself with the Buddha's teachings to understand the actions that are harmful to oneself or others and those that are beneficial or helpful to oneself or others, which is essential for keeping the precepts. And even when cultivating wisdom through Vipassanā meditation, one needs to have a standard or criteria to know how to understand oneself and the world to see them as they are, and to know whether or not what they see is correct.

In a broad sense, the flow of Buddhist meditation presented in the Noble Eightfold Path consists of learning the Buddha's teachings, acquiring Right View (Pāli: sammā-diṭṭhi), observing the precepts (Pāli: sīla), and on this foundation developing concentration (Pāli / Sanskrit: samādhi) and cultivating wisdom (Pāli: paññā). The ultimate goal of Buddhist meditation is the complete cessation of all suffering, or Nirvana (Pāli: Nibbāna). Since the cause of suffering is greed, hatred, and ignorance, the goal of Buddhist meditation can be seen as eliminating these causes. Upon reaching the state of complete liberation where one is no longer reborn, all mental and physical suffering disappears 'permanently.' In 400–300 BCE as India became mostly unified under Chandragupta at the beginning of the Mauryan dynasty, Buddhism began to flourish. The religion experienced its golden age in India when Ashoka, the grandson of Chandragupta came to power.

However, following Ashoka's death and the collapse of the Mauryan dynasty, Buddhism declined in India and only remained as a subject of study, giving rise to Hinduism as the prominent religion that has continued until today.

Afterwards, one tradition of Early Indian Buddhism centered around monks was transmitted southward to Sri Lanka and Southeast Asia, whereas the Mahāyāna Buddhism focused on methods of practice for ordinary people, spread northward to China, Korea, Japan, and eventually Tibet. In Korea, Buddhism was introduced through China during the Three Kingdoms period around 372 CE.

The Various Meditation Practices That Emerged After Early Buddhism

In addition to the Vipassanā, the main method of meditation of the early Buddhist era, there are many methods of meditation in Buddhism, including the unique practices developed in the Tibet region, Hwadu Seon (話頭禪, Huàtóu Chán, Japanese: Huatou Zen) or Mukjo Seon (默照禪, Mòzhào Chán) developed in Northeast Asia, and various chanting practices developed in later Buddhism. [Hwadu Seon: a practice that focuses the mind on puzzle-like Hwadus or Gong'ans (公案, Gōng'àn, Japanese: Koan). Mukjo Seon: a form of Vipassanā developed in Northeast Asia that involves silently observing the mind. In Korea, Ganhwa Seon (看話禪, Kànhuà Chán, Japanese: Kanhua Zen) is a famous meditation practice that was developed from Seon (Zen) Buddhism within Mahāyāna Buddhism. Ganhwa Seon employs a 'Hwadu,' a puzzle or question that cannot be answered by mere logical reasoning. In the case of Vipassanā, as the method that was practiced in Myanmar and Thailand spread to the West, it became famous in Western psychiatric and psychological fields as it was shaped and transferred into 'mindfulness meditation.'

Other Forms of Meditation in Various Religions Aside from Buddhism

Around the fifth and sixth centuries BCE, various forms of meditation were practiced not only in the Hindu, Jain, and early Buddhist traditions of India and Nepal, but also in Confucianism and Daoism of China. In Hinduism, meditation is practiced by constantly reciting mantras, which are sacred sounds. Other religions aside from Buddhism and Hinduism also used meditation as a practice, and among them there is 'Kabbalah' in Judaism and 'Dhikr' in Islam's Sufism. In Judaism, ancient prophets and rabbis practiced 'Kabbalah' to communicate with Yahweh by deepening their consciousness, and Christian monks also practiced meditation in the form of contemplative prayer and a practice called 'the prayer of the heart' to more fully experience the presence of God. In Islam, Sufis also practiced meditation to directly experience Allah. And in Daoism of China, there is a meditation method using deep hypogastric breathing and intense mental focus to achieve a state of immortality beyond simply being in good health. Finally, even in Confucianism, which values social ethics, there is a meditation method that is used to recover the innate morality by resisting the temptations of external influences.

The Popularization and Scientification of Meditation

In 1893, meditation was popularized through the Parliament of the World's Religions, held during the commemoration of the World's Columbian Exposition in Chicago. The representative of Hinduism Paramahansa Yogananda and the representative of Japanese Zen Buddhism D.T. Suzuki were both in attendance during this conference. Suzuki exchanged ideas with philosophers such as Erich Fromm, while Paramahansa Yogananda traveled throughout the United States giving lectures on meditation. In the 1960s, as the counterculture and New Age movements gained momentum, meditation expanded in earnest, and it emerged as a hot trend of the times as the Beatles went to India to practice meditation. Science also played a role here, and as meditation gained attention as a method to cope with stress, related studies in the fields of neuroscience and medicine followed. In 1967, Professor Herbert Benson of Harvard Medical School introduced the term 'relaxation response' through his research on transcendental meditation, and argued that this term was the opposite of the 'fight or flight response.' As a result of studying many meditation methods based on the experience gained from his research on transcendental meditation, Benson found a basic common ground and announced a relaxation technique that could be easily applied to induce relaxation. It is said that the technique stabilizes the heart rate and respiratory rate, and primarily stabilizes the parasympathetic nervous system, which helps to relax the autonomic nervous system. It was discovered that meditation relaxes the mind and body. Through his experiments with Tibetan Monks, Professor Richard J. Davidson of the University of Wisconsin also discovered that meditation relieves stress and activates the left prefrontal cortex of the brain. From the 1990s, Buddhist insight meditation (Vipassanā) began to be applied to psychotherapy under the name of 'mindfulness meditation.' Professor Jon Kabat-Zinn of Massachusetts State University created the Mindfulness-Based Stress Reduction (MBSR) program. MBSR is used in many medical institutions around the world to treat chronic diseases such as depression and cardiovascular disease. In addition, Kabat-Zinn discovered that meditation is also effective in strengthening the immune system. According to a report in Neuroscience in 2005, Sara Lazar, a psychologist at Harvard Medical School, also discovered that meditation had an age-delaying effect. As people age, the cortex of their brain thins and their cognitive ability deteriorates. However, this was not the case for practitioners of meditation. In the religious world, the Dalai Lama was the first non-scientist to give a keynote speech at the 2005 Annual Meeting of the American Neuroscience Association, and he helped with research on meditation.

Conclusion

The origins of meditation can be found in various religious practices of India. The methods of meditation developed in India are largely classified into 'concentration meditation' (Samathā) and 'insight meditation' (Vipassanā). Concentration meditation was popular even before Buddhism. It is a method of meditation where one achieves a peaceful state by focusing the mind on a specific object or the breath. Insight meditation has its origins in Buddhism. Unlike concentration meditation, it is a method of meditation where one gains insight by observing the thoughts and phenomena that appear in the body and mind as they are. These Indian religious practices were transmitted to China along with Buddhism, where they were accepted in various forms such as Zen Buddhism, and were eventually transmitted to the West. In recent years, meditation's contact with Western culture has expanded to various fields, including medicine.

Bibliography

Feuerstein G. The history of meditation: a brief timeline of practices and traditions. 2018. Retrieved from: https://get2meditate.com/author/george/page/2/

Hahm BJ, Kwon JS, Rhi BY. Korean Neuropsychiatr Assoc. 1997;36(6):1125–37.

Jin YS. Mind-body medicine in integrative medicine. Hanyang Med Rev. 2010;30(2):84–90.

Mead, E. The history and origin of meditation. 2020. Retrieved from: https://positivepsychology.com/history-of-meditation/

Park S. The Understanding of Meditation. Korean J Str Res. 2006;14:247–57.

The history of medication. 1~12. 2019. Retrieved from: http://www.kbulgyonews.com/

Wynne A. The origin of Buddhist meditation. London: Routledge; 2007.

What Is Mindfulness?

3

Kyung-Seung Kim

If you define meditation philosophically or religiously, it can be said that it is 'accessing the activities of a consciousness which does not distinguish between subject and object and which knows we are one with the world, a level of consciousness that is deeper than a surface-level consciousness which distinguishes self and other.' It is an ultimate finality inherent in all finite beings that surpasses being or non-being. It is called 'emptiness' (空, Śūnyatā) or 'Buddha nature' (佛性, buddha-dhātu) in Buddhism, 'tao' (道) in Taoism, 'heaven' (天) or the 'Supreme Ultimate" (太極) in Confucianism, 'existence itself' in Neo-Platonist philosophy, or the 'divine intellect' in Christian mysticism. On the other hand, scholars who study meditation scientifically define it as a 'collection of complex emotional and attention control training with various purposes including psychological stability and balance.'

As a form of meditation, Mindfulness refers to a practice, a state of mind-body complex that can be attained through practice, or is also used as a concept of traits that appear in daily life even without practice through neuroplastic changes as a result of repetitive practices. Mindfulness is a translation of the word 'sati,' the most important concept in Buddhist meditation. However, in order to understand it clearly we need to be careful as the meaning of sati used in ancient religious traditions is slightly different from the concept used in modern secular or clinical mindfulness. In truth, there is no clearly agreed-upon definition of mindfulness. The Buddhist tradition has itself debated for centuries on the meaning of sati without reaching a consensus. Buddhist scholars in Korea, where Seon (Zen) Buddhism, which traditionally centers on Ganhwaseon (看話禪), is popular, have translated mindfulness, a concept related to the tradition of Vipassana meditation of Theravada Buddhism that started to become popular at the end of the twentieth century, into various terms, including mind-keeping, awareness, and passive attention.

In this chapter, we will examine the meanings of mindfulness from its classical meaning through the process of its modern interpretation to its meaning in clinical practice.

The Classical Definition of Mindfulness: Sati

Mindfulness is a term translated from 'sati' in Pali and 'smṛti' in Sanskrit. Literally, it means 'to remember.' In 1881, Thomas William Rhys Davids, a professor at the University of London who translated Early Indian Buddhist scriptures into English, first translated the term 'sati' as 'mindfulness.' From there, mindfulness was gradually absorbed into English vocabulary, at first within the Theravada Buddhist society in the

K.-S. Kim (✉)
Department of Psychiatry, Maya Mental Hospital, Kyung-Buk, Republic of Korea

J.-H. Chae, H.-Y. Lee (eds.), *Meditation in Psychiatry and General Medicine*, https://doi.org/10.1007/978-981-95-7147-5_3

West, and was eventually recognized in general society by 1910.

There is actually no clear definition of Sati in the Nikāyas, the scriptures of Early Indian Buddhism. For more than 400 years after the Buddha's death, Buddhist scriptures were passed down through oral transmission, which led their core tenets to be narrowed down into simple and repetitive formulas to make it easier to remember. Therefore, within the Nikāyas one can only find references to how sati functions in Buddhist psychology and the practice of meditation instead of a clear definition of the term.

There are two metaphors for sati in the Nikāyas. One is that of taming a wild elephant, and the other is that of the gatekeeper of a city. In the metaphor of taming a wild elephant, sati is likened to a pole firmly planted on the ground with a rope tied around a wild elephant's neck to tame it. Here, sati's role is to firmly calm our mind, which is like a wild elephant rampaging around. Like a pillar that is firmly planted on the ground, sati functions to have us directly face objects that we experience. By directly facing objects that we experience in the present moment, sati captures and binds six kinds of 'wild animals' (sensory organs), stabilizing and calming the mind.

Sati also watches over and protects the mind with this calmness by keeping an eye on everything that enters and exits the mind, much like a gatekeeper who guards the gate of a city.

> Suppose, bhikkhu, a king had a frontier city with strong ramparts, walls, and arches, and with six gates. The gatekeeper posted there would be wise, experienced, and intelligent; one who keeps out strangers and admits acquaintances. (Kimsuka Sutta, SN 35:245)

Here, the gatekeeper is sati, the six gates are the six sense organs (eyes, ears, nose, tongue, body, and mind), and the king is our consciousness. With wisdom, competence, and intelligence, sati helps our consciousness assess what is admitted and what is turned away. Sati is not merely observation, but discerning friends vs foes. This characteristic of discerning is what connects sati with wisdom (pañña).

Mindfulness as Bare Attention

It was the German monk and Buddhist scholar Nyanaponika Thera (1910–1994) who established the basis for popularizing mindfulness among Westerners. As a disciple of the Mahasi Sayadaw (1904–1982), a leading figure in Myanmar's insight meditation movement who worked to spread meditation outside of the monastery to the general public through standardized methods that ordinary people could practice, Nyanaponika presented mindfulness to the general public as the Buddha's core philosophy and method of liberation. Under the influence of the Mahasi Sayadaw, he explained sati or mindfulness as 'bare attention,' devoid of any habitual judgments or mental projections towards an object. Our minds tend to react to objects automatically and reflexively with craving, aversion, or indifference. Bare attention means solely paying attention to an object as it is presented through the five senses and the mind, rather than automatically or reflexively reacting to it with actions, words, or thoughts. If this kind of automatic reaction occurs, it too becomes the object of bare attention. This is primarily how mindfulness was understood, taught, and refined by modern Western meditation teachers. Jon Kabat-Zinn's concept of mindfulness was also inherited through this genealogy.

According to Nyanaponika, in order to obtain freedom of the mind, we must be free from the automatic and obsessive tendency to conceptualize our experiences according to what we like and dislike. To do this, we limit the scope of our attention to what is happening right now. Rather than habitually and automatically judging and evaluating things as good or bad and then relating them to past memories or future expectations, we simply pay attention to what is happening right now and observe our experiences and reactions. This is mindfulness (sati) as bare attention. Through this, we are able to reach a state of non-reactive equanimity, and we will be able to be free from the habitual reactions of holding onto what we like and pushing away what we dislike.

Mindfulness as the Ability to Retain an Object

In response to Nyanaponika's view of mindfulness as bare attention, the philosopher and Buddhist scholar William Dreyfus suggested the concept of mindfulness as the 'ability to retain an object' by stating that 'bare attention' misses this core aspect of mindfulness. The concept of bare attention reveals an important aspect of the practice of mindfulness rather than a perfect definition of sati. Rather than being non-judgmental awareness of an object centered around the present moment, mindfulness uses close attention to preserve information about an object in order to understand information transmitted through our cognitive mechanisms. Thus, Dreyfus sees mindfulness as a cognitive activity closely linked to the original meaning of mindfulness as memory and, in particular, a working memory that activates related information to integrate it into meaningful categories and is used for the purpose of goal-oriented action. Rather than just passively paying attention to an object, understanding mindfulness as a function of holding onto and preserving an object in one's consciousness fits very well with the function of mindfulness to present an object without drifting away, as stated in the Abhidhamma. It is holding onto an object with the mind and remembering it later, that is, mindfulness as the ability to preserve an object.

Dreyfus believes that according to the Abhidhamma, attention begins with orienting the mind (manasikāra). Orienting the mind refers to the mental factor that allows the mind to pay attention to an object, and it is through this that an object appears in our consciousness. The process of attention that begins with orienting the mind is maintained along with 'sati' (mindfulness) and concentration (samādhi). Here, orienting directs the mind towards an object, while mindfulness (sati) is the ability of the mind to pay close attention so that it does not drift away or lose an object. Concentration (samādhi) completes this attention with the ability to maintain focus and become one with an object. Mindfulness and concentration work together to strengthen and enhance attention.

At the most basic level, precise mindfulness is to preserve an object and not disengage from the mind, allowing one to focus on the object. It attempts to develop a clear understanding (sampajañña) and evaluates various aspects of one's experience, such as distinguishing between a wholesome mind and an unwholesome one. Dreyfus calls this wise mindfulness. Wise mindfulness is different from precise mindfulness because it includes the ability to understand and discern an object. Precise mindfulness is limited to preserving an object, and it is seen as providing the basis for clear understanding (sampajañña). Taking the two metaphors in the Nikayas, the pillar that binds the elephant can be understood as precise mindfulness, whereas the gatekeeper can be understood as wise mindfulness. The main point of wise mindfulness is to not only obtain a calm and focused state of mind, but also to gain a deeper understanding of the body and mind, through which we are able to free the mind from the habits and tendencies that bind us in suffering.

Dreyfus says that bare attention, which is paying attention to whatever arises, is only one aspect of mindfulness. The meaning of mindfulness is much broader, and it includes the cognitive ability to clearly assess the state of the mind and body. If you understand mindfulness only as bare attention, you may devalue the cognitive implications of mindfulness that combine the various aspects of one's experience together to create a clear understanding of the state of the mind and body. In addition, if you overemphasize the non-judgmental aspect of mindfulness, you run the risk of understanding it merely as a form of therapeutic and relaxed stillness. Mindfulness is not merely a therapeutic technique, but also an intrinsic function that plays a key role in the cognitive process. It is not merely bare attention, but a foundational cognitive ability that brings about a liberating transformation of knowing.

Mindfulness as Lucid Awareness

Bhikkhu Bodhi was a disciple of Nyanaponika, who described mindfulness as bare attention, and spent 12 years with him in a temple in Sri Lanka. According to Bodhi, his teacher Nyanaponika did not intend to explain Sati solely as bare awareness, but used the term as a practical concept for beginners of vipassanā meditation practice. Though the concept of bare attention can serve as a practical, educational, and procedural set of instructions for beginners who practice mindfulness, it can be difficult to regard it as a valid theoretical description. Mindfulness can be conceptualized as bare attention for some methods of practice. Since it is a faculty of the mind that can take on various appearances, however, Bhikkhu Bodhi suggests 'lucid awareness' that vividly and clearly presents an object to the consciousness as a concept of mindfulness that can comprehensively explain all forms of practice, including the practice of paying attention to images of the disgusting body, contemplation of death, and loving-kindness, etc.

Sati returns the light of consciousness to the experiencing subject to illuminate the physical, sensory, and psychological dimensions. By shedding light on these areas through the act of returning, sati allows perception that is hazy, like the dawn, to become clear. Mindfulness is explained as lucid awareness because it allows us to investigate clearly by facing an objective area of a phenomenon.

Mindfulness (sati) as lucid awareness usually occurs in the early stages of practice, and as mindfulness is strengthened, it is accompanied by clear understanding (sampajañña), where cognitive elements are added. A clear understanding is not just observing phenomena but interpreting the phenomena presented to us within a meaningful context. As one's practice deepens, this sampajañña becomes more and more important, ultimately leading to direct insight (vipassanā) and wisdom (pañña). The role of sati, or mindfulness, is to reveal the contents of our experience. On the other hand, the role of sampajañña, or clear understanding, is to figure out and investigate its contents. When one is able to contemplate the arising and passing away of the patterns of objects, clear understanding (sampajañña) begins to turn into wisdom (pañña).

Bhikkhu Bodhi criticizes the explanation of mindfulness as pure attention in two ways. In the Buddhist psychological analysis of the mind, attention is understood as a concept that includes orienting the mind (manasikāra). Manasikāra refers to automatically and naturally turning the mind towards an object at the beginning of the process of recognition. On the other hand, sati creates a clear and vivid knowledge of an object through sustained conscious attention. Therefore, it can be said that a more accurate definition of sati is conscious attention rather than simply bare attention that includes automatic one.

As for the word 'bare' itself, although it can serve as a practical concept for beginners, Bodhi believes that no mental activity can be strictly speaking 'bare.' As seen in the Noble Eightfold Path, in order for there to be right awareness (sammā-sati), it must be accompanied and conditioned by right view (sammā-diṭṭhi), right thought(sammā-saṅkappa), the three ethical factors of right speech (sammā-vācā), right action (sammā-kammanta), and right livelihood (sammā-ājīva), right effort (sammā-vāyāma), and right concentration (sammā-samādhi).

Clinical Mindfulness

Mindfulness cannot exist on its own. It exists as part of a wider phenomenological network. However, as it was transmitted over to modern clinical contexts such as MBSR (Mindfulness-Based Stress Reduction), rather than being a concept accompanied and conditioned by other factors, mindfulness was understood through the concept of a container or umbrella that contains all of these factors. It was understood not as a singular concept, but as a collective and plural concept. This is evident in the definition of mindfulness by Jon Kabat-Zinn, who was the first to redefine and apply mindfulness to clinical practice through his MBSR program in 1979. He says, 'mindfulness is the awareness that emerges through paying attention on purpose, in the present moment, and non-judgmentally to the unfolding of experience moment by moment.'

Here Hwang et al. understand mindfulness as defined by John Kabat-Zinn as a collective concept that contains at least four aspects, including awareness, attention, intention, and having a particular attitude. As a whole, it is a concept that contains the 'what' and 'how' of mindfulness. In terms of 'what' (its identity), mindfulness is the awareness emerging from a specific process. And in terms of 'how' (its process), it includes the concept of the process of intentionally paying attention to one's experience as it unfolds in the present moment without judgment.

On the other hand, according to Pollock et al., sati is defined as awareness, attention, and memory, and they understand it to mean continuously remembering that one needs to be aware of and pay attention to, with another key dimension of acceptance or non-judgment. t.

By combining the three elements of attention, awareness, and acceptance, Germer defines mindfulness as the awareness with acceptance of the experiences of the present moment. It is a state of paying attention to and accepting what is happening in the present moment.

Hayes et al. explain mindfulness by dividing it into four processes. The first is the awareness of the present moment. Above all, mindfulness consists of coming in contact with the experiences of mind and body in the present moment and being aware of these experiences. The second is acceptance. It is acknowledging and accepting one's experience in this moment without judging whether one likes it or not. Not clinging onto craving or hatred, one allows one's experiences as they are without holding onto them or pushing them away.

The third is cognitive defusion. When you accept and are aware of experiences in the present moment as it is, you are not caught up in the internal experiences of thoughts, emotions, and impulses. Instead, you are able to simply let the experience come and go. The fourth is the perspective of 'self-as-context.' Through the previous three processes, the contents of your consciousness such as sensations, thoughts, emotions, and impulses gradually become a temporary 'I' that merely comes and goes. The transcendental 'I' of awareness itself that is witnessing the consciousness in the background is called 'self-as-context.' These four processes are the concepts of mindfulness understood in Acceptance and Commitment Therapy (ACT). They are useful in that they can be understood as simultaneous processes that occur when practicing meditation, or as those that can be used individually and separately as needed in psychotherapy sessions.

The State, Traits, and Practice of Mindfulness

Contemporary clinical, therapeutic, or secular mindfulness is a concept that points to all of the following three aspects, namely its state, traits, and practice. The mindfulness state can be experienced spontaneously. From time to time, especially if we go to a new place or walk alone in the mountains, or experience beautiful scenery, we are able to have an experience where all of a sudden everything seems to stand still, the mind becomes peaceful and calm, and everything feels vivid and intimate. This is called a spontaneous mindfulness state. Then, in a state of metacognitive awareness, we are able to easily be aware of sensations, emotions, thoughts, etc. that arise moment to moment, and are able to reach a state of awareness where we do not judge these experiences as good or bad. This is called the mindfulness state. The method of reaching this state of mindfulness artificially to experience it more often and for longer is called mindfulness practice. Here there are both formal practices that take place at a specific time and place with specific methods, and informal practices where we strive to be aware of the moment-to-moment experiences in our daily lives, regardless of what we are doing, with acceptance. Formal practice includes practices like sitting meditation, walking meditation, body-scan meditation, and loving-kindness meditation. Informal practice consists of the practice of paying close attention and being aware of the movements of the body, changes in sensation, and thoughts and emotions that arise while repetitively doing habitual and automatic activities in our daily lives, including showering, washing one's face, and brushing one's teeth. Thus, through repeated practice, neuroplastic changes occur in the brain, and by being more aware of experiences in each moment, even when not actively practicing, the mind develops the trait to be aware of and choicefully respond with awareness, rather than being caught up in our automatic and habitual reactions. This mindfulness trait can be measured in various ways, such as through tools like the FFMQ (Five Facet Mindfulness Questionnaire) or the MASS (Mindful Attention Awareness Scale). Because the mindfulness trait can serve as an antidote to negative emotions, stress, as well as impulsive, compulsive, and addictive behaviors, mindfulness can become a basis that is widely used in clinical practice.

Focused Attention

At least three major techniques are used to cultivate mindfulness in clinical practice. They are focused attention, open monitoring, and compassionate acceptance. Focused attention refers to the technique of focusing on one object and paying intentional attention to it. It is the act of turning one's attention towards an object such as one's breathing, the feeling of the soles of one's feet, sounds, visual stimuli, etc. with an attitude full of interest and curiosity and being aware of it. Inevitably, our minds will be distracted by thoughts, sounds, and uncomfortable sensations felt in the body. Your concentration improves by gently and kindly returning your attention repeatedly to the original object once you realize that you have been distracted. As you spend more and more time paying attention to one object, physical relaxation and a calm and serene mind find you. If you are not able to reach a certain level of concentration, it is difficult for the metacognitive awareness that is able to clearly see the movements of the mind to arise. Being caught up in your thoughts and feelings, you will be unable to choose your actions but will react instead compulsively based on impulsive automaticity. Therefore, because it is difficult to practice open monitoring and compassion without it, focused attention is a cornerstone of mindfulness meditation.

Focused attention uses three techniques to control attention. The first technique is monitoring a chosen object while observing and being alert when the mind becomes distracted. The second is disengaging your attention from objects that distract your focus. The third is quickly redirecting your attention back to the original object. As they are more easily distracted, beginners will more frequently use these three techniques to control their attention. As practice deepens, changes in the mindfulness trait will occur due to neuroplasticity, allowing you to remain more easily and calmly attentive to your chosen object of focus with less and less effort. Through this, an increase in physical lightness, vitality, and serenity as well as a decrease in emotional reactivity will follow.

Open Monitoring

Once a certain level of focused attention and concentration is developed, you can practice open monitoring. Rather than repeatedly returning your attention to a single chosen object, this consists of focusing on and being aware of anything that stands out in your consciousness at that moment. At this time, your attention may shift away from breathing to sounds, bodily pain, the flow of air brushing your face, or a feeling of sadness in your eyes and throat. Rather than thinking about or analyzing these phenomena, you simply practice being with them with an attitude of interest, curiosity, and acceptance. It is like sitting next to a small spring inside a quiet forest. What animals come to visit and when they leave is completely out of our control, but we welcome them all. Pollack et al. likened the relationship of focused attention and open monitoring to taking pictures with a manual camera. The better the focus, the clearer the quality of the picture that is produced. Here, focused attention refers to the effort to focus the camera, and through this, being able to see an object clearly can be called open monitoring.

The practice of open monitoring includes several key aspects. At the beginning of the practice, you use the practice of focused attention to reduce distractions and calm the mind. As the ability to monitor improves through the development of focused attention, you are able to switch to practicing open monitoring. Here the goal is not to focus on any particular object, but to simply remain in a state of attentiveness and be aware of whatever object you are experiencing moment to moment. This can be called 'wakefulness.' In order to reach this state, practitioners gradually reduce their focus on a particular object, which is the goal of focused attention. At the same time, by strengthening their metacognitive awareness through more emphasis on the function of monitoring, they will come into contact more with aspects such as the intensity of their experience, their emotional state, and their activated cognitive schema. Unlike with focused attention, with open monitoring there is no sharp distinction between chosen and unchosen objects. For example, in focused attention, emotional atmospheres are noticed in the background of a chosen specific object, such as the sensation of breathing, whereas in open monitoring, emotional moods can be noticed without paying conscious attention to a particular object. Thus, the practice of working hard to choose and focus on an object is gradually replaced by a continuous and comfortable awareness without a specifically chosen object. Here, if an object that you encounter at a given moment causes a strong sense of attachment or aversion, leading the mind towards disarray, you can recover your mind's balance by practicing focused attention on a single object.

A key objective of the practice of open monitoring is to cultivate a clear self-reflective awareness of the normally obscured cognitive and emotional aspects of one's own mental processes. Metacognitive awareness makes it easier to control the thoughts and emotions that occur automatically and habitually through the mechanisms of cognitive defusion, decentering, and de-identification. In addition, the practice of open monitoring allows for a clearer but less emotionally reactive awareness of the so-called autobiographical identity that is projected into the past and future, such as 'I am this kind of person.' On the other hand, through open monitoring, our everyday lives become richer as we savor more deeply the richness of the present moment.

Compassionate Acceptance

Acceptance is acknowledging and allowing things as they are in the present moment. We waste a lot of energy denying and resisting that which is already true at this moment. This is trying to force situations into our liking, and only creates tension and inhibits positive change. Acceptance does not mean we have to like everything. You do not have to give up your principles and values and take up a positive attitude, nor do you have to be content with the way things are. Acceptance simply refers to an attitude of willingly acknowledging and allowing things as they are. It is about opening yourself to the thoughts, emotions, sensations, and feelings that come to you in the present moment without forcing your own thoughts and feelings onto them every moment.

To do this, we must take a step back and be aware of the flow of our mind, which constantly judges and reflexively reacts to internal and external experiences. When we begin to practice paying attention to our own minds, we are surprised to find that we are constantly judging our experiences. If you want to know how to cope effectively with stress, you need to be able to be aware of these automatic judgments. In order for us not to get caught up in the intense contents of our minds or fall into the trap of self-critical rumination, we need to practice embracing and comforting ourselves through the skills of loving-kindness, self-compassion, and equanimity so that we can accept whatever experience we face. This is compassionate acceptance. A common method used in the practice of compassionate acceptance is to imagine a person or animal for whom you feel love and compassion and direct loving-kindness and care towards them. Then, after you have felt these feelings, you redirect them back to yourself, to those you love, and to the wider community. It is repeating the mantras that wish happiness in your mind such as 'may you be happy,' 'may you be free from suffering,' 'may you be peaceful' in line with your breathing There are also a variety of techniques of loving-kindness that can be used to help you feel safe during times of emotional distress, as well as several practices of equanimity that can be used to increase your ability to endure and embrace difficult experiences as well as feel a sense of security in the face of difficult emotional storms. Literally, compassion means 'to be in pain together.' It connects us to others and challenges the assumption that we are separate and alone. In the state of compassion, we feel wholeness and inner strength. A mind full of compassion cannot be destroyed or broken in the face of suffering. Compassion is a therapeutic factor in most forms of psychotherapy.

As we have seen above, the practice of focused attention (concentration) helps us maintain connection with the present moment, open monitoring expands and deepens our awareness of what is actually happening in that moment, and the practice of loving-kindness and compassion helps us approach everything that happens in our minds with acceptance. It is therefore important to find the optimal balance between the practices of concentration, awareness (open monitoring), and acceptance. If the mind is confused, unfocused, or lost in thought, practicing more concentration can be helpful. If the mind is overflowing with difficult emotions, memories, or thoughts of self-blame, the practices of loving-kindness, compassion, and equanimity can be helpful. When the mind is more stable and receptive, you can be aware of and accept a variety of thoughts, emotions, and memories through open monitoring, and this will lead you to more insight and integration.

Concentration, awareness, and acceptance all need each other. In order to focus better with conscious attention, you need to be aware of when you are distracted, and on the other hand, you need to accept things as they are. In order to be well aware, you need to have focused attention and you need the acceptance to be able to let go of aversion and craving. Acceptance also requires the qualities of being well aware that the mind is clinging onto craving and aversion, and returning attention intentionally back to the original object.

Although focused attention, open monitoring (awareness), and compassionate acceptance can all be practiced separately, formal practices such as sitting meditation and walking meditation include all three of these elements. For example, it can be said that these three elements are already present in the practice of being aware of one's breath during sitting meditation, which is one of the most basic forms of mindfulness meditation. Consciously paying attention to the sensation of breath is practicing focused attention. Acknowledging and allowing that things are not going our way as they are when our attention is distracted by thoughts, sounds, or uncomfortable sensations is practicing acceptance. Finally, noticing and briefly observing these phenomena that arise is practicing open monitoring (awareness).

The Mechanisms of Mindfulness and its Application in Psychotherapy

'Mindfulness is an incredibly simple way to change one's relationship with one's experience.'

An experience, whatever it is, and our mind's reaction to that experience (thoughts, emotions, impulses, senses, etc.) make up the contents of our consciousness, and we have a tendency to sink into the swamp of our experiences by identifying and fusing ourselves with them. At this time, if we are able to be aware of the contents of our consciousness with acceptance, we can reduce our habitual and automatic reactions by de-identifying and de-fusing with them. From here, we can go from being slaves of our mind bound to the contents of our consciousness to being the masters of our mind, able to choose our own responses. Through this we can reduce suffering and stress and can coexist with them.

The more we can be aware of the contents of our consciousness through metacognition, the more we are no longer fused with them and bound to them. Whether it is pain, depression, or fear, when we can see these contents of our consciousness, we are no longer one with them. We transcend them. We are no longer defined, manipulated, conditioned, or determined by them. Instead, we simply exist alongside them. We realize, 'this pain is not me,' 'this depression is not me,' 'this thought is not me.' The stories of our past traumas, which we have firmly identified ourselves with for so long, simply become a 'story' of the past.

In essence, this is accomplished by being aware of the 'autopilot reactions' to our experiences. Autopilot reactions refer to automatic and habitual reactions that automatically divide all internal and external objects we experience into pleasant, unpleasant, and neutral, and which try to hold onto pleasant experiences (craving), push away unpleasant experiences (aversion), and ignore or overlook neutral experiences. Although attachment is the cause of suffering, it can be said that it is inevitable for an individual's survival. Autopilot reactions are a concept that corresponds to the 'Noble Truth of the Origin of Suffering' within the Four Noble Truths taught by the Buddha. Because the autopilot reaction seeks immediate gratification, it can be described as a kind of addictive reaction. It becomes the root of addictions and sufferings that we attach to, the craving which seeks to immediately hold onto things that we like and the aversion which seeks to immediately push away things we dislike. The more we are able to be aware of our minds, which are attached to craving and aversion, the more we are able to choose whether we allow ourselves to be dragged on by our autopilot reaction or to stop it. Once we are aware of our autopilot reaction, we can choose to stop it. Viktor Frankl said there was a space between stimulus and response. The power to choose how we responded existed in that space. Our development and freedom depended on how we chose to respond. Here, the space between stimulus and response is the space of mindful awareness. The more we are aware of the impulses of our automatic and habitual reactions, the more we can choose whether we allow them or not. Up to this point we have examined the psychological mechanisms related to the clinical effects of mindfulness. The neurobiological mechanisms will be addressed in other chapters of this book.

Meanwhile, mindfulness in psychotherapy can have various functions. Here these include (1) practicing therapists, (2) mindfulness-informed psychotherapy, (3) mindfulness-based psychotherapy.

Through the practice of mindfulness, therapists themselves begin to relate to patients in a different way than before. First, by improving intentional attention, it becomes easier for a therapist to focus on and be aware of both the patient and their own thoughts and feelings at every moment during psychotherapy. In addition, a therapist can improve their affective tolerance that allows them to be present with and accept their patient's painful emotions, and this, in turn, improves the therapeutic relationship between therapist and patient.

On the other hand, in mindfulness-informed psychotherapy, therapists gain insight into the universal cause of emotional pain as their own practice deepens, and they are able to utilize during therapy sessions the four processes of mindfulness in ACT to reduce emotional pain. As described above, contact with the contents of one's consciousness in the present moment, acceptance of them, their defusion, and a view of self-as-context can not only be explained and taught as a concept that can reduce a patient's emotional pain in the process of psychotherapy, but can also be used as a skills training. In addition, a therapist will become able to know that resisting certain contents or experiences that occur in their minds will cause them to actually persist and expand, and they will learn how attempting to cling to pleasure, avoid pain, and expand the egocentric self causes pain. Through this, the therapist will proceed in a way of treatment that helps patients open up to and accept themselves regarding their various experiences.

Mindfulness-based psychotherapy suggests that patients directly practice mindfulness at the appropriate time during the treatment process and introduces relevant techniques of mindfulness practice. Therapists take time to practice with the patient during therapy sessions, and assign homework for patients to practice alone afterwards. The primary examples of this include MBSR, MBCT (Mindfulness-Based Cognitive Therapy), MBRP (Mindfulness-Based Relapse Prevention), and MORE (Mindfulness-Oriented Recovery Enhancement).

Conclusion

Through its involvement in mental health issues, mindfulness therapy is changing the landscape of mental health treatment around the world. Psychotherapists use mindfulness therapy second only to cognitive behavioral therapy, and prefer it over classical psychodynamic therapy. In the UK, MBCT is recognized as an effective treatment for major depression, and hundreds of papers related to mindfulness are being published every year worldwide. In addition, mindfulness is being used in many fields, including psychiatry, clinical psychology, health psychology, cognitive therapy, neuroscience, education, law, business, and leadership. Although the understanding of the mechanisms that drive the efficacy of meditation is still in its infancy, evidence is emerging that mindfulness meditation can lead to neuroplastic changes in the structure and function of the brain's regions that are involved in controlling attention, emotion, and self-awareness. Therefore, the practice of mindfulness meditation can contribute not only to the treatment of clinical diseases but also to an improvement in mental health and wellbeing. I hope that conversations and research between ancient and modern, East and West, will enrich each other and open the way for new insights and research on mindfulness in various fields.

Bibliography

Korean Sources

Heesung G. 신앙과 이성 사이에서 (In between faith and reason). Seoul: Sechang Publishing House; 2016.

Jagyeong H. 명상의 철학적 기초 (The philosophical basics of mindfulness). Seoul: Ewha Womans University Press; 2008.

Joonyoung J. 사띠 논쟁 (Debates on Sati). Buddh Rev. 2015;62

English Sources

Baer RA, Smith GT, Hopkins J, Krietemeyer J, Tony L. Using self-report assessment methods to explore facets of mindfulness. Assessment. 2006;13:27–45.

Bodhi B. What does mindfulness really mean? A canonical perspective. Contemp Buddhism. 2011;12(1):19–39.

Bowen S, Chawla N, Marlatt GA. Mindfulness-based relapse prevention for addictive behaviors: a clinician's guide. New York/London: The Guilford Press; 2014.

Brown KW, Ryan RM. The benefits of being present: mindfulness and its role in psychological well-being. J Pers Soc Psychol. 2003;84(4):822–48.

Dreyfus G. Is mindfulness present-centred and non-judgmental? A discussion of the cognitive dimensions of mindfulness. Contemp Buddhism. 2011;12(1):41–54.

Dunne JD. Buddhist styles of mindfulness: a heuristic approach. In: Ostafin BD, Robinson MD, Meier BP, editors. Handbook of mindfulness and self-regulation. 2015th edition. Springer; 2015.

Garland E, Howard MO. Mindfulness-based treatment of addiction: current state of the field and envisioning the next wave of research. Addict Sci Clin Pract. 2018;13:14.

Germer CK. The mindful path to self-compassion: freeing yourself from destructive thoughts and emotions. New York/London: The Guilford Press; 2003.

Gethin R. On some definitions of mindfulness. Contemp Buddhism. 2011;12(1):263–79.

Grabovac AD, Lau MA, Willett BR. Mechanisms of mindfulness: a Buddhist psychological model. Mindfulness. 2011;2(3):154–66.

Hayes SC, Plumb JC. Mindfulness from the bottom up: providing an inductive framework for understanding mindfulness processes and their application to human suffering. Psychol Inq. 2007;18:242–8.

Hwang YS, Kearney PK. A mindfulness intervention for children with autism spectrum disorder, mindfulness in behavioral health. Cham: Springer; 2015.

Kabat-Zinn J. Full catastrophe living. Using the wisdom of your body and mind to face stress, pain, and illness. New York: Dell Publishing; 1990.

Kabat-Zinn J. Mindfulness-based interventions in context: past, present and future. Clin Psychol Sci Pract. 2003;10(2):144–56.

Lutz A, Slagter HA, Dunne JD, Davidson RJ. Attention regulation and monitoring in meditation. Trends Cogn Sci. 2008;12(4):163–9.

Nyanaponika Thera. The heart of Buddhist meditation. London: Riders; 1962.

Nynaponika T. The power of mindfulness. Kandy: Buddhist Publication Society; 1968.

Pollack SM, Pedulla TM, Siegel RD. Sitting together: essential skills for mindfulness-based psychotherapy. New York/London: The Guilford Press; 2016.

Rhys Davids TW, Stede W, editors. The Pali text society's Pali-English dictionary. Oxford: The Pali Text Society; 1999.

Shapiro SL, Carlson LE, Astin JA. Benedict freedman. Mechanisms of mindfulness. J Clin Psychol. 2006;62:373–86.

The Anthropological Approach to Meditation

4

Seongkeun Lee

Humans practiced meditation in the process of adapting to the ecosystem. There is a lack of archaeological evidence pointing to when and how meditation was first practiced. Records of meditation began around 1500 BC. Experiences of meditation before written records can be indirectly inferred through fossil artifacts, cave paintings and the lives of hunter-gatherers. After splitting off from the last common ancestors of the chimpanzees, hominins walked upright, controlled fire, held funerary rites, and, through language, established knowledge and created various cultures. It is speculated that during this evolutionary process, meditation helped humans transform their consciousness and adapt to the ecosystem. This chapter was written in the hope that it will help solve the problems facing our time, which people call the Anthropocene.

Prologue

The Application of Meditation

Meditation is being applied in an increasing number of fields of medicine and education. It is measured using various metrics to verify its state and effectiveness. Physiologically, it is called an awake low metabolic state, a scientific expression of the 'meditative state' (惺惺寂寂) in the old days. In one psychological tool, the Five Facet Mindfulness Questionnaire (FFMQ), variables such as non-judgment and awareness are measured as factors of meditation. Clinically, these two factors are being studied in relation to the treatment of addiction. For example, in Mindfulness-Based Relief Prevention for Addictive Behaviors (MBRP), relapse into addiction is prevented by training patients to be aware of and to ride along the waves of their cravings as if they are surfing. Despite the increase in research on the subject, meditation has been criticized for not being scientifically rigorous in its definition and effects. Examining how meditation started and developed may help the complementary research to understand meditation.

Early Records on Meditation

Meditation was first recorded in the Hindu Vedas around 1500 BCE. Since there is no empirical data preceding 1500 BCE, we have no choice but to make inferences when conducting research on meditation before the Vedas. Fossils, artifacts, cave paintings, and the lives of hunter-gatherers can indirectly tell us when human beings began to practice meditation.

S. Lee (✉)
Department of Psychiatry, Hyungju Hospital,
Yangsan-si, Gyungsangnam-do, Republic of Korea

J.-H. Chae, H.-Y. Lee (eds.), *Meditation in Psychiatry and General Medicine*,
https://doi.org/10.1007/978-981-95-7147-5_4

The Evolution from Breathing Life Forms to Mammals

Breathing is an anchor that is often used in meditation. We observe the coming and going of breath like the process of a life form's birth and death. We carry out the practice while facing the universe with a confident and dignified posture. The Big Bang Theory explains the origin of the universe as having started with a big explosion 13.8 billion years ago. According to this theory, the Earth was formed about 4.5 billion years ago. The first life forms on Earth appeared about 3.8 billion years ago, evolving and adapting from asexual organisms to sexual organisms with distinctions between males and females. About 500 million years ago, the Cambrian eruption occurred, leading to the appearance of numerous species, and about 200 million years ago, mammals that held fetuses in their placenta rather than as eggs first appeared. At that time, mammals were well adapted to the darkness underground, and after the extinction of the dinosaurs, they began to increase their activity above ground.

From the Advent of the Hominin to the Discovery of Fire

About 7 million years ago, human ancestors branched off from their last common ancestor with the chimpanzees. Although humans and chimpanzees differ genetically by only about 2%, the size of the human brain is approximately 1400 cubic centimeters, more than three times the size of the chimpanzee brain at 400 cubic centimeters. In addition, while chimpanzees mainly eat vegetables, humans are omnivorous. While humans are generally monogamous, alpha male chimpanzees have several female companions. At the time when humans branched off from chimpanzees, the Great Rift Valley in East Africa had become dry due to the foehn phenomenon. As trees decreased, species descended from them and began walking upright on open ground. The group of the last common ancestors that branched off from the chimpanzee and evolved into humans is called hominins.

About 3 million years ago, there lived among the hominins the Australopithecus Afarensis, whose remains are relatively well preserved. They walked in groups and these footprints still remain in the Laetoli volcanic zone, providing evidence that supports upright walking. In competition with the Australopithecus, there lived the Homo habilis of the genus Homo, who possessed a brain the size of approximately 600 cubic centimeters and whose remains and stone tools were discovered to date back to around 2.3 million years ago. As the species of the genus Homo evolved, Homo erectus first appeared 1.7 million years ago, and the hearths they used to control fire, dating back 800,000 years, were discovered in Israel. Controlling fire is associated with the evolution of cognitive functions such as working memory, and we can infer that meditation was involved in these changes.

Darwin's Theory of Evolution and Dawkins''Meme'

Charles Darwin and Richard Dawkins are among the key scholars who developed the theory of evolution. In his 1859 book, *The Origin of Species*, Darwin argued that life survives and reproduces through natural and sexual selection. Dawkins, who inherited Darwin's theory, stated that emotions and cognitive functions emerged as gene phenotypes, and he called genes that were culturally replicated through learning 'memes.'

In order to approach meditation anthropologically, we briefly examined the time after the Big Bang up to the remains of our ancestors who controlled fire. Hominins, our ancestors, controlled fire, held funeral rites, and developed diverse cultures as language evolved. In addition, humans are the only species to live and adapt widely across the Earth. The evolutionary process was not linear, but rather consisted of various species appearing and becoming extinct. Although humans also underwent our own crisis of extinction, we overcame it to reach the present day.

If we imagine a scene where the state of focused attention and awareness, along with relaxation, is repeated during the intense process of hominins controlling fire in their hearths, we can presume that a transformation of consciousness that served as the embryo of meditation took place here. We can assume that the accumulation of these experiences mediated the process of evolution by bringing about cognitive flexibility and variability.

The Control of Fire and Human's Meditation

Homo Erectus

Although there were several species that used fire, here we will only look at Homo erectus, for which there is a relatively large amount of research data. It is speculated that although Homo erectus was less sophisticated than Homo sapiens, they would have accumulated and passed on more diverse cultures than their previous human ancestors. Homo erectus survived from 1.7 million years ago to 100,000 years ago, and the size of their brains increased from the early stages to the later stages of their existence. At that time, due to the change in climate, the number of trees decreased, leading to an increase in life in open areas. Stone tools necessary for protection against predator attacks and the provision of food were developed and produced. Stout reviewed the linguistic origins in making stone tools, and given that the use of language facilitates more diverse experimental manipulations, he speculated that communication at this time would have at least improved compared to earlier, even if there is controversy over whether Homo erectus used language. In addition, female Homo erectus' bodies increased in size while their sexual dimorphism decreased, which suggests a change in their role in families and groups. These changes were mediated by fire, and many scholars agree that fire was controlled and used by Homo erectus 1 million years ago.

Controlling Fire

Controlling and using fire can protect against attacks from predators during the day and night. It is argued that the use of fire to cook meat and absorb a high amount of calories led to the increase in the size of the brain and body. Meanwhile, bringing meat back from the hunt to the hearths to cook and eat it together suggests an increase in social interaction. In addition, we can also speculate that Homo erectus lit fires in hearths in their caves to prevent attacks from predators at night, and they shared stories of hunting during the day as their time awake increased. These activities are also related to cognitive development.

Effects of the Campfire

Experiments show that looking into the flames of a campfire lowers blood pressure. One becomes relaxed due to the activation of the parasympathetic nervous system. In particular, it is said that the campfire strengthened the psychological characteristics of absorption and prosociality. There is a possibility that, along with relaxing, Homo erectus meditated by paying attention to the crackling sound of the flames while looking at the flames of the hearths in their caves. And meditation may have helped them adapt to the ecosystem during this time.

Evolutionary Psychiatry

Evolutionary psychiatry assumes that most human psychology was formed in the primitive era. When dividing human behavior into its proximate and ultimate causes, proximate causes see the relationships with direct causes that influence individual behavior, where ultimate causes see relationships with evolutionary environments at the species level. Evolutionary psychiatry deals with the latter. If we assume that the genus Homo appeared 2.3 million years ago and that the era of agricultural settlement began around 10,000 years ago, we can presume that meditation mediated the emotions and cognitive functions, such as anxiety and depression, of long-ago primitive life, and influenced its adaptation in later generations.

Funeral Rites and Meditation in Humanity

Homo Sapiens

It is estimated by genetic analysis that Homo sapiens appeared in South Africa about 350,000 years ago, but fossil remains and stone tools estimated to be about 300,000 years old were found in Morocco in Northern Africa. Although we do not know which part of Africa humans originated from, we are certain that they originated in Africa. They left the continent while moving around in search of food, and began to adapt to the ecosystems of Europe, Asia, and the Americas.

Since about 30,000 years ago, Homo sapiens have been the only remaining species to survive, with their other subspecies all becoming extinct. The genes that include not only those of the Neanderthal and Denisovan, but also those believed to be ancient humans, suggest that hominins existed and hybridized in various ways. The brain of Homo sapiens is known to be a very expensive tissue, using only 2% of their body weight but 20% of their metabolism. Comparing the size of the brain of early Homo sapiens from 300,000 years ago to that of modern humans, we find that its shape gradually became round, decreasing by about 10% 40,000 years ago.

In addition, Homo sapiens' prefrontal lobe and the precuneus, which is conscious of self, are relatively larger than those of the Neanderthals. On the other hand, there are examples in the evolution of the hominin brain where its structure is more important than its size. Homo naledi, who lived in South Africa 250,000 years ago, was unusually small in size and had a brain of about 500 cubic centimeters. However, like modern humans, their brain structure had the frontal operculum associated with language, and we expect that Homo naledi had a high level of intelligence. As for Homo sapiens, the size of male and female bodies is identical or within the range of 15%. Due to this, it is hypothesized that there have been changes in their sexual and social roles from previous species that exhibit sexual dimorphism. Less than 5% of mammals are monogamous. Humans, in contrast to chimpanzees, do not show any outward appearance during ovulation since they conceal their ovulation. It is argued that this induces paternal investment, which is advantageous in rearing children that require a long parenting period. And unlike other species, as groups of humans grew larger, they developed social intelligence and passed on accumulated knowledge through generations. We will examine how meditation has functioned in religion and art to create a symbolic culture shown in modern activities such as religion, art, and language.

Funeral Rites

In terms of animals, both wild and domestic animals are said to exhibit behaviors of mourning. However, animals do not attempt to connect with the world beyond death through rituals. We can find the origins of funeral rites in sites where burial was intentional. Artifacts believed to depict the first acts of burial, dating back 120,000 years ago, were discovered in Israel's Tabun Cave for Neanderthals, and 92,000 years ago in Israel's Qafzeh Cave for Homo sapiens. The shells found for the latter were brought from the Mediterranean Sea, 35 km away. When performing burials, humans brought relics from far away to connect with the world beyond death and expand their consciousness.

Shamans and Meditation

Shamans lead rituals that attempt to use supernatural powers through the conversion of consciousness. And this kind of shamanism was present in all hunter-gatherer societies throughout the ancestral cultures of mankind. In Sunghir, Russia, a roughly 30,000-year-old skeleton of a supposed shaman was discovered buried with a ring made of mammoth ivory and over 13,000 beads. In contrast to the argument that class inequality was more severe in settled societies with surplus goods, this can be seen as evidence showing discrimination according to the social division of labor since the Paleolithic era. 15,000 years ago, a shaman wearing a bird mask and carrying a bird cane was depicted in a cave in Lascaux, France. Next to that mural is an image of a bison being stabbed by a spear with its intestines sticking out, which suggests that the shaman attempted to connect with the world beyond death. Rossano argues that shamans maintained their meditative practice by transforming their consciousness through dancing and reciting incantations, and he argues that meditation facilitated the evolution of mankind by explaining the Baldwin effect in which these kinds of practices can affect genes. Through the rituals of shamans, humanity cultivated solidarity within its groups by attempting healing and expressing grief for the dead.

Social Intelligence

The difference between humans and other social animals such as ants and whales is that while other social animals adapted biologically through various mutations in their genes, humans adapted as one species by diversifying their culture and transmitting accumulated knowledge. The working memory of the brain and linguistic communication play an important role in the manifestation of intelligence embedded in such cultural diversity, and it can be assumed that there is a high probability that meditation was involved here.

There is a social intelligence hypothesis that states that language evolved as the number of groups increased. Dunbar argued that primates perform the intimate act of grooming each other to remove parasites, and that as the number of groups increased, language that facilitated interaction evolved in proportion to the increase in the neocortex. Humans also developed cognitively to process information while reading others' minds and carrying on conversations, and language is seen to have evolved and played a pivotal role here.

The Evolution of Language and Meditation in Humanity

The Emergence and Evolution of Language

The process of maturity is longer for humans than for chimpanzees, and they grow up learning language during a long period of care. Contrary to the opinion that the emergence of human language was a byproduct of brain development in the process of evolution, there are cognitive scientists who claim that it is instead the result of evolutionary adaptation, much like wings on a bird. They explain that the reason why natural selection carries more weight than cultural factors in the emergence of language is that it was already at work before cultural learning occurred, and because complex grammar was already at work even in primitive societies. Modern and symbolic activities in humanity include the use of pigments such as ochre and the use of adhesives, bows and arrows, etc., since humans were in Africa, and these are seen to have been related to the evolution of language. Although it is argued from genetic evidence that the FOX2P gene appeared in modern humans 200,000 years ago and that language began to develop in earnest at this time, there are also arguments that genes alone cannot explain the development of language since Neanderthals also shared this gene, and that the development of language must be viewed in relation to culture. In other words, language emerged and evolved through the interaction of both biological and cultural factors. There are some arguments that ancestral languages evolved to become languages through the reduction of errors in communication. However, despite being a single species, there are approximately 6000–8000 human languages, which shows that humans have conducted various cognitive experiments that surpass simply genetics.

Although it is still debated whether universal grammar exists innately in the use of various languages, the sign language of Nicaragua can be suggested as a representative example of human grammar. Deaf children in Nicaragua had difficulty adapting to a foreign language while learning Spanish, and in the process of communicating with each other, they created a new language system for themselves.

With these characteristics, humans created cultures and spoke a variety of languages in regions all over the world. However, scientists predict that many languages that are currently in use will disappear due to various reasons, including those languages that are not being passed down through the generations when young people from those regions leave to live in big cities.

Spells, Mantras, and Acceptance and Commitment Therapy (ACT)

The Sapir-Whorf hypothesis suggests that language may influence thinking. Although it is still difficult to prove, it is also difficult to argue that language has a minimal and limited effect on human thought. For example, during an experiment on color, it is possible to distinguish colors without using any words for them. However, it was found that Russian speakers who use two separate words depending on the brightness and darkness of the color blue can distinguish colors better than people in English-speaking countries who do not use two separate words to distinguish the color blue. This demonstrates a difference in human perception according to the language used. In other words, language can have some degree of influence on thinking, which contributes to the creation of diverse cultures.

When meditating, a shaman recites a spell. This is to use the magical power of connecting with the world beyond death. In Hinduism and Tibetan Buddhism, mantras are used to connect with and invoke cosmic forces. Results of tests showed that heart rate variability increased when reciting mantras. Studies on brain activity related to the recitation of mantras have shown an increase in hippocampus activity. There was also an evidence-based pilot study of the efficacy of reciting mantras when nursing beside dying patients.

On the other hand, mindfulness meditation is used in the Acceptance and Commitment Therapy (ACT) program to act directly on the mind without going through language. It is a process to directly enter into the mind by de-emphasizing language and emphasizing images and experience. It shows that language can be used as an anchor to meditation by being a window into various cultural differences.

Language and the Culture of Ethnic Minorities

We can speculate that language helped the imagination unfold in the form of stories and contributed to the emergence of culture and religion. In cross-cultural studies of ethnic minorities, spells can be viewed as an aspect of evolutionary adaptation. In one example, sociocultural gender roles can be seen in spells with obscene content. By controlling fire and consuming a high volume of calories, the bodies and brains of humans grew, and through funeral rites and connecting with the world beyond death, groups of humans were organized and grew in size. When language had not yet been developed, Homo sapiens would have engaged minimally in modern activities such as art, religion, and science. It should be seen that language contributed to the creation and spread of religion and literature through to the modern age. As a result, we can speculate that humanity created its own collective culture by attaching emotions and stories to the symbols of language.

Meditation provides insight into life and death. We can assume that meditation, along with the control of fire, was involved in working memory and helped to develop creative ideas in the creation and development of tools. In addition, there is a high probability that meditation, along with religious rituals, was involved in working memory related to life, death, and the afterlife. In this very process, meditation is considered as seeing the birth and death of the tribalistic collective culture that used language. Linguistic anthropology examines the evolution of human culture through this process.

Conclusion

The Anthropocene

Geologically, the present age is also called the Anthropocene. This is because Homo sapiens, who appeared about 300,000 years ago on Earth, which erupted from space 5 billion years ago, has had a great influence on Earth's geology. The Industrial Revolution in the 1800s is seen as the beginning of the Anthropocene, the nuclear tests in 1945 as an important milestone, and global warming, environmental pollution, and the breeding of livestock as its defining characteristics. Although the period from the formation of the Earth to the modern age is extremely insignificant from the perspective of the universe, the impact of humanity has been significant, drastically changing the environment and driving many species to extinction.

Self-Domesticated Humanity

Homo sapiens mobile lives, evolving their brains, developing cognitive functions, and creating modern symbolic cultures. It is said that humans domesticated wolves about 30,000 years ago. And while settling down, they domcsticated and raised many animals and plants. However, like domesticated animals, humans continue to exhibit the phenomenon of neoteny, where rearing takes a long period of time according to the human self-domestication hypothesis. Mismatches have occurred due to cultural and informational changes, where biological adaptations have changed rapidly as a result of living mobile lives. Some claim that this has led to diseases such as diabetes and alcoholism. It will be possible to investigate the evolution of the human species through further studies on developmental biology.

Meditation as a Regulator of the Human Evolutionary Processes

Just as we see the breath coming in and going out through meditation, if we examine the process of human evolution, we can see various cultures emerge and disappear. In this process, meditation provided the awareness to adapt to these changes. Without the process of awareness in meditation, it is possible to speculate that the problems in the Anthropocene would have proliferated much further. If we can be aware of this, we can make different choices and shape the direction and speed of the Anthropocene. The physiological and psychological effects of meditation influence our genes and culture, and now I believe that experiments in various forms will be conducted in relation to virtual reality.

Meditation as a Regulator in the Age of Civilizational Conflict and Artificial Intelligence

Historically, various species and cultures appeared and disappeared. Even now, civilizations continue to be in conflict with one another while at the same time trying to cooperate with one another. In addition, the use of artificial intelligence has been a double-edged sword for humanity. While reactive violence may decrease, premeditated violence may paradoxically increase. In this situation, we have no choice but to ask the question, What is evolution for exactly? If humanity can develop concentration, awareness, and insight through meditation, we will be able to contribute to controlling the direction and speed of the Anthropocene by making flexible choices.

Challenges Ahead

Future research should more closely analyze how mediation, along with molecular biology, genetics, and archeological data, contributed to the process of evolution. We are mapping out the brain and genes as they adapt to the ecosystem, and this will help us understand the role of meditation in more detail. The problem is how humans with their biological limitations can create a culture to solve problems in the face of unpredictable changes in circumstances. If we proceed while looking at the ecosystem and humanity through the lens of meditation, we may be able to move forward while making other choices.

Bibliography

Abrams DM, Strogatz SH. Modeling the dynamics of language death. Nature. 2003;424(6951):900.

Aiello LC, Wheeler P. The expensive-tissue hypothesis: the brain and the digestive system in human and primate evolution. Curr Anthropol. 1995;36(2):199–221.

Antón SC. Natural history of Homo erectus. Am J Phys Anthropol. 2003;122(S37):126–70.

Bernardi L, Sleight P, Bandinelli G, Cencetti S, Fattorini L, Wdowczyc-Szulc J, Lagi A. Effect of rosary prayer and yoga mantras on autonomic cardiovascular rhythms: comparative study. BMJ. 2001;323(7327):1446–9.

Brüne M. Textbook of evolutionary psychiatry & psychosomatic medicine: the origins of psychopathology. Oxford: Oxford University Press; 2008.

Bruner E, Iriki A. Extending mind, visuospatial integration, and the evolution of the parietal lobes in the human genus. Quat Int. 2016;405(A):98–110.

Bunting K, Hayes SC. Language and meaning: acceptance and commitment therapy and the EI model. In: Schneider KJ, editor. Existential-integrative psychotherapy: guideposts to the core of practice. Routledge/Taylor & Francis Group; 2008. p. 217–34.

Burchett PE. The 'magical' language of mantra. J Am Acad Relig. 2008;76(4):807–43.

Darwin C. The origin of species: by means of natural selection of the preservation of favoured races in the struggle for life. Kennebec Large Print; 2010.

De Bruin EI, Topper M, Muskens JGAM, Bögels SM, Kamphuis JH. Psychometric properties of the Five Facets Mindfulness Questionnaire (FFMQ) in a meditating and a non-meditating sample. Assessment. 2012;19(2):187–97.

Dirzo R, Young HS, Galetti M, Ceballos G, Isaac NJB, Collen B. Defaunation in the anthropocene. Science. 2014;345(6195):401–6.

Dobrovolskaya M, Richards M-P, Trinkaus E. Direct radiocarbon dates for the Mid Upper Paleolithic (eastern Gravettian) burials from Sunghir, Russia. Bull Mém Soc Anthropol Paris. 2012;24(1–2):96–102.

Dunbar RIM. The social brain hypothesis. Evol Anthropol Issues News Rev. 1998;6(5):178–90.

Engström M, Pihlsgärd J, Lundberg P, Söderfeldt B. Functional magnetic resonance imaging of hippocampal activation during silent mantra meditation. J Altern Complement Med. 2010;16(12):1253–8.

Everly GS Jr, Lating JM. A clinical guide to the treatment of human stress response. 3rd ed. New York: Springer; 2013.

Goren-Inbar N, Alperson N, Kislev ME, Simchoni O, Melamed Y, Ben-Nun A, Werker E. Evidence of hominin control of fire at Gesher Benot Yaaqov, Israel. Science. 2004;304(5671):725–7.

Groucutt HS, Petraglia MD, Bailey G, Scerri EML, Parton A, Clark-Balzan L, Jennings RP, Lewis L, Blinkhorn J, Drake NA, Breeze PS, Inglis RH, Devès MH, Merdith-Williams M, Boivin N, Thomas MG, Scally A. Rethinking the dispersal of Homo sapiens out of Africa. Evol Anthropol Issues News Rev. 2015;24(4):149–64.

Haig D. The gene meme. In: Grafen A, Ridley M, editors. Richard Dawkins: how a scientist changed the way we think. New York: Oxford University Press; 2007. p. 50–65.

Holloway RL, Hurst SD, Garvin HM, Schoenemann PT, Vanti WB, Berger LR, Hawks J. Endocast morphology of Homo naledi from the Dinaledi Chamber, South Africa. Proc Natl Acad Sci. 2018;115(22):5738–43.

Hublin JJ, Ben-Ncer A, Bailey SE, Freidline SE, Neubauer S, Skinner MM, Bargmann I, Le Cabec A, Benazzi S, Harvati K, Gunz P. New fossils from Jebel Irhoud, Morocco and the pan-African origin of Homo sapiens. Nature. 2017;546(7657):289–92.

Hussein BAS. The sapir-whorf hypothesis today. Theory Pract Lang Stud. 2012;2(3):642–6.

Johanson DC, Edey MA. Lucy: the beginnings of humankind. Simon and Schuster; 1990.

Kang Y. 'Open desire, close the body': magic spells, desire and the body among the Petalangan women in Indonesia. In: Language and sexuality: contesting meaning in theory and practice. CSLI Publications; 2001. p. 251–73.

King BJ. Animal mourning: précis of how animals grieve (King 2013). Anim Sentience: Interdiscip J Anim Feeling. 2016;1(4):1.

Larsen CS. Equality for the sexes in human evolution? Early hominid sexual dimorphism and implications for mating systems and social behavior. Proc Natl Acad Sci. 2003;100(16):9103–4.

Leakey MD, Hay RL. Pliocene footprints in the Laetolil Beds at Laetoli, northern Tanzania. Nature. 1979;278(5702):317–23.

Leakey LSB, Tobias PV, Napier JR. A new species of the genus Homo from Olduvai Gorge. Curr Anthropol. 1964;6(4):424–7.

Lukas D, Clutton-Brock TH. The evolution of social monogamy in mammals. Science. 2013;341(6145):526–30.

Lynn CD. Hearth and campfire influences on arterial blood pressure: defraying the costs of the social brain through fireside relaxation. Evol Psychol. 2014;12(5):983–1003. https://doi.org/10.1177/147470491401200509.

Marlatt GA, Bowen S, Chawla N, Wikiewitz K. Mindfulness-based relapse prevention for substance abusers: therapist training and therapeutic

relationships. In: Hick S, Bien T, editors. Mindfulness and the therapeutic relationship. New York: Guilford Press; 2008. p. 107–21.
Mayer DEBY, Bandermeersch B, Bar-Yosef O. Shells and ochre in Middle Paleolithic Qafzeh Cave, Israel: indications for modern behavior. J Hum Evol. 2009;56(3):307–14.
McBrearty S, Brooks AS. The revolution that wasn't: a new interpretation of the origin of modern human behavior. J Hum Evol. 2000;39(5):453–563.
Mellars P. Why did modern human populations disperse from Africa ca. 60,000 years ago? A new model. Proc Natl Acad Sci. 2006;103(25):9381–6.
Neubauer S, Hublin JJ, Gunz P. The evolution of modern human brain shape. Sci Adv. 2018;4(1):eaao5961. https://doi.org/10.1126/sciadv.eaao5961.
Nowak MA, Krakauer DC. The evolution of language. Proc Natl Acad Sci. 1999;96(14):8028–33.
Pinker S, Bloom P. Natural language and natural selection. Behav Brain Sci. 1990;13(4):707–27.
Purdy IB, Melwak MA. Implementing evidence-based practice: a mantra for clinical change. J Perinat Neonatal Nurs. 2009;23(3):263–9.
Rossano MJ. Did meditating make us human? Camb Archaeol J. 2007;17(1):47–58.
Ryan RE. The strong eye of shamanism: a journey into the caves of consciousness. Inner Traditions/Bear & Co; 1999.
Senghas A, Kita S, Özyürek A. Children creating core properties of language: evidence from an emerging sign language in Nicaragua. Science. 2004;305(5691):1779–82.
Singh M. The cultural evolution of shamanism. Behav Brain Sci. 2018;41:1–62.
Stout D, Chaminade T. Stone tools, language and the brain in human evolution. Philos Trans R Soc B Biol Sci. 2012;367(1585):75–87.
Strassmann BI. Sexual selection, paternal care, and concealed ovulation in humans. Ethol Sociobiol. 1981;2(1):31–40.
Stringer CB. Replacement, continuity and the origin of Homo sapiens. In: Bräuer G, Smith FH, editors. Continuity or replacement. Rotterdam: A. A. Balkema; 1992. p. 9–24.
Theofanopoulou C, Gastaldon S, O'Rourke T, Samuels BD, Messner A, Martins PT, Delogu F, Alamri S, Boeckx C. Self-domestication in Homo sapiens: insights from comparative genomics. PLoS One. 2017;13(5):e0185306.
Wallace RK, Benson H, Wilson AF. A wakeful hypometabolic physiologic state. Am J Physiol-Legacy Content. 1971;221(3):795–9.
Winawer J, Witthoft N, Frank MC, Wu L, Wade AR, Boroditsky L. Russian blues reveal effects of language on color discrimination. Proc Natl Acad Sci. 2007;104(19):7780–5.
Wrangham R. The goodness paradox: the strange relationship between virtue and violence in human evolution. New York: Pantheon; 2019.
Wrangham R, Carmody R. Human adaptation to the control of fire. Evol Anthropol Issues News Rev. 2010;19(5):187–99.

Meditation and Spirituality

5

Jeong-Ho Chae

We are spiritual beings that have human experiences, not human beings that have spiritual experiences.

—Pierre Teilhard de Chardin

Introduction

It is very difficult to arrive at a precise definition of the term "spirituality" that everyone can agree with. Spirituality has been used in a variety of ways depending on different contexts, positionalities, backgrounds, and speakers' identities. Due to the historical development, transformation, and expansion of the meaning of spirituality over time, the word now carries a wide variety of complex meanings. Spirituality is both distinct from and a broader concept than religion. Spirituality involves finding a transcendental purpose in life. Many individuals pursue spirituality through religious activities, but non-religious individuals can also explore or express spirituality through avenues such as music, art, philosophy, and relationships with others. Religion is an array of religious beliefs and activities that are specialized methods and systems of pursuing transcendental values. Thus, not everyone has a religion. By contrast, spirituality—the pursuit of transcendental values—can be present in everyone. According to some points of view, spirituality is one of many positive psychological factors such as peace, harmony, meaning, purpose, and fulfillment. However, one must note that spirituality has a transcendental and immaterial nature beyond these other concepts, is distinct in that it connotes a pursuit of the sacred aspects of the universe and human existence and can be understood as a personal investigation to reach answers to the ultimate questions regarding a human's relationship with a divine or transcendental being. Incipient religious traditions considered spirituality as "a process of reformation for the purpose of recovering the inherent original human form" and as a process of orientation towards a life devoted to a god or an absolute being. Thereafter, the meaning of spirituality has expanded to include all of life's invisible elements. Accordingly, in the present day, spirituality is largely understood as "the ultimate profound values and the meaning of life," "beliefs in supernatural realms," or "an investigation into ultimate or divine significances." Sometimes, the word is used simply as an alternative phrase for "religious experiences," or to express "one's encounter with one's own interior dimension." Popular meanings of this term in the present day include the following similar yet various definitions: "the ultimate and immaterial reality," "the inner path that leads to discovery of the essence of existence," "the most profound values and meanings among the principles according to which one should live," "finding one's self in a larger sense through experiencing a connection or union with a reality bigger than oneself," "experiencing a connection

J.-H. Chae (✉)
Department of Psychiatry, The Catholic University of Korea, Seoul, Korea (Republic of)
e-mail: alberto@catholic.ac.kr

J.-H. Chae, H.-Y. Lee (eds.), *Meditation in Psychiatry and General Medicine*,
https://doi.org/10.1007/978-981-95-7147-5_5

or union with others or the community," "experiencing a connection or union with nature or the cosmos," and "experiencing a connection or union with the divine realm" Wikipedia (2020a). For example, Dr. Christina Puchalski defined spirituality as "the aspect of humanity that refers to the ways in which individuals pursue and express meaning and purpose, and a way of experiencing a connection between the self and the moment, others, nature, and what is divine." Mario Beauregard and Denyse O'Leary stated that spirituality means "any experience that allows the experiencer to come in contact with a divine being." Therefore, spirituality is sometimes experienced as a source of inspiration that informs one's direction of life. In addition, it can also mean faith in immaterial realities or experiencing the immanent or transcendent natures inherent in the world and the universe.

To fully experience and maintain one's spirituality, a variety of spiritual practices have been developed and passed down. Representative examples of such practices include meditation, prayer, and contemplation. Broadly speaking, any method of practice that allows one to attain spirituality can be considered meditation. Such spiritual practices allow for the precise perception and development of one's internal life, and ultimately allow the experience of spirituality in one's life. Therefore, in this chapter, we will investigate the meaning of spirituality in the temporal, religious, and modern contexts, and inquire into the significance of meditation as a method of practicing such spirituality.

Spirituality

Spirituality—How Its Meaning Has Changed Over the Years

Originating from the term spirit, which signifies the breath, vitality, the wind, the soul, etc., spirituality is a holistic concept that refers to the all-encompassing and complex experiences relating to an absolute being or realm in which the soul participates, where the "soul" is a fundamental and essential element of human life and existence. However, since the term spirituality is used by many religions of divergent backgrounds and perspectives, and even routinely used by laypeople outside of religious traditions, it is almost impossible to present a universally agreed-upon definition. Moreover, it is important to precisely identify the contexts in which the term spirituality is used, because this concept is sometimes used expansively, not only to indicate spirituality on its own, but also to indicate self-transcendence, asceticism, and connection to all humanity and sometimes to all living beings. Keith Weissman presented a relatively traditional definition, stating that spirituality is a "process of reformation with the aim of restoring humanity's original image, i.e., the image of God." In other words, this defines spirituality on the level of traditional religious concepts, indicating a return to its original state as defined by the various religious traditions, such as Torah in Judaism, Jesus in Christianity, the Buddha in Buddhism, and Muhammad in Islam. From the beginning of the contemporary era, however, contents from fields such as humanistic psychology, mystic traditions, and Eastern religions began to merge with the term spirituality. Through this process, spirituality has expanded and developed into a term that means, at its core, "the most profound values and meanings of human life," which also encompasses individual growth and transformation in forms outside of traditional religions.

Linguistically, the word spirituality has widely been used to refer to "the roots of life and vitality present in humans or animals." The word spirit, like its French counterpart esprit, has its linguistic roots in the words *spiritus* and *spirare* in Latin, the former meaning "the soul, courage, energy, the breath," and the latter meaning "to breathe." In the context of Christianity, these Latin words have been used to translate the Greek word *pneuma* and the Hebrew word *ruah* as they appear in Paul's Letters. The English term spirituality is considered to have derived from *spiritualis* in Latin, *spiritualitatem* in Late Latin, and *spiritualité* in Middle French. In the religious context, the Latin word *spiritualitas* became widely known as used by Hieronymus in the fifth century to connote "to hold onto the good and to progress." In other words, this term indicated the activities of the absolute God. At its origins, then, spirituality referred to the act of following the good as according to God in spirit. By the eleventh century, however, the term was used to refer to the mind-related aspects of life, as opposed to material or sensual aspects. Befitting the Middle Ages, spirituality came to indicate the realm of internal life as opposed to worldly possessions or pleasures, to indicate "light" as opposed to "darkness." With the birth of Scholasticism after the twelfth century, monasteries were no longer the center of theology; rather, universities took on the research and study of theology alongside other disciplines, developing a culture of persuasion and argument. Gradually, as scholars distinguished material reality from the spiritual realms, they came to use the term "spiritual being" to refer to intellectual beings as opposed to creatures that lacked the power of reason. As the term spirituality increasingly embodied such a dichotomy that distinguished the spiritual realms from material reality, it was sometimes even used to refer to phenomena that could not be understood with reason alone, straying far from its original meaning. Therefore, in some religious circles, different terms such as devotion, perfection, and piety were emphasized to distinguish them from these developments, in an effort to faithfully represent the original meaning of spirituality. Moreover, some circles used spirituality as a concept that distinguished the clergy from the laity, further complicating the implications of the term. When used in a positive light, spirituality was used to connote having a relationship with God on a personal and experiential level. On the other hand, when used in a negative light, spirituality was used in a disparaging way to connote irrational emotions and fanaticism. Therefore, spirituality was considered a special and distinct virtue that could not be obtained from everyday life. Even afterwards, controversy has continued over the relationship between a life of asceticism as a part of one's everyday routine and a life consisting of a mystical and transcendental grace. In the present day, it may seem obvious that anyone could attain transcendence. However, for quite a long time, the mystical was considered distinct from the everyday. In fact, even in theological circles, ethical or ascetical theology was considered separate from spiritual or mystical theology. Following such discussions, spirituality came to be used as a comprehensive term that included both ascetical and mystical theologies. As a result, spirituality developed into a term that examines the complex mysteries of human growth and maturity, unfettered by any specific religious traditions or tenets. Over the nineteenth and twentieth centuries, the term was infused with elements from Western mystical traditions and Asian, especially Indian, religions. Spirituality therefore became tied to movements such as liberalism, feminist theology, and green politics, in a form different from traditional religions. Thereafter, emphasis was placed on transcendence, focused on intuitive and experiential approaches. The concept was then expanded as previously lesser-known elements such as Hindu religions were incorporated into its discourse, followed by pantheistic universalism. Finally, a concept was born that spoke to a connection among all living beings. Further major influences incorporated into spirituality include the development of the Theosophical Society with an interest in Asian mysticism, the Neo-Vedanta school that sought to philosophically consummate traditional Indian beliefs, and Theravada Buddhism.

Accordingly, the term spirituality used today integrates all aspects of human life and existence, and it considers the connections of all such aspects. To cite an example of such a definition, spirituality can be considered as "the ultimate or immaterial reality, the inner path that allows one to discover one's essence of existence, and the most profound values and meanings among the principles to abide by in life." As such, it is of course conceivable that a person may not be religious but at the same time possess a high level of spirituality. A person may be considered spiritual if he or she possesses an intuition of a larger existence beyond material realities. By definition, spirituality is not an optional virtue that is simply good to have if one can afford it. Rather, spirituality itself is the ultimate existence, and it is therefore indispensable to seek and work towards attaining spirituality. Unfortunately, most people in this day and age generally live their lives focused on handling everyday matters that need immediate attention, as opposed to directing their interest towards matters concerning the ultimate existence. Therefore, when people encounter certain situations that are impossible to deal with practically—moments that are defined by existential psychology as those in which one cannot help but face questions of death, freedom, isolation, meaninglessness, etc.—it is likely difficult for them to overcome such overwhelming situations without a connection with spirituality. On the other hand, we also see an abundance of cults or pseudo-religions that target people who ordinarily lack spiritual experience in their lives and provide them with opportunities to practice spirituality or engage in spiritual experiences. Even in the cultural realm, spirituality-related content is gaining great popularity. For example, the film Avatar captured the public's interest by describing the presence of spirituality in the "Na'vi," an alien species with an emphasis on the "Hometree" that symbolizes the most sacred soul, and how the "Na'vi" engaged in prayer and were connected to each other and to a higher being through their antennas. In this way, spirituality in the present day is used, at least in non-religious contexts, to refer to having faith in immaterial realities, or experiencing an existence that is transcendental or that exists in the world and the universe since their inception.

Spirituality and Religion

While spirituality was previously closely tied to the category of religion, the concept became increasingly divorced from religion after World War II. Rather than referring to "attempts to align the self within the context of a larger existence," the term came to place a greater emphasis on the individual's subjective experience Gil (2004). With the incorporation of influences from humanistic psychology, supernatural or mystic traditions, and Asian religions, the concept of spirituality was expanded to signify the theme of finding the "real self" or "true self" through practices such as meditation or self-expression. In the twentieth century, the discourse was further expanded with the advent of secularism and the New Age movement. As a result, spirituality became entrenched in popular discourse as a general term to such a degree that sometimes "spiritual" would be used in contexts that would have previously been described as "religious." However, it is impossible to consider spirituality as distinct and separate from religion, because the concept has always been approached in the context of religious traditions since the beginning of history. Therefore, this section seeks to provide an overview of the meaning of spirituality and spiritual practices in the contexts of major religions, as well as how such meanings have changed leading up to the present day Wikipedia (2020b).

Judaism

Judaism, which is based on the Torah centered on the laws directly received from God, emphasizes the practice of spirituality through religious rituals, such as moral codes, prayer, religious garments, sabbath, pilgrimage, studying the Torah, and food restriction. Meaning "transmission" or "reception" in Hebrew, the term Kabbalah refers to Judaism's mystic aspects, which do not exist in any text but were instead passed down orally amongst a small number of people. Over the ages, this oral transmission took place only amongst qualified disciples who had observed certain strict rites of passage according to tradition. As seen in Judaism, humans are created as collaborators of God at the intersection of the celestial and terrestrial realms. Through asceticism and the memorization of the names of God and the angels, humans can enter into a spiritual state of ecstasy and obtain the mystical experience of relating to the secret workings of the celestial realm. In other words, humans can serve God intimately and relish in the presence of God. After Abraham received the celestial secrets and Moses received God's prophecies, Moses recorded God's laws, but for those he could not express in writing, it is known that Moses passed them on through the vehicle of Kabbalah. Starting from early efforts in mysticism to participating in celestial spheres by replicating Ezekiel's experience of seeing visions, Kabbalah was further developed in the Middle Ages with efforts to revive it as a way to connect spiritual experiences with everyday life. Thereafter, the influence of Kabbalah extended into Christianity, and even into secret societies that had no direct connection with Christianity, such as the Rosicrucians and the Freemasons. The Kabbalistic philosophy is realized in the form of the "Tree of Life," where "Keter" at the top means the original present form of "God," and "Malkuth" at the very bottom means the ultimate present form of "God," in other words, the material realm. A practitioner of Kabbalah is considered to freely navigate the various levels between "Keter" and "Malkuth," and refers to a person who possesses a spirituality that allows connection to the secrets that underlie the entirety of humanity and the universe. Therefore, Kabbalah presents a method to achieve spirituality through providing explanations to various existential questions such as the essence of humanity and the universe, and the essence and purpose of existence. In addition, there were some trends in Judaism that encouraged spiritual practices as a way to publicize and internalize mysticism and thereby cultivate spirituality through piety.

Christianity

The core purpose of Christianity, including both Catholicism and Protestantism, is union with Jesus Christ. Christian spirituality asks individuals to practice their faiths and engage in spiritual practices in their everyday lives. Such practices include reading spiritual texts (Lectio Divina), prayer, and contemplation. For many centuries, ancient monasteries in the Middle Ages incorporated spiritual training and practice as a part of everyday life, attempting to relate to God through prayer. Prayer brings forth self-awareness and attention, through which an individual concentrates on the absolute Being. Within this interaction, the individual experiences the presence of God and enters a spiritual experience in which the ordinary divisions between the sacred and profane, body and soul, and the world and the church become blurred. Contemplation, a word often used in Christian circles in the place of meditation, itself signifies experiencing the presence of God in the templum, i.e., the place that the prophets reserved for God. In progressive Christian circles, we have also seen contemporary movements to remove the supernatural arguments from Christian faiths and replace them with a critical understanding of biblical spirituality based on historical and scientific research. Nevertheless, even these progressive groups still remain focused on the vivid experience of spirituality and accept that faith is a true and humane foundation and that spiritual experiences are psychologically and neurologically real and effective. In Christian traditions, individuals are encouraged to continue spiritual practices through internal practices such as contemplation, prayer, fasting, and study, external practices such as simplicity, obedience, and service, and communal practices such as confession, worship, spiritual guidance, and celebration.

Islam

The five pillars of Islam are the five basic actions required of believers, which are *shahadah* (confession of faith), *salat* (prayer), *hajj* (pilgrimage to Mecca), fasting during Ramadan, and *zakah* (relief and charitable giving). It is through these actions that Muslims experience spirituality Islam presents several different forms of spirituality, one of which is Sufism. Popularized by famous masters such as Rumi and Hafez, Sufism is a well-known tradition of spiritual training and practice, referring to the internal and mystical realms of Islam. Regarding the origins of the word *ṣufı*, the dominant theory is that the word refers to donning *ṣūf* (wool) as a garment, but there are also alternative theories. For example, there is a theory that it originated from the Greek word *sophia*, meaning wisdom. Sufism requires strict self-discipline and asceticism, and through such spiritual practices, individuals can attain the stage of preeminence in a state of rapture or an ecstatic trance. Terms used in Sufism such as *tawakkul* (faith), *ma'rifa* (knowledge), and *fana* (self-oblivion) illustrate this approach. Sufi philosophy is communicated in the form of poetry and is expressed through works of poets such as Ibn al' Arabi, Ibn al' Farid in Arabic, Rumi,

Hafez, and Jami in Persian, and Nizami or Nezāmiin Turkish. Many Sufi schools (such as *tariqa*) surfaced, including the Turkish Sufi Dervishes that utilize whirling dances as a method of reaching the state of rapture. Dikhr, which is a sort of incantation, is also often used as a method of spiritual practice. Among the Islamic religions, the Sunni branch regards Sufism as un-Islamic and nontraditional and does not acknowledge Sufism as a part of Islam. On the other hand, some groups regard Sufism as the true supporters of Islam in its pure and original form. These groups are characterized by their emphasis on tolerance and peace, and opposition to all forms of violence. Such groups define Islam as "the science of restoring the mind by turning away from everything but God," argue that the core of Sufism is the process of cleansing oneself and getting closer to God and consider spiritual practice as a very important element.

Buddhism

The word Buddhism has two meanings: the religious tenets as preached by Sakyamuni Buddha (Siddhartha Gautama), and the principles to be followed in order to become a Buddha. The word "Buddha" means "the enlightened one" in Sanskrit and Pali, and was used as a general term in ancient India, whereas afterwards the term mainly referred to Sakyamuni. To pursue enlightenment, one must inevitably focus on spirituality. Buddhist practices are centered around *bhavana*, which the word itself signifies "development," "cultivation," "creation," etc. *Bhavana* generally means both *citta-bhavana*, which refers to the development of the mind, and *metta-bhavana*, which refers to the development of love, kindness, and compassion. In general usage, *bhavana* signifies "spiritual cultivation," and is very important in Buddhist practice (*patipatti*). Through the "Four Noble Truths," i.e., the truth of suffering, the truth of the origin of suffering, the truth of the cessation of suffering, and the truth of the path to the cessation of suffering, one awakens to the truth of life and the solution to suffering. Among the Four Noble Truths, the truth of the path to the cessation of suffering employs the Noble Eightfold Path as a method of practice, which comprises the right view, right intention, right speech, right action, right livelihood, right effort, right mindfulness, and right concentration. Notably, as opposed to Hinduism and other traditions, Buddhism does not encourage asceticism but employs the practice of moderation (the Middle Way) to pursue wisdom and compassion. The core contents of wisdom comprise the truths of "transience" (the temporal principle that vertically cross-sections the universe) and "dependent arising" (the spatial principle that horizontally connects the universe). It is understood that the root of all suffering comes from desire and obsession over illusions that always change and have no real substance. To rid oneself of such desires and obsessions, Buddhists emphasize spiritual practice and meditation, through which they strive to discard illusions, to behold objects with an unwavering focus, and to face the truths of reality. Pāramitās, or "perfections" are used in Buddhist practice, which include the Six Paramitas of Dāna, Śīla, Kṣānti, Vīrya, Dhyāna, and Prajñā. Dāna refers to generosity, Śīla refers to adherence to the rules, Kṣānti refers to enduring and overcoming adversity, Vīrya refers to diligence and effort, and Dhyāna refers to concentration that stabilizes the mind, in accordance with the "right concentration" of the Noble Eightfold Path. Prajñārefers to truthful and proper wisdom, which becomes the foundation of the other five Pāramitās. There is also a reference made to Ten Pāramitās, which include the four additional Pāramitāsof Upāya (skillful means), Praṇidhāna (resolution or determination), Bala (spiritual power), and Jñāna (knowledge). Through a quiet, relaxed, and steady state of awakening, practitioners seek to attain Nirvana. Contemporary psychology utilizes various Buddhist terms and practices regarding meditation in the context of a variety of psychological treatments.

Hinduism

Hinduism is quite distinct from other religions in that it is difficult to pin down, comes in a variety of forms, and does not have a traditional church order, central religious organization, religious court, prophets, or a particular religious text.

Structured in an open and expansive way, Hinduism allows a practitioner to choose between polytheistic, pantheistic, monistic or atheistic approaches to individually experience Hindu philosophy and spirituality, referred to as ksaitrajña, to attain self-awareness, discovery of higher truths, the true nature of reality, and a free and self-sufficient consciousness. Hinduism traditionally employs three methods or paths (marga) of spiritual practice: Jñāna-marga is the method of knowledge, Bhakti-marga is the method of devotion, and the self-effacing Karma-marga is the method that utilizes yoga. Since the nineteenth century, Rāja yoga has also been added, which refers to contemplation and meditation. There are also movements that consider all of the above collectively as yoga. Jñāna refers to receiving instructions and assistance from a leader or teacher, called a "guru," during spiritual practice. Bhakti refers to the act of faithful devotion in front of a sacred idol, sometimes using hymn-like music and songs such as *kirtans*. Karma refers to spiritual liberation from the body in everyday life through diligent practice, or *vartta*. Rāja emphasizes various spiritual practices, such as necessary virtues, self-discipline, and *tapas*, which refers to meditation, contemplation, and self-reflection, as the foundations to attain the experience of the climactic state of *Samādhi*, in which the self is separated from, and then united with, the universe.

Sikhism

Sikhism was born in the fifteenth century in Northern India, and it combines the Bhakti religion in Hinduism and Islamic mystic ideologies. The word *Sikh* is said to have originated from the Sanskrit word *sisya*, meaning "education" or "learning", or *siksa*, meaning "teaching." In both cases, the term connotes education. At its core, the purpose of Sikhism is deliverance through cultivating one's mind in the name of God Vahiguru and according to his message. Sikh practitioners follow the teachings of Nanak the founder and his nine guru disciples, and conform their actions to the scripture called "Guru Granth Sahib," which discusses various aspects of the society, economy, and religion. The Sikh God is formless, infinite, and invisible. Therefore, the only way to approach God and obtain deliverance is through spiritual practices relating to God. In addition, because practitioners in a state of advanced spiritual communion can actually see God, the development of one's individual internal spirituality is emphasized. Nanak, the founder of Sikhism, stressed the importance of living an "active, creative and practical life" as a higher mode of practice rather than engaging solely in meditation, which focuses on "truth, devotion, self-control and purity." Through engaging in such spiritual practices, an individual could cultivate their own spirituality and reach deliverance.

African Religions and Other Spiritualities

Spirituality is not limited to the major religions discussed above. Rather, it is recognized as a common element in every corner of humanity, no matter what belief system or religion a culture may have. However, the understandings and methods of practice of spirituality in some cultures may not be well-known. For example, cultures in Africa have spirituality as a belief system that protects society and people from evil demons and misfortune. More than any other continent, Africa has distinct animism-related faiths that survive to the present day. Traditional African religions consist of a great variety of faiths that have interacted and combined among themselves. Belief in spirits and ancestor worship has even been used in traditional African medicine. Practitioners of traditional African religions pray not only to their ancestors but also to various spirits and attempt to connect with God through these spirits as intermediaries. Regardless of whether one believes in one God (e.g., Chukwu, Nyame, Olodumare, Ngai, Roog), a dual God (e.g., Mawu-Lisa), or a female God, there is definitely a belief in a transcendental being or existence. The environment and natural elements are deeply connected with spiritual experiences in traditional African religions. Theories of the universe and transcendental beliefs are intertwined with natural phenomena and the environment in a complex way. Every element of nature such as the weather, thunder, lightning, rain, day, moon, sun, and stars is connected with Africans' cosmologies, and individuals engage in spiritual practice through their connection with such a cosmic existence.

Contemporary Spirituality

In the contemporary era, the term "spiritual" is now more widely and expansively used than the term "religious." Contemporary spirituality is also referred to as "post-traditional spirituality" or "new age spirituality." A narrow definition of "new age" designates the trend originating from Britain in the twentieth century in the fields of theosophy and anthroposophy; a broader definition understands "new age" to indicate the post-1970s era. In any case, as it is now possible to conceive of a person who is spiritual but not religious, we are clearly in an era in which it is no longer a novelty to approach spirituality in aspects beyond traditional religious categories. Contemporary spirituality focuses on "the deepest values and meanings by which people live." As such, it encompasses concepts about the ultimate and immaterial realities. It is about finding one's internal way towards the discovery of the essence of one's own human existence. It is not always the case that all contemporary understandings of spirituality necessarily involve transcendental elements. In a secular vein, spirituality also emphasizes humanist values relating to morality (qualities such as love, compassion, patience, generosity, forgiveness, contentment, responsibility, harmony, and regard for others). Even without applying beliefs about supernatural realities or the existence of God, it is possible to go beyond the purely materialistic perspectives of the world and deal with the immaterial and communal experience aspects in life and human existence. However, there is a concern that such conceptualization may lead to an excessive broadening of the term spirituality. The definition of spirituality continues to expand so that it can encompass discussion about supernatural and invisible phenomena, and at the same time it can also be explained via secular morality and philanthropy.

Spirituality and Mental Health

We define health as not simply an absence of disease or disability, but a state of psychological, physical, social, and spiritual well-being. Likewise, if we regard a human being not only as a psychological being but in a holistic and comprehensive perspective, we must approach the subject with a combination of all approaches and consider all areas of social, cultural, psychological and physical influences. This means we must necessarily include a spiritual approach. The current definition of "health" according to the World Health Organization (WHO) is "physical, mental, and social well-being." The need to add spiritual health to this definition is clear, but due to the broad categories of spirituality and difficulties in formulating a scientific definition of spiritual health, an official inclusion of spiritual health has not yet been made. Nevertheless, one cannot help but recognize the importance of understanding the spiritual dimensions of health. Furthermore, instead of considering spirituality as but one aspect of human existence, one should proceed with the recognition that spirituality is at the core of being human. It is especially appropriate that spirituality is incorporated in mental health and medical diagnosis and treatment, which considers human beings in a holistic and integrated perspective. Moreover, even though post-Freudian psychotherapy is considered to be the origin of mental health and medical practice, a broader view could trace the beginnings of mental health treatment to the role of ancient priests in prehistoric cultures. As such, it perhaps makes obvious sense to use the framework of spirituality to approach human beings' treatment and recovery. Indeed, it would be strange not to consider spirituality at all. Humans are essentially spiritual beings, and so spirituality is tied to the nature of being human. "Becoming human" can also be defined as developing one's spirituality as befits the nature of humans as spiritual beings.

In approaching spirituality, it is impossible not to consider the mind. In many contexts, human beings are categorized in a dichotomy of the body and mind. In other perspectives, the mind is divided into psychology and spirit(soul). More recently, some have recognized that a clear division among such elements is impossible and have instead argued for a unified perspective considering the body, mind, and spirit as an indivisible whole. In either approach, spirituality is closely related to mental health. There have been many scholars who attempted to formulate a psychological understanding of spirituality by separating the mind into psychology and spirit Mcminn (2001). For example, scholars such as Daniel A. Helminiak and Bernard Lonergan have contributed to explaining spirituality in psychological terms. There are many studies that have investigated the relationship between mental health and spirituality or religion. In spite of the inherent limitations in evaluating spirituality using scientific tools, results indicate that spirituality in particular, and especially spiritual well-being in general, are positively associated with other positive indicators of mental health. It is said that spirituality develops inner peace and forms the foundation for happiness. Spirituality exhibits a close positive correlation with broad-ranging factors of psychological well-being, including optimism, hope, self-esteem, the purpose and meaning of life, social support, internal locus of control, and marital satisfaction Scazzero (2015). On the other hand, studies consistently report a negative correlation between spirituality and depression symptoms, although the effect size is moderate. In situations of extreme stress, in particular, spirituality exhibits a higher negative correlation with depression symptoms. Likewise, in cases of moderate or severe depression, spirituality shows a higher negative correlation with depression symptoms than in cases of light depression. In addition, spirituality shows a clear negative correlation with drug use and/or abuse. Students who have not received religious or spiritual education in their youth are more likely to engage in drug abuse than students who have, and an absence of spiritual training during one's teenage years is directly related to an increase in drug use. Spirituality is also closely related to suicide. Individuals with relatively higher levels of spirituality exhibit a lower likelihood of committing suicide. Individuals with no religion, compared to individuals with religion with identical levels of depression, make more attempts at suicide throughout their lifetimes, feel less purpose in life, and hold fewer moral objections towards the idea of suicide. Moreover, spirituality is even related to symptoms of serious mental illnesses such as schizophrenia. Higher levels of spirituality were correlated with lower levels of schizophrenia symptoms. In a study that involved participants engaging in weekly prayer and bible lectures, subjects showed noticeable improvements in their psychopathological conditions and their abilities to function in their daily lives. In cases of PTSD where traditional methods of treatment may have limited effects, enhancing spirituality sometimes plays a key role in treatment. A series of studies conducted by the author's research team have also confirmed this close relationship between spirituality and mental health Jeon et al. (2020). Min et al. (2013) measured optimism and clinical data in individuals diagnosed with depression and/or anxiety disorder, and investigated the relationship between spirituality and resilience, i.e., the strength to overcome and recover from the various adversities that one encounters in life. As a result, the study found that individuals with lower levels of spirituality showed lower levels of resilience. Such results are evidence that spirituality is a critical factor in experiencing and recovering from despair. Song et al. (2012) studied patients diagnosed with depression and found a significant negative correlation between spirituality and symptoms of depression and/or anxiety (i.e., lower levels of spirituality indicated higher severity of symptoms). Furthermore, positive affect—a factor unrelated to symptoms—increased with higher levels of spirituality, and negative affect increased with lower levels of spirituality. Yi et al. (2012) also investigated patients diagnosed with depression and found that spirituality critically influenced hope, which is a key element in the treatment of depression. In sum, spirituality can prevent mental illnesses such as depression, can assist recovery from such disorders, can alleviate symptoms, and can increase hope, which is a key factor in treatment and recovery. Together, these studies illustrate the importance of incorporating spirituality in mental health and medical diagnosis and treatment, particularly in the context of depression and anxiety disorders. Continuous research by Min et al. (2012, 2013) reveals that elements such as the purpose of life and spirituality play an important role in recovering from mental illnesses such as depression and anxiety disorders. More recently, Kim et al. (2015) investigated the factors associated with the successful treatment of patients diagnosed with depressive disorder. Factors related to successful treatment included maintenance of marital relationship, sufficient length of treatment, relatively mild symptoms, etc. Also related to successful treatment were spirituality and whether the subject considered their religious life to be important. Even after using regression analysis to control for other factors such as marital maintenance, length of treatment, and level of symptoms, spirituality and the importance placed on religion were significantly correlated with responsiveness to treatment. The final model revealed that spirituality was the strongest factor associated with treatment response. As outlined above, evidence is accumulating that shows the importance of a spiritual approach to patients endorsing mental illness symptoms.

Many theories have been proposed to explain the beneficial effects of spirituality on physical and mental health. First, most spiritual practices encourage sound and healthy actions and lifestyles. Barring excessively radical and/or extreme religious activities, most spiritual practices are beneficial to one's health. Second, spiritual practices and religious activities can be a source of social support, due to the fact that one can belong to a group and derive support from the group. Third, spiritual beliefs that go beyond visible realities can bring forth peace, self-confidence, a sense of purpose, and forgiveness, etc., and enable the exercise of acceptance and patience. Fourth, spirituality enables one to discover the meaning and purpose of life, and thereby fosters individual development and increases one's capacity to handle adversities. Finally, spiritual practice carries benefits in and of itself, such as transforming one's personality through meditation, contemplation, prayer, etc., decreasing tension, anxiety, and self-deprecating thoughts, decreasing emotional fluctuation, and developing insight into oneself. This can cause improvements in various symptoms, including anxiety, depression, insomnia, stress, and chronic pain. Spiritual practice can incorporate all of the aforementioned elements and cause a comprehensive transformation of one's beliefs, actions, and environment that operates favorably towards one's mental health Korean Christian Counseling Psychology Association (2018). Sometimes spirituality could even result in effects that go beyond what is scientifically explainable. Care must be taken, however, as the scientific definition of spirituality itself can be ambiguous and difficult to pin down; such findings can be perceived as an unscientific or pseudo-scientific opinion.

Spiritual Practice and Meditation

Spiritual practice can be pursued in a variety of ways that can be broadly categorized into the following: first, there are physical practices. This refers to deprivation and reduction. Deprivation cleanses the body and reduction makes one confront one's egotistical impulses. Many cultures, since antiquity, have used fasting and practicing poverty for spiritual training. Examples include fasting in the wilderness and self-discipline through asceticism. Second, there are social practices, such as obedience and engagement in community life, which seek to reorient one's egocentric life towards a life centered on others. Representative examples include monasteries and convents of the Middle Ages. Third, there are practices such as meditation that seek to cleanse egocentrism and pursue true existence. Following the era of the ascetic, meditation has become the most certain and definite method of spiritual practice in the contemporary era. Spiritual practice is defined as any and all methods that help one's spiritual transformation and growth. It refers to encountering or participating in real existence, or one's internal truth. In other words, it is the process through which a human being achieves insights into real existence through interactions between the self and others, society, nature, and an absolute being. Meditation is a common element of such practices that seek true existence. Although meditation is commonly perceived to be closely linked to Hindu or Buddhist religious traditions, a variety of religious and philosophical traditions have continuously used meditation since the beginning of history as a method of introspection and spiritual training. Simply put, meditation is akin to a vessel, and spirituality is the contents that are placed in this vessel. Thus, spirituality matures within the vessel of meditation.

Meditation is a difficult word to define, as is spirituality. Widely known definitions include Howard Clinebell's definition of silencing and centering one's consciousness and entering a realm of unwavering clarity, and Eknath Easwaran's definition of a skill that maximizes and focuses the potential of the mind so that one can travel from the surface of consciousness to its depths. Still, meditation is defined by each person in a wide variety of terms. Meditation can emphasize religious meanings such as enlightenment and peace. However, meditation can also be seen as a skill to simply lead an effective life, unrelated to any religious purpose. Regardless, meditation in whatever form is a good method with which one may approach spirituality Jang (2018).

To perceive true existence, one must first direct one's attention towards true existence. True existence is what is truly real. Most perceptions are manufactured by the world, and are far from "real." Through news and media, these perceptions are reinterpreted according to someone else's point of view, in which bias and preconceptions may enter. It is an indispensable challenge for everyone to figure out how to perceive one's own true existence through one's own perspective, not through the eyes of another person or through the world's perspective. However, to someone who has not been living a meditative life, peering into one's true existence is not an easy task. Therefore, it is best to begin with simply engaging in self-reflection in a method that is different from one's ordinary mode of life. Eastern philosophy and religions have continuously emphasized meditation, and Christianity has encouraged practices such as *Lectio Divina*, the spiritual exercises of Ignatius of Loyola, and contemplative prayer, for purposes of spiritual training. In Christianity, the word *contemplation* is preferred to the word *meditation*. Contemplation originates from *temple*, where the Gods reside in, and means to enter the place of the presence of God. Compared to "Quiet Time (QT)," a common practice in contemporary Christianity which refers to cognitive reflection, *contemplation* goes one step further and involves a purposeful gaze into the realm of spirituality. In South Korean Christian circles, contemplation is commonly translated into QT. Technically speaking, however, QT refers to traditional practices in Christianity from the Middle Ages of meditating on the word of God in thought. On the other hand, *contemplation* refers to a state of transcendence beyond the level of thought. Thus, meditation is a state in which the self remains intact, whereas *contemplation* is a state of unity with God in transcendence of the self. Thomas Keating referred to this state as "pure awareness," beyond any consciousness of the self. According to one definition, contemplation is "a long loving look at the real," which is analogous to the methods commonly used in practicing meditation. Therefore, regardless of the exact terminology or methods used, any and all means to approach the contents of spirituality can be called *meditation*. Enlightenment through meditation is the precondition for spiritual growth, so it is impossible to speak of meditation that does not reach spirituality, or spirituality that does not make use of meditation. Therefore, it is indispensable to learn and practice meditation as a means for spiritual formation and growth Chae (2025). In contrast with traditional religions, which placed an emphasis on doctrine and ritual, contemporary modes of spirituality place a great focus on the "spiritual experience." Spiritual experience connects an individual to a larger reality and brings forth a more comprehensive sense of self, and allows an individual to experience connection or unity with others, the community, nature, the cosmos, and/

or God. Regardless of which religion one's practice is based on, and even if one has no religion at all, it is a natural conclusion that spirituality should be approached through meditation.

Among the principles of Buddhism, there is a concept called "vijñāna," or consciousness. This concept refers to the understanding that there is a consciousness of the object itself, and another consciousness that perceives the subject that is being conscious of the object. One can perceive seeing a material thing, and also perceive the self that is perceiving that thing. Thus, there is a consciousness that perceives a thing as an objective other, and also a consciousness that perceives that a subjective self exists that is perceiving that thing. Once the subject becomes an object of observation, however, it has already disappeared—the subjective self, then, must remain as experience. On the act of reading this text, as an example, we perceive the letters on the page as objects and simultaneously perceive ourselves as the subjects that perceive. When these two perceptions occur at the same time, we become one and the same with the objects of perception and thereby obtain the knowledge that is contained in the text. As such perception is repeated with these types of actions, we can also understand the subject of this perception as the *spirit*. This spirit can be experienced as a subjective existence, not as an objective other. This process can exemplify how spirituality can be approached through "awareness meditation," a method widely used in the present day.

Conclusion

Even though ours is an era of increasing skepticism towards religion, interest in seeking a spiritual life has actually increased. As long as humanity exists, human beings' inherent curiosity towards the internal self and practices to reach self-fulfillment will continue to be explored. In either religious or non-religious contexts, spirituality has an aspect of pursuing what is more true, more real, more good, towards an existence that transcends limitations Gil (2018). Meditation is a way of approaching such goals. Of course, some argue that one must be able to scientifically approach spirituality itself. Within this logic, however, there is a risk of being trapped in reductionism in interpreting all that is transcendental as simply another type of psychological phenomena.

Philosophical currents that emphasize the uniqueness of human beings point to the spirit, or spirituality, as the distinguishing quality of humans. As the word *spirit* originated from terms meaning the wind or air, civilizations have understood the spirit as something that definitely exists even if invisible, such as the wind or the air, and that the spirit, by entering the body, brings forth the phenomena of life. This image of the wind related to the breath, and therefore the mystery of life, was thought to lie with the breath. When a life ceases to be, it no longer breathes. Some languages use idioms such as "take one's last breath," or "one's breath was cut off" to signify death. As such, the wind and the breath were considered the vital energy of life bestowed on human beings by the Gods. Almost all varieties of meditation practice emphasize, or at least utilize, the breath. Considering this connection, it is perhaps an obvious conclusion that meditation is used as a means to attain spirituality.

Regardless of whether one is religious or nonreligious, questions regarding the meaning, connection, and values of human life—such as *Who am I?*, *Why does pain exist?*, *What is the relationship between me and other people and the world at large?*, *What is the reason behind everything that happens?*, and *What does it mean to live a good life?*—cannot be answered without spiritual considerations. Human beings are certainly made of flesh. However, human beings refuse to remain within the boundaries of the body, with its temporal and spatial limitations. Human beings have the transcendental ability to seek a greater realm, beyond the self, that cannot be perceived within such limitations. Through seeking such greater realms, human beings approach spiritual existence, and meditation is the road that leads to such existence. Therefore, meditation is not our ultimate goal. Rather, it is the means—the road that leads—to ultimate reality, the ultimate existence. To not engage in meditation means to not incorporate such means into one's own life. If spirituality is "the ability to transcend oneself," one will not be able to go beyond the self or discover one's true identity without engaging in meditation. Moreover, instead of remaining on the level of simply disconnecting with the world or being immersed within oneself, meditation can be more appropriately used to transcend the self in the pursuit of ultimate values and involve a purposeful integration of one's life. Spirituality refers to the real, true existence of a human being that cannot be accessed solely by humans' emotions or cognitive reason. Human beings cannot attain fundamental fulfillment without encountering such true existence. Therefore, meditation in pursuit of spirituality, i.e., spiritual practice, must involve continuous self-transcendence. Such reflection, cultivation, and training are not to be "completed," but rather continuously developed throughout our lifetimes. Only through ceaseless efforts to place our minds within the sphere of spirituality can we reach our true and inherent state of being. Such a state is a spiritual realm accessible only to those who have actually gone through a profound spiritual experience. This is more than just a subjective psychological state, but one that reaches transcendental existence that cannot be perceived through the eye or mind in one's ordinary life. In longstanding religious traditions, states such as Nirvana in Buddhism or the Kingdom of God in Christianity do not refer to a transformation of the world at large. Rather, they are referring to a spiritual revolution within oneself. In practicing meditation, it is to be expected that a variety of methods will be used according to different cultures and/or situations. Buddhist prayer, contemplative prayer, mantra, ajna chakra, scriptures, divine lecture, breathing, perception, philosophical approaches, encounter groups, artistic media, physical movements, etc., are all methods that can be used to go beyond the self and be oriented towards spirituality through decentering the self, through which one can ultimately recover one's true form of life.

Bibliography

Korean Sources

Chae JH. Spiritfulness: a journey to discover the light within. Gyeong-gi: Seonyul; 2025.

Gil H. Bodhisattva Jesus. Seoul: Hyeon-Am Publishing; 2004.

Gil H. From religion to spirituality. Gyeong-gi: Bookscope; 2018.

Jang H-G. The answer is in meditation. Seoul: Dam & Books; 2018.

Jeon WT, Min SG, Han SI, Chae JH, Kim DH. Psychiatry and christianity. Seoul: Park-Yeong Publishing; 2020.

Korean Christian Counseling Psychology Association. Christian (pastoral) counseling and spirituality. Seoul: Hak-Ji Publishing; 2018.

Song JM, Min JA, Yi NB, Chae JH. Effects of spirituality on the positive and negative affect in patients with depressive disorders. Mood Emot. 2012;10(3):159–64.

Yi NB, Min JA, Chae JH. Difference of the effects of spirituality on the Hope in early adults and middle aged patients with depression. Mood Emot. 2012;10(1):31–6.

English Sources

Kim NY, Huh HJ, Chae JH. Effects of religiosity and spirituality on the treatment response in patients with depressive disorders. Compr Psychiatry. 2015;60:26–34.

Mcminn MR. Psychology, theology, and spirituality in Christian counseling. Tyndale House Publishers; 2001.

Min JA, Lee NB, Lee CU, Lee C, Chae JH. Low trait anxiety, high resilience, and their interaction as possible predictors for treatment response in patients with depression. J Affect Disord. 2012;137(1–3):61–9.

Min JA, Jung YE, Kim DJ, Yim HW, Kim JJ, Kim TS, Lee CU, Lee C, Chae JH. Characteristics associated with low resilience in patients with depression and/oranxiety disorders. Qual Life Res. 2013;22(2):231–41.

Scazzero P. Emotionally healthy spirituality: unleash a revolution in your life in Christ. Thomas Nelson, Inc; 2015.

Wikipedia. (2020a). https://en.wikipedia.org/wiki/Spirituality.

Wikipedia. (2020b). https://en.wikipedia.org/wiki/Religion.

The Brain and Meditation

6

Hwa-Young Lee, Jeongjae Bak, Hyeon-Ah Lee, and Jae Hyun Han

Meditation can be defined as a method for an individual to relieve tension or reach self-growth or liberation by intentionally controlling their attention and concentration. All methods of meditation are based on inward-facing attention or focused attention, and this is called 'awareness' or 'mindfulness.' Through this, meditation induces the so-called 'relaxation reaction,' which functions as a physiological antagonist to what appears in a stressful reaction. This aspect is where we expect to see the clinical effects of meditation, and it has been observed to have an effect on stress-related diseases including cardiovascular, immune, and inflammatory diseases, as well as neurological disorders including anxiety-related disorders and depression.

The practice of meditation and mindfulness is focused on the effects of reducing physiological, psychological, and neurophysiological stress, and is attracting much attention in medical and health fields due to its various clinical effects. Amid such trends, many studies have recently been published on its molecular and neurophysiological mechanisms. This chapter aims to present useful information about the brain and meditation based on the results of current neuroscience research findings.

H.-Y. Lee (✉) · H.-A. Lee
Department of Psychiatry, Soonchunhyang University Cheonan Hospital, Cheonan, Republic of Korea

J. Bak
Mauman Psychiatry Clinic, Incheon, Republic of Korea

J. H. Han
Department of Psychiatry, Seoul National University Bundang Hospital, Seongnam, Republic of Korea

Fundamental Concepts of Meditation and Mindfulness Practice for Understanding Biology

Mindfulness practice is a method of meditation practice through which one carefully accepts the whole or fully accepts existence. According to Jon Kabat-Zinn, who first introduced mindfulness in Western academia, mindfulness is turning one's attention non-judgmentally and continuously towards all states and changes of the mind and body. It is concentrating on the present moment and paying constant attention to the thoughts and sensations that arise in one's mind without any evaluation or judgment. People have a tendency towards automatic thinking in situations of stress, which is a cognitive stress response. These tendencies in thinking not only manifest themselves in negative automatic thoughts, ruminations about the past, or worries about the future, which occur in stressful situations, but also as patterns of the mind that function in boring or challenging situations. If you practice mindfulness systematically, you can escape from this loop of automatic thinking. Skilled meditators can focus their minds on the present by concentrating on experiences that are occurring 'here and now' or on their breathing, and through this they can will-

J.-H. Chae, H.-Y. Lee (eds.), *Meditation in Psychiatry and General Medicine*,
https://doi.org/10.1007/978-981-95-7147-5_6

fully suppress automatic thinking. Even this alone has the effect of relieving physiological and mental stress. While practicing mindfulness, we experience that we are not in danger at this very moment, and through this we realize that there is no real life-threatening danger at this moment and there is no particular 'reason' to be stressed or anxious. By intentionally focusing on the present moment that is absent of any danger, our 'mindset' such as our inner capacity or our attitude can be trained and developed through systematic mental practice.

In order to provide a clearer definition of mindfulness in a scientific way, Bishop and others developed a model that considered two aspects. The first is mindfulness expressed as self-regulation of attention. It is self-regulating the turning of one's attention to the present and to intrinsic experiences. The second is striving to know something continuously and actively, having an open mind, and accepting all experiences. Through this one's ability to accept improves, which makes it possible to 'let things be' without judging. Likewise, by cultivating empathy and orientation towards the external world and inner senses such as mental and physical experiences, one comes to realize one's own existence and 'connectedness.' In this process, we acquire the ability to accept 'that which comes up from within' and better ways to deal with stress and challenges, and these characteristics resemble important elements in previously known studies on positive psychology or on living a happy and healthy life. Thus, it is not surprising that the concepts mentioned so far and the various methods of practice overlap in many areas. This is because it is affected by and is shared with activities of various concepts in specific areas such as the mechanisms of intrinsic reward and motivation in the brain. These activities not only share the ability to self-regulate attention, but also the areas of the brain responsible for empathy and altruistic behavior, as well as areas where mirror neuron activity occurs.

The Molecular Neurological Aspects of Meditation

Meditation appears in every way to be associated with the central limbic system, the mesolimbic system, or the striatum. This area is where the motivational and reward systems of the brain are located, and where dopamine is the main neurotransmitter. Numerous studies have shown that the presence of dopamine in the brain and plasma is directly connected to meditation. Although it is affected by the practitioner's individual proficiency, personal characteristics, or emotional state at the moment of practice, meditation is associated with short highs or special moments, an ecstatic state, a deep sense of joy, contentment, and inner peace. Today, substances such as dopamine are discussed as neurotransmitters related to these phenomena.

In stress physiology, there have also been multiple reports that detected the metabolism and secretion of the enzymes norepinephrine and epinephrine, which regulate stress. When compared to the control group, a lower concentration of plasma norepinephrine was reported amongst practitioners of meditation. The enzymatic systems associated with it are simultaneously associated with the metabolism of dopamine and morphine. Additionally, meditation decreases the concentration of cortisol in the peripheral part of the brain and increases the concentration of melatonin. At the same time, the responsiveness of the sympathetic nervous system is reduced, and hyperactivity in the parasympathetic nervous system can be seen. Although there have been no real-time measurements of the metabolism of morphine in the body during meditation so far, it is presumed to be related to meditation. Stress (particularly chronic stress) is known to increase the activity of acetylcholine-degrading enzymes, lower the concentration of acetylcholine, and activate several genes that molecularly regulate stress/anti-stress mechanisms. Practicing relaxation/meditation also shows individual gene activation. Acetylcholine and morphine increase the activity of the enzyme that produces nitrogen oxide, which is presumed to be the reason for the high concentration of nitrogen oxide in the breath of practitioners of meditation. Nitrogen oxide has an anti-inflammatory effect of inhibiting 'NFkappaB,' an inflammatory nuclear transcription factor, whereas chronic stress promotes an inflammatory response. Although there may be genetic differences, there have also been reports of brain-derived neuropathic factors that are sensitively tied to stress. These aspects suggest that meditation's ability to regulate stress and its positive effects on health may be related to the neurophysiological basis, though more research is needed in the future.

Meditation also appears to have an effect on the concentration of serotonin in the central and peripheral areas of the brain. Although it shows tendencies to increase the concentration of serotonin, its effects are still unclear. This may be due to the circadian rhythm and its interaction with other hormonal systems, and it could be caused by the antagonism of melatonin and tryptophan itself.

When gamma band oscillations appear synchronized in all areas of the brain with a high amplitude, there have been reports of mystical experiences such as 'the experience of being one with the world.' At this moment, it was expressed as a change in the spatial expression of self and the proprioception of the body. Although this phenomenon has only been reported by experienced practitioners who have meditated for a long time, if we consider that a similar phenomenon occurs when psychotropic drugs are used or when one is in a psychopathic situation, we can infer that there is a molecular mechanism here. This state is controversial because it may correspond to side effects that can occur in meditation-based treatment.

The Neuroscientific Aspects of Mindfulness Meditation

Mindfulness-based techniques emphasize consciously focusing on perceptible emotions and sensations in the present moment. It acknowledges emotions but does not try to evaluate them or deliberately change them. For example, you can train your own senses using mindfulness by contemplating your breath, posture, bodily tension, pain, etc., and these senses can be seen as being 'separate' from you. In addition to psychological and physical explanations, there are increasing attempts to explain the mechanisms of meditation and mindfulness through neuroscientific methods.

The Neurophysiological Aspect

According to the model of frontal lobe alpha band symmetry in cortical activation, brain activity in the left anterior region is associated with the enhancement of positive emotions and improved immune function. Based on this assumption, Davidson et al. found that there was a correlation between the high antibody titer produced during flu vaccination and a higher level of activity of the left frontal lobe in the group that had undergone mindfulness training than in the control group. As cortical activity increased, the antibody titer also increased. This demonstrates that the mind and body are related to each other, just as the center and the periphery are on a continuum.

In terms of functional changes in brain activity, Lutz et al. observed an increase in synchronized gamma band activity among EEG activity when a specific method of meditation was practiced for many years. These oscillatory patterns are the same as those seen when performing high-level conscious functions and cognitive tasks, such as the process of functional learning that requires a high degree of attention. However, in this study, gamma band activity was observed in a much wider area compared to synchronized high-frequency EEG activity that typically appear in the brain. The level of gamma band activity can be said to be a measure of the quality of one's meditation practice. However, changes associated with this can be observed in EEG activity even after a relatively short period of practice. In addition to the changes in alpha and gamma bands mentioned above, modulations in beta and theta bands may also appear in some areas of the brain. However, there are significant differences in EEG activity and brain physiology between long-term and short-term or beginner practitioners. Therefore, differences in proficiency, duration of individual practice, individual characteristics, and meditation techniques should all be considered.

Gamma bands in the parietal lobe, parieto-occipital lobe, and temporal lobe seem to be associated with experiencing the 'dissolution of boundaries' or transcendental experiences. To assess the quality of an individual's experience of meditation, theta bands (prominent in the frontal lobe, midline region) can be used to measure the depth of relaxation or 'inner reflection.' The synchronization or synchronicity of EEG patterns that start at a specific location and extend to other areas is generally considered to be a positive signal. It has been consistently confirmed that these EEG bands increase in experienced meditators. Changes in alpha band were primarily seen in beginners, and it seems to be related to non-meditation-specific relaxation that occurs when the eyes are closed.

Looking at the EEG patterns that appear in various methods of meditation, first the traditional meditation practice in Tibetan Buddhism, one of the intensive forms of practice, is associated with high gamma band activity. In a study that compares beginners and experienced meditators, a high ratio of gamma-band/theta and alpha-bands was observed in experienced meditators. Gamma-band in parietal, temporal, and frontal lobes were more than 30 times higher, and researchers observed gamma band tuning in the high frontal-parietal region. Other studies have also shown increased activity of gamma band or high beta2 band. Second, Vipassanā meditation, the practice of open monitoring, is associated with theta band of the frontal lobe and gamma band of the occipital lobe. Zen meditation leads to high theta band in the midline region of the frontal lobe. The longer the period of practice, the higher the theta band was observed. High theta band were also observed in other methods of meditation such as Sahaja meditation and Qigong. Third, studies on transcendental meditation repeatedly observed high alpha band and low beta and gamma band in the frontal lobe. Studies on Qigong meditation, which is practiced in a similar manner to transcendental meditation, observed an overall increase in alpha band.

Newberg and Iverson found results similar to those previously observed in neurophysiological changes occurring during meditative states. According to this, during meditation, changes occur in major cerebral structures, hormones, and the autonomic nervous system that are responsible for overall brain activity that affects cognition, sensory reception, emotions, endocrine system-hormones, and autonomic nerve activity.

The Neuroanatomical Aspect

The most important finding related to mindfulness meditation is that it activates the insula, frontal lobe, and anterior cingulate regions of the brain. These include not just functional changes but also structural changes. Creswell et al. reported that in cases of people who have practiced mindfulness meditation for a long time, there was increased activity in the prefrontal cortex and inactivity in the amygdala, which classifies emotions. A recent study can be seen to support this, wherein there was a structural change in the amygdala that 'shrunk' after subjects underwent 8 weeks of mindfulness practice. The structural changes seen in this study showed a positive correlation between reducing the degree of one's subjective experience of stress and coping better with it. These results show mindfulness practice's potential to have a positive effect on the neural pathways that regulate affect and emotions.

In addition, the effects of meditation on brain structure show that various areas of the cortex thicken in those who practice meditation regularly. These areas are responsible for attention and memory, internal sensation, sensory processing, and self-regulation.

Classification by Mechanism of Action

Attention Control

Mindfulness techniques can help you focus your attention in one place or spread it out widely. Regular practice cultivates the ability to maintain focus on a single object, and to notice and respond when the mind is swept away by some thought. On the other hand, by expanding the 'stem of consciousness,' mindfulness allows us to widely recognize and accept things that arise in our present circumstances. It has been confirmed that these phenomena appear not only in research conditions but also in everyday life. The areas of the brain that are connected to this are the prefrontal cortex and the anterior cingulate cortex. Just as the saying goes, 'the more you use it, the sharper it gets,' it is reported that as you practice controlling your attention, you can slow down the aging of the brain. As functional and structural differentiation occurs in the corresponding regions of the brain and neural connections are strengthened, it appears that there is not only an increase in the density and size of gray matter, but also a strengthening of white matter. Cultivating the habit of maintaining a 'beginner's mind,' can also slow down the aging of the brain. This phenomenon appears to be related to a decrease in the default activity of the default mode network in the brain. This is still an area that requires further research. We know that memory is generally improved when attention is enhanced. This includes not only the working memory in the prefrontal cortex, but also explicit memory in the hippocampus. Thus, the practice of meditation not only enhances stimulus or task-specific learning, but also learning such as procedure or pattern recognition. In addition, it improves mental function.

In modern neurophysiology, the limbic system can be functionally divided into three layers that regulate internal emotion and motivation, called limbic autoregulation. The lower and middle areas are generally difficult to control consciously, and this includes the amygdala, which evaluates emotions and feelings. However, the upper region is one that has an impact on the regulation of emotions. This area, sometimes called the paralimbic region, is a part of the prefrontal cortex and is associated with the anterior cingulate cortex, orbitofrontal cortex, and insular lobe. It functions as a bridge between the limbic system and the cortex and is responsible for motivation and self-regulation. On the one hand, it connects reason and cognition, and on the other hand, it connects affect and emotion. These functions can be strengthened through mindfulness practice. Although it is debatable, these connections can be used to recognize and correct strongly connected negative emotions and perceptions that lead to a vicious cycle. However, a strong connection can also mean the negative link is strong. In other words, since this area connects the mind with reason and emotions with the body, techniques that activate this area can affect the integrative tasks of the brain. The connection between body and mind is real and can be observed and evaluated through this area. Since there is a clear area, it is also possible to improve the self-regulation ability that manages stress and emotions. Mindfulness practice can achieve systematic desensitization of negative affects and emotions. By inhibiting the function of the amygdala, it is possible to strengthen the parietotemporal junction of the hippocampus and the posterior cingulate cortex junction. This can be seen as improving the ability to recognize what is important. However, its relationship with the posterior cingulate cortex junction remains a subject of debate.

Through meditation, you can suppress unpleasant external stimuli such as 'unwanted' automatic thought patterns or stress, and enhance the integrative function of higher neural structures. Through this, new behavioral patterns will emerge, and you will be able to cultivate the ability to control stress or reduce the amount of stress that you feel. This also improves the ability to cope with pain.

Bodily Awareness

It is generally known that mindfulness practice helps to improve the function and structure of somatosensory areas and the insular cortex. From this point of view, while training bodily awareness, meditation can expand the precision of the 'body map,' and can enhance the function of internal senses to the same level as external senses. The cingulum of the brain is involved in this process, and this is an area that helps us quickly recognize and filter out 'errors' in our current experience. A person who practices meditation continuously through this area can get in contact with their positive emotions more closely and feel 'good.' One can improve their intuitions or instincts with bodily awareness through the process of more clearly feeling the sensations in the body. Procedural memory skills associated with the dorsal striatum are also improved. These improvements help you not only notice more quickly what is happening to your body, such as its response to stress, but also determine an appropriate and effective response. It can also help you effectively notice warning signs.

In addition, mindfulness also helps us to maintain close relationships with others. This is because the area of the brain that bodily awareness improves overlaps with the area of the brain needed when dealing with others. In general, mirror neuron areas are considered to be located in temporal and parietal-temporal areas that are closely synaptic with the prefrontal cortex. Empathy and compassion are both the emotional function of empathizing with others as well as the cognitive function of noticing how others think and accept things, and it has been reported that these abilities also improve with bodily awareness. Compassion and altruism can be cultivated through meditation, and it appears that the strengthening of the prefrontal lobe, orbitofrontal lobe, midbrain dopamine area, and prefrontal-limbic connectivity are all related to this.

Self-View

Several studies have shown that mindfulness practice leads to a more organized self-view. It allows us to be able to distinguish more clearly between ideas of the self and actual self-perception. This phenomenon was also observed in studies on pain control. During the process of practicing meditation, practitioners learn to not be discriminatory towards any thoughts, sensations, or emotions. This attitude is called 'decentering' or 'non-judgment' and can be practiced through mindfulness. Through this, you will be able to better handle mental stress, thoughts, or emotions. You will also be able to reduce excessive negative self-beliefs and reduce bringing up negative past results. This can be said to be an experience of self-efficacy or an experience of true inner control. Neurophysiologically, this process can be seen as a change in the way we deal with pain ('I will not try to do anything about this pain but accept it as it is.' 'This pain does not make me uncomfortable.') rather than staying on the same level as primary cognitive control ('I do not want to be in pain anymore.' 'I am able to cope with this pain'). By engaging sensory systems and interoceptive areas such as the anterior cingulate cortex and the insular lobe, mindfulness appears to regulate nociception and anticipation of pain. This experience of positive regulation allows one to take responsibility for their own health. Some studies claim that mindfulness practice strengthens coherence and connectedness by reducing inner judgment and instead increasing self-awareness and integrative capacity. In a variety of literature, 'the self' includes self-attributed attributes such as self-reference and self-image as well as egocentric perspectives such as 'the evaluation framework.' The egocentric view is neurologically associated with central line regions of the brain, including the medial prefrontal cortex. By focusing on non-judgment towards oneself through practicing mindfulness, one activates the lateral areas of the brain, such as the insular lobe and somatosensory cortex. It is generally known that mindfulness has a tendency to reinforce the 'self' rather than the ego, and reduces one's evaluation or judgment of their experiences. Among the various ways of managing one's experience, it can be said that it is a practice that deals with one's experience in a flexible manner and transforms it into a way of recognizing. As a resting state network that can be identified in structures along the midline of the brain, the 'default mode' is associated with things such as fantasies of internal representation and self-association. This can be adjusted through the self-regulation approach of mindfulness practice. Mindfulness practice maintains a resting state by remaining in a 'natural state of mind' regardless of what arises in the mind. On the other hand, mindfulness has the effect of suppressing the activity of the basic synaptic state, such as reducing daydreaming. Although follow-up studies are needed to evaluate these aspects, it can be said that mindfulness enhances the function of self-view and improves mental/internal flexibility.

In the same context as regulating brain activity, mindfulness can ultimately reveal a more positive direction in behavioral regulation. Improving one's ability for internal control can improve self-efficacy and 'inner strength.' Playing an important role in the healthcare system, it is particularly closely related to the treatment of addiction and lifestyle control. In addition, by functionally integrating the synapses of the midline and lateral regions of the brain, mindfulness affects mirror-image neurons and has a positive effect on the functions of harmony and empathy.

The Neurobiology of Innate Mindfulness and Meditation Practice

Most studies describe the neural mechanisms underlying different levels of mindfulness by comparing novice and experienced practitioners. However, it is important to understand that individuals with varying levels of innate mindfulness also have different neuroanatomical characteristics. Interestingly, individuals with high levels of innate mindfulness who have not engaged in meditation practices exhibit certain brain mechanisms similar to those who have practiced meditation.

Innate mindfulness is associated with cognitive reappraisal processing and interoceptive awareness. These behaviors involve top-down regulation of the amygdala by activation of the PFC and diminished activity in the DMN. This is explained by decreased amygdala activity at rest and enhanced top-down control by the vlPFC over the right amygdala during emotion regulation tasks in individuals with high levels of innate mindfulness. Similarly, higher levels of innate mindfulness correlate with increased activity in the dmPFC, which is also linked to reduced amygdala activity.

Novices in mindfulness meditation showed activation of the insula, while experts showed activation of the medial prefrontal gyrus and globus pallidus. The activation of the insula seen in novices might be explained by the findings that more than half of them used a focused breathing technique that targeted the awareness of the physiological sensation of breath and the right insula was associated with respiratory function and interoception. The activation regions observed in the experts, the medial frontal gyrus and globus pallidus, are involved in the regulation of attention and emotion. Repeated practice improves the attentional control, so that over time, experts can more quickly identify periods of mind wandering, shift their focus, and refocus their attention on the mindfulness practice. The different activation patterns related to the amount of mindfulness practice support mindfulness as a learned skill. In other words, the process of engaging in mindfulness can become habitual through repeated practice and experience.

Conclusion

To summarize, meditation acts as an antagonist to stress at the mental, physical, and molecular levels. Although these effects may be subjective evaluations by researchers, they can be objectively demonstrated through appropriate methods. Practitioners of meditation have reported improvements in mood and emotion, as well as the subjective experience of relaxation, happiness, and simple joy. Based on this, we can infer that internal circuits of motivation and reward are connected to meditation and have a direct relationship with self-regulation.

Bibliography

Aftanas LI, Golocheikine SA. Human anterior and frontal midline theta and lower alpha reflect emotionally positive state and internalized attention: high-resolution EEG investigation of meditation. Neurosci Lett. 2001;310:57–60.

Aftanas LI, Golocheikine SA. Non-linear dynamic complexity of the human EEG during meditation. Neurosci Lett. 2002;330:143–6.

Benson H, Klipper MZ. The relaxation response. New York: Harper Collins; 2000.

Bishop SR, Lau M, Shapiro S, Carlson L, Anderson ND, Carmody J, Segal ZV, Abbey S, Speca M, Velting D, Devins G. Mindfulness. A proposed operational definition. Clin Psychol Sci Pract. 2004;11(3):230–41.

Brand S, Holsboer-Trachsler E, Naranjo JR, Schmidt S. Influence of mindfulness practice on cortisol and sleep in long-term and short-term meditators. Neuropsychobiology. 2012;65:109–18.

Cahn BR, Delorme A, Polich J. Occipital gamma activation during Vipassana meditation. Cogn Process. 2010;11:39–56.

Cahn BR, Delorme A, Polich J. Event-related delta, theta, alpha, and gamma correlates to auditory oddball processing during Vipassana meditation. Soc Cogn Affect Neurosci. 2012;8:100–11.

Creswell JD, Way BM, Eisenberger NI, Lieberman MD. Neural correlates of dispositional mindfulness during affect labeling. Psychosom Med. 2007;69:560–5.
Critchley HD, Melmed RN, Featherstone E, Mathias CJ, Dolan RJ. Brain activity during biofeedback relaxation: a functional neuroimaging investigation. Brain. 2001;124:1003–12.
Davidson RJ. Anterior electrophysiological asymmetries, emotion, and depression: conceptual and methodological conundrums. Psychophysiology. 1998;35:607–14.
Davidson RJ, Kabat-Zinn J, Schumacher J, Rosenkranz M, Muller D, Santorelli SF, Urbanowski F, Harrington A, Bonus K, Sheridan JF. Alterations in brain and immune function produced by mindfulness meditation. Psychosom Med. 2003;65:564–70.
Desbordes G, Negi LT, Pace TWW, Wallace BA, Raison CL, Schwartz EL. Effects of mindful-attention and compassion meditation training on amygdala response to emotional stimuli in an ordinary, non-meditative state. Front Hum Neurosci. 2012;6:292.
Ernst S, Welke J, Heintze C, Gabriel R, Zöllner A, Kiehne S, Schwantes U, Esch T. Effects of mindfulness-based stress reduction on quality of life in nursing home residents: a feasibility study. Forsch Komplementmed. 2008;15:74–81.
Esch T, Stefano GB. The neurobiology of pleasure, reward processes, addiction and their health implications. Neuroendocrinol Lett. 2004;25:235–51.
Esch T, Stefano GB. The neurobiology of love. Neuroendocrinol Lett. 2005;26:175–92.
Esch T, Stefano GB. The neurobiology of stress management. Neuroendocrinol Lett. 2010;31:19–39.
Esch T, Stefano GB. The neurobiological link between compassion and love. Med Sci Monit. 2011;17:RA65–75.
Esch T, Stefano GB, Fricchione GL, Benson H. An overview of stress and its impact in immunological diseases. Mod Asp Immunobiol. 2002;2:187–92.
Esch T, Stefano GB, Fricchione GL. The therapeutic use of the relaxation response in stress-related diseases. Med Sci Monit. 2003;9:RA23–34.
Esch T, Guarna M, Bianchi E, Stefano GB. Meditation and limbic processes. Biofeedback. 2004a;32:22–32.
Esch T, Guarna M, Bianchi E, Zhu W, Stefano GB. Commonalities in the central nervous system's involvement with complementary medical therapies: limbic morphinergic processes. Med Sci Monit. 2004b;10:MS6–MS17.
Esch T, Duckstein J, Welke J, Braun V. Mind/body techniques for physiological and psychological stress reduction: stress management via Tai Chi training—a pilot study. Med Sci Monit. 2007;13:CR488–97.
Esch T, Sonntag U, Esch SM, Thees S. Stress management and mind-body medicine: a randomized controlled longitudinal evaluation of students' health and effects of a behavioral group intervention at a middle-size German University (SM-MESH). Forsch Komplementmed. 2013;20:129–37. https://doi.org/10.1016/j.ctcp.2009.01.003.
Farb NAS, Segal ZV, Mayberg H, Bean J, McKeon D, Fatima Z, Anderson AK. Attending to the present: mindfulness meditation reveals distinct neural modes of self-reference. Soc Cogn Affect Neurosci. 2007;2:313–22.
Fjorback LO, Arendt M, Ornbøl E, Fink P, Walach H. Mindfulness-based stress reduction and mindfulness-based cognitive therapy: a systematic review of randomized controlled trials. Acta Psychiatr Scand. 2011;124:102–19.
Gard T, Hölzel BK, Sack AT, Hempel H, Lazar SW, Vaitl D, Ott U. Pain attenuation through mindfulness is associated with decreased cognitive control and increased sensory processing in the brain. Cereb Cortex. 2012;22:2692–702.
Grossman P, Niemann L, Schmidt S, Walach H. Mindfulness-based stress reduction and health benefits. A meta-analysis. J Psychosom Res. 2004;57:35–43.
Hölzel BK, Ott U, Hempel H, Hackl A, Wolf K, Stark R, et al. Differential engagement of anterior cingulate and adjacent medial frontal cortex in adept meditators and non-meditators. Neurosci Lett. 2007;421:16–21.
Hölzel BK, Ott U, Gard T, Hempel H, Weygandt M, Morgen K, Vaitl D. Investigation of mindfulness meditation practitioners with voxel-based morphometry. Soc Cogn Affect Neurosci. 2008;3:55–61.
Hölzel BK, Carmody J, Evans KC, Hoge EA, Dusek JA, Morgan L, et al. Stress reduction correlates with structural changes in the amygdala. Soc Cogn Affect Neurosci. 2010;5:11–7.
Hölzel BK, Carmody J, Vangel M, Congleton C, Yerramsetti SM, Gard T, Lazar SW. Mindfulness practice leads to increases in regional brain gray matter density. Psychiatry Res. 2011a;191:36–43.
Hölzel BK, Lazar SW, Gard T, Schuman-Olivier Z, Vago DR, Ott U. How does mindfulness meditation work? Proposing mechanisms of action from a conceptual and neural perspective. Perspect Psychol Sci. 2011b;6:537–59.
Infante JR, Torres-Avisbal M, Pinel P, Vallejo JA, Peran F, Gonzalez F, et al. Catecholamine levels in practitioners of the transcendental meditation technique. Physiol Behav. 2001;72:141–6.
Jung YH, Kang DH, Jang JH, Park HY, Byun MS, Kwon SJ, Jang GE, Lee US, An SC, Kwon JS. The effects of mind-body training on stress reduction, positive affect, and plasma catecholamines. Neurosci Lett. 2010;479:138–42.
Jung YH, Kang DH, Byun MS, Shim G, Kwon SJ, Jang GE, Lee US, An SC, Joon HJ, Kwon JS. Influence of brain-derived neurotrophic factor and catechol O-methyl transferase polymorphisms on effects of meditation on plasma catecholamines and stress. Stress. 2012;15:97–104.
Kabat-Zinn J. Full catastrophe living: using the wisdom of your body and mind to face stress, pain, and illness. New York: Delta; 1990.
Kang DH, Jo HJ, Jung WH, Kim SH, Jung YH, Choi CH, Lee US, An SC, Jang JH, Kwon JS. The effect of

meditation on brain structure: cortical thickness mapping and diffusion tensor imaging. Soc Cogn Affect Neurosci. 2013;8:27–33.

Kerr CE, Jones SR, Wan Q, Pritchett DL, Wasserman RH, Wexler A, Villanueva JJ, Shaw JR, Lazar SW, Kaptchuk TJ, Littenberg R, Hämäläinen MS, Moore CI. Effects of mindfulness meditation training on anticipatory alpha modulation in primary somatosensory cortex. Brain Res Bull. 2011;85:96–103.

Lazar SW. The meditating brain. Berlin: 4. Europäischer Kongress für Integrative Medizin; 2011.

Lazar SW, Bush G, Gollub RL, Fricchione GL, Khalsa G, Benson H. Functional brain mapping of the relaxation response and meditation. Neuroreport. 2000;11:1581–5.

Lazar SW, Kerr CE, Wasserman RH, Gray JR, Greve DN, Treadway MT, McGarvey M, Quinn BT, Dusek JA, Benson H, Rauch SL, Moore CI, Fischl B. Meditation experience is associated with increased cortical thickness. Neuroreport. 2005;16:1893–7.

Lustyk MK, Chawla N, Nolan RS, Marlatt GA. Mindfulness meditation research: issues of participant screening, safety procedures, and researcher training. Adv Mind Body Med. 2009;24:20–30.

Lutz A, Greischar LL, Rawlings NB, Ricard M, Davidson RJ. Long-term meditators self-induce high-amplitude gamma synchrony during mental practice. Proc Natl Acad Sci USA. 2004;101:16369–73.

Manoch R, Gordon A, Black D, Malhi G, Seidler R. Using meditation for less stress and better wellbeing: a seminar for GPs. Aust Fam Physician. 2009;38:454–8.

Marchand WR. Mindfulness-based stress reduction, mindfulness-based cognitive therapy, and zen meditation for depression, anxiety, pain, and psychological distress. J Psychiatr Pract. 2012;18:233–52.

Mendelson T, Greenberg MT, Dariotis JK, Gould LF, Rhoades BL, Leaf PJ. Feasibility and preliminary outcomes of a school-based mindfulness intervention for urban youth. J Abnorm Child Psychol. 2010;38:985–94.

Modinos G, Ormel J, Aleman A. Individual differences in dispositional mindfulness and brain activity involved in reappraisal of emotion. Soc Cogn Affect Neurosci. 2010;5(4):369–77.

Newberg AB, Iversen J. The neural basis of the complex mental task of meditation: neurotransmitter and neurochemical considerations. Med Hypotheses. 2003;61:282–91.

Newberg A, Alavi A, Baime M, Pourdehnad M, Santanna J, d'Aquili E. The measurement of regional cerebral blood flow during the complex cognitive task of meditation: a preliminary SPECT study. Psychiatry Res. 2001;106:113–22.

Newberg AB, Wintering N, Waldman MR, Amen D, Khalsa DS, Alavi A. Cerebral blood flow differences between long-term meditators and non-meditators. Conscious Cogn. 2010;19:899–905.

Ott U. Meditation für Skeptiker. München: O. W. Barth; 2010.

Petermann F, Vaitl D. Entspannungsverfahren: Das Praxishandbuch. Weinheim: Beltz; 2009.

Rossano M. Did meditating make us human? Camb Archaeol J. 2007;17(1):47–58.

Salzberg S, Kabat-Zinn J. Achtsamkeit als Medikament. In: Goleman D, editor. Die heilende Kraft der Gefühle. München: Dt. Taschenbuch-Verl; 2000. p. 134–81.

Schmidt S, Grossman P, Schwarzer B, Jena S, Naumann J, Walach H. Treating fibromyalgia with mindfulness-based stress reduction: results from a 3-armed randomized controlled trial. Pain. 2011;152:361–9.

Stefano GB, Esch T. Integrative medical therapy: examination of meditation's therapeutic and global medicinal outcomes via nitric oxide. Int J Mol Med. 2005;16:621–30.

Stefano GB, Benson H, Fricchione GL, Esch T. The stress response: always good and when it is bad. New York: Medical Science International; 2005.

Stefano GB, Fricchione GL, Esch T. Relaxation: molecular and physiological significance. Med Sci Monit. 2006;12:HY21–31.

Thees S, Gobel J, Jose G, Bohrhardt R, Esch T. Die Gesundheit von Studierenden im Bologna-Prozess: Untersuchungen zu Gesundheitsverhalten, Stress und Wohlbefinden zei-gen Handlungsbedarf. Pravent Gesundh. 2012;3:196–202.

van Leeuwen S, Müller NG, Melloni L. Age effects on attentional blink performance in meditation. Conscious Cogn. 2009;18:593–9.

Vestergaard-Poulsen P, van Beek M, Skewes J, Bjarkam CR, Stubberup M, Bertelsen J, Roepstorff A. Long-term meditation is associated with increased gray matter density in the brain stem. Neuroreport. 2009;20:170–4.

Vøllestad J, Nielsen MB, Nielsen GH. Mindfulness- and acceptance-based interventions for anxiety disorders: a systematic review and meta-analysis. Br J Clin Psychol. 2012;51:239–60.

Wang DJ, Rao H, Korczykowski M, Wintering N, Pluta J, Khalsa DS, Newberg AB. Cerebral blood flow changes associated with different meditation practices and perceived depth of meditation. Psychiatry Res. 2011;191:60–7.

Yu X, Fumoto M, Nakatani Y, Sekiyama T, Kikuchi H, Seki Y, Sato-Suzuki I, Arita H. Activation of the anterior prefrontal cortex and serotonergic system is associated with improvements in mood and EEG changes induced by Zen meditation practices in novices. Int J Psychophysiol. 2011;80:103–11.

7 The Psychological and Physiological Mechanisms of Meditation

Hye-Geum Kim

Improvement of Metacognitive Awareness

One of the important elements of mindfulness meditation is based on the fact that 'nothing is eternal and unchanged,' which is considered to be at the heart of Buddhist psychology. With mindfulness meditation practice, all experiences are observed as they arise and pass away. The practitioner notices things constantly changing along the way, and so they understand that all experiences are temporary. This mindfulness and non-judgmental observation promotes a separation from identifying oneself with the content of one's consciousness. In the literature dealing with mindfulness-based therapy, the following terms are used interchangeably as terms referring to 'the ability to observe one's thoughts or feelings as temporary events of the mind rather than as true and accurate in themselves': metacognitive awareness, decentering, defusion, distance, and reperceiving.

Through meditation practice, it becomes possible to see the content of consciousness—that is, one's own moment-by-moment experience—with a clearer and more objective view without equating oneself with one's own thoughts. Through this process, it becomes a therapeutic process that introduces a 'space' between one's 'perception' and 'reaction' wherein one escapes from one's own immediate experience in order to obtain insight and analysis on habitual patterns of emotions and behavior. Insights achieved through meditation have been reported to provide awareness that thinking is subjective and transitory, promoting 'non-attachment' and enhancing well-being and satisfaction with interpersonal functioning.

Emotion Regulation

Emotion regulation is divided into two types based on their mechanism. The first is an antecedent-focused strategy. It is a mechanism that regulates the factors that induce emotions, which are often accompanied by cognitive reappraisal. The second is a response-focused strategy, which is a method of suppressing the expression of emotions that have already occurred. The former emotion regulation through cognitive re-evaluation focuses on controlling the selection or change of context in the process of emotional processing. That is, they actively reinterpret emotional stimuli in a way that modifies their emotional impact. It is related to the top-down regulation of the lateral prefrontal region and the inhibitory function of the orbitofrontal cortex.

H.-G. Kim (✉)
Department of Psychiatry, Yeungnam University College of Medicine, Yeungnam University Medical Center, Daegu, South Korea
e-mail: psykhg@yu.ac.kr

J.-H. Chae, H.-Y. Lee (eds.), *Meditation in Psychiatry and General Medicine*,
https://doi.org/10.1007/978-981-95-7147-5_7

In that case, conflicting results are being reported at the same time as the results of studies on how meditation controls emotions. First of all, there are reports of a bottom-up process claiming that it is effective by fully experiencing the emotionally significant, particularly unpleasant, stimuli in an uncritical attitude rather than an attempt to cognitively reevaluate them. According to the actual results of studies, mindfulness meditation training was associated with reduced activation of the limbic system (amygdala and striatum) without activation of prefrontal cortex regions, particularly the lateral prefrontal cortex and orbitofrontal cortex, in response to emotionally significant stimuli. On the other hand, it has been argued that emotion regulation in mindfulness meditation is a top-down process. It has been reported that mindfulness meditation is an important factor in promoting positive reappraisal and that mindfulness meditation training is associated with activation of the prefrontal cortex area, which is associated with reappraisal, which is related to emotional regulation. There are also studies that claim that it depends on the skill level of meditation training. In other words, it was argued that short-term mindfulness trainees use the mechanism through the process of reappraising emotions more, and more experienced trainees have the ability to observe in a more detached manner. Even in actual neurobiological evidence, beginners of mindfulness meditation observed slightly more activity in the prefrontal cortex during meditation. Another study reported that the activity of the ventrolateral prefrontal cortex was increased after mindfulness-based stress reduction (MBSR) training. On the other hand, in the case of mindfulness meditation masters, the activity of the medial prefrontal cortex was rather decreased, and it can be seen that they can more accept this in emotional situations and the need for efforts for reappraisal is reduced.

Reduction of Automatic Thoughts and Self-Referential Thinking

Automatic thoughts begin unconsciously and are not easy to stop or prevent. In other words, when the conscious mind fails to draw attention consciously, the default mode network (DMN) starts involuntarily. Objective awareness of thinking through mindfulness meditation prevents interpreting thoughts as 'mere thoughts' and believing irrational negative thoughts as facts. Objective recognition of these automatic thoughts through mindfulness meditation is known to be a major mechanism by which mindfulness-based therapy reduces depression, anxiety, and stress.

Among thoughts about the past and the future, repeated negative thoughts are mainly worries about the future and rumination about the past. These two are said to be closely related to each other and are a symptom that accompanies a wide range of psychopathological and psychiatric disorders. In mindfulness meditation, the practitioner is trained to be aware of all the thoughts, feelings, and bodily sensations that occur to them here and now. They are aware of any concerns or ruminations that arise and allow them to return to the present moment, through awareness of breathing or bodily sensations. There was a study that reported finding the effect of rumination as a mediator of the effectiveness of mindfulness-based cognitive therapy (MBCT) for depression. In addition, in a recently reported meta-analysis, it was reported that repeated negative thoughts significantly mediate the mental health outcomes of mindfulness-based treatment according to the results of analysis, including five randomized controlled studies and three quasi-experimental design studies.

Part of the DMN, particularly cortical midline structures (CMS), includes the medial prefrontal cortex, anterior cingulate cortex, and posteromedial cortices (PMCs). It is known that the region plays an important role in automatic thinking, and it has been reported that a decrease in the activity of this region is associated with a decrease in automatic thinking. CMS is also involved in self-referential thinking, a type of automatic thinking known to be associated with mood and anxiety disorders. Mindfulness meditation weakens the non-adaptive habitual self-view by affecting the DMN domain, especially the CMS. In fact, MBSR is reported to increase positive views of the self, and when a person has a negative self-view, an increase in dorsomedial prefrontal cortex activity during MBSR is significantly associated with a decrease in social anxiety and an increase in mindfulness.

Control of Attention

Improving attention is one of the key elements of mindfulness meditation training. A general guideline for focused meditation aligned with the tradition of mindfulness meditation is: 'Focus on the incoming and outgoing breath. Stay focused, not distracted. If you become distracted, quietly turn your attention to your breath and start over.' Attention training improves the ability to maintain uncritical awareness of thought patterns, emotions, and sensory perceptions. This awareness helps you distance yourself from your thoughts and emotions so that you don't become overly intense.

Attention consists of three components, namely alerting, orienting, and executive control. In the first alerting stage, the right lateralized frontal-parietal-thalamic network functions as an important part in maintaining the alert state in preparation for incoming stimuli. The second orienting phase is the phase of selectively focusing on one or more among many stimuli. The posterior parietal lobe, the superior colliculus of the midbrain in charge of the eye area, the pulvinar, and the reticular nucleus of the thalamus play important functions in this stage. The last stage is the executive control stage, and it is responsible for execution functions such as monitoring, error detection, conflict resolution, and overcoming habitual behaviors. The anterior cingulate cortex, lateral frontal cortex, and basal ganglia, known as the anterior attention system, are responsible for this.

Research results on the mechanism by which mindfulness meditation affects attention improvement have been reported in various ways. This is because the type of meditation and training durations differ for each study, and it varies depending on which part of the attention component is affected. A study that showed that short-term intensive mindfulness meditation training helped improve attention and self-regulation, including conflict monitoring, reported that mindfulness meditation for 3 months was associated with improved attention related to executive function. A cross-sectional study and a study reported in 2010 reported that Samatha mindfulness training for 3 months improved the ability to maintain an alerting state as well as the ability to orient to a visual target compared to the control group. In a randomized control study reported in 2014, when MBSR was administered for 8 weeks, no significant improvement in sustained attention maintaining an alerting state was found compared to the control group, but improvement in orientation ability was reported to have been found. In a study in which 14 meditators performed brain scans during breathing meditation, DMN activity was shown when the mind was wandering, and the salience network was activated when the mind was aware of this state. When transferring or maintaining attention, the executive network is activated.

The brain region related to the effect of mindfulness meditation on attention is reported most consistently in the anterior cingulate cortex. Other attention-related brain regions where functional changes are observed by mindfulness meditation include the dorsolateral prefrontal cortex, parietal attention region, and putamen. In addition, mindfulness-based therapy promotes the improvement of interoceptive attention to intrinsic bodily sensations as well as attention to extrinsic stimuli. In this regard, changes in the activity of the insula, an important site for visceral sensation, have also been reported.

Self-Compassion

The concept of self-compassion is closely related to mindfulness. According to Neff's definition, self-compassion consists of three components. The first is self-kindness, which is an attitude that allows one to have a kind and understanding attitude rather than being harsh and critical of oneself. The second is common humanity, the perception of one's own experience as part of a greater human experience rather than being separate and isolated. The third is mindfulness, the ability to experience one's painful feelings and thoughts with balanced awareness rather than over-identifying with them.

As the concept itself suggests, mindfulness and self-compassion are highly related, and one study reported a correlation between total scores on the mindfulness scale and total scores on the self-compassion scale. It has also been reported that changes in mindfulness can predict changes in self-compassion, and it has been argued that self-compassion partially mediates the relationship between mindfulness and well-being. Kuyken et al. found that the positive effect of Mindfulness-Based Cognitive Therapy (MBCT) on depressive symptoms was mediated by the improvement of self-compassion through treatment. A more recent study found that in patients with anxiety disorders, scores on the Self-Compassion Scale were more strongly associated with symptom severity and quality of life than scores on the Mindful Attention Awareness Scale.

Mindfulness meditation is generally practiced intentionally (implicitly or explicitly) to foster self compassion as well as compassion for other beings. These levels vary somewhat depending on the type of meditation, but general guidelines for mindfulness meditation are as follows: 'Come back kindly whenever you realize that your mind is wandering' and 'If you encounter pain in your body or mind, take care of them.' In fact, many studies show that after mindfulness-based therapy, it has been reported that scores on the compassion scale significantly increased and self-compassion is considered as a mediator of the effectiveness of mindfulness-based therapy. One study asserted that the effect of mindfulness-based treatment for depression in patients with recurrent depression was through self-compassion, and two other studies reported self-compassion as a mediator of effects on anxiety traits and anger expression respectively. Thus, seeing one's own difficult experiences as part of the larger human experience rather than seeing them as separating and isolating ultimately results in a change in one's view of the self. However, the neurological evidence of the neurobiological link of self-compassion in the context of mindfulness is still lacking.

Improving Values Clarification and Behavioral Self-Regulation

Mindfulness meditation can help people recognize what is meaningful to them and what is truly valuable. When we can observe our values in isolation and reflect on our objectivity, we rediscover more genuine values in ourselves and have the opportunity to choose. In other words, we can reflectively choose what was previously adopted or adjusted reflexively. Previous literature reports that automatic processing limits our consideration of options consistent with our needs and values. However, open and intentional awareness through mindfulness meditation allows us to choose behaviors that are consistent with our needs, interests, and values. The actual study results also reported that a high level of the self-reported mindfulness scale had a significant effect on the selection of valuable actions or interests and that it was related to the ability to take more goal-oriented behaviors even in emotionally upsetting situations. In addition, mindfulness meditation training was associated with improved behavioral control and decreased self-discrepancy, which in turn was associated with adaptive self-regulation after recovery in patients with a history of depression and suicidal thoughts. In another study, value clarification was reported as a mediating factor between the improvement of mindfulness and the reduction of psychological discomfort in subjects who performed MBSR.

Exposure, Extinction, and Reconsolidation

Exposure is another process suggested by several authors that may occur during mindfulness meditation training. By intentionally participating in the experience in a non-critical, open-minded way, the individual engages in a desensitization process that makes unavoidable emotions less painful. By attending carefully to negative emotional states, we find empirically and phenomenologically that we do not need to fear or avoid those feelings and that they eventually go away. One study found that the degree of exposure significantly increased after MBSR training. Exposure, extinction, and reconsolidation are important mechanisms for reducing habituated anxiety and fear. Mindfulness acts as a self-regulating mechanism for efficiently integrating from maladaptive trajectories to more positive and adaptive trajectories. This type of transformation appears to use circuits related to extinction and reconsolidation. It is suggested that biases for attention and memory associated with habitual distortions are dissipated and reconstructed. Phelps et al. emphasized the moment of reconsolidation as a way to modify memories of fear. In the process of reconsolidation, if the contingency of the contextual cues and their meanings are changed, new cues are generated. The hypometabolic state through mindfulness meditation creates a new parasympathetic association with the previous anxiety-inducing stimuli and thus the extinction process. That is, noticing and new labeling of sensory, cognitive, and sensory states during hypometabolic states lead to more positive rehardening of the nature of the conditioned response. In addition, in the process of mindfulness meditation, positive reappraisal strategies can be used to examine specific emotions and determine whether they are desirable or undesirable, warranted or unfair. If you want to change something about an emotional state, you can intentionally modify it. Important brain regions in this process are the hippocampus, amygdala, rhinal cortices, and ventromedial prefrontal cortex. In particular, the dorsolateral prefrontal cortex plays a role in controlling the response of the amygdala and suppressing the expression of fear. Neuroimaging studies have been reported to reveal changes in the structure and function of the brain region through mindfulness-based therapy.

The Physiological Effects of Meditation

Experienced meditators showed physiological changes in a 'wakeful hypometabolic state' during mindfulness meditation. The activity of the sympathetic nervous system is decreased, and the activity of the parasympathetic nervous system, which is important for relaxation and rest, is increased. In other words, in addition to relaxing the body, meditation aims to reduce mental activity, thus relaxing the mind, and mental relaxation can give feedback to the body, leading to deeper physical relaxation. This part has been proven in studies that measure physiological changes in the body while practicing mindfulness meditation. Body relaxation, such as simple muscle relaxation, is associated with activation of primary and secondary motor regions. The activity of paralimbic brain regions mediating sympathetic nerve stimulation, such as the anterior cingulate and insula, is known to be a change that occurs in both relaxation and mindfulness meditation. It is known that specific areas are additionally activated, and many experienced meditators report activation of fronto-limbic and fronto-parietal neural networks. More interestingly, more enhanced activation was observed in the fronto-parietal attention networks in experienced meditators compared to novice meditators with little experience. If mindfulness meditation is not different from simple general relaxation, it is expected that short-term and long-term meditators will relax similarly and there will be no differences in physiological or neurophysiological characteristics. However, specific differences in physiology and brain activation were found in long-term meditators, demonstrating that mindfulness meditation can induce experience-dependent 'dose'-effects in neurofunctional networks. One study also found a direct correlation between individual variability in the subjective quality of mindfulness meditation and the degree of brain activation. The intensity of activation of the frontal-parietal and frontal-limbic neural networks was induced by subjectively reported states of reduced thinking and meditation. There was a linear relationship with the intensity of happiness.

During mindfulness meditation, subjects showed more happiness and less mental activity when compared to normal rest. In one study that proved this by measuring actual EEG, long-term meditators reported that low-frequency EEG activity of theta and alpha was increased, especially in the left frontal area. Also, the intensity of happiness was positively correlated with the theta activity of the left frontal lobe. An increase in fronto-parietal theta activation was significantly associated with an increase in attentional neural network activity and inhibition of task-irrelevant processes. This means that reduced mental activity during meditation triggers activity in regions that mediate positive emotions (left prefrontal cortex) while activation of internalized attentional networks that reduce external attention and irrelevant networks is mediated. In other studies using EEG, it was reported that increased activity of alpha waves was associated with a decrease in anxiety levels, and there was also a report that MBSR and MBCT help to correct frontal alpha asymmetry.

Recently, there have been reports that meditation also affects the activity of telomerase, which can prevent the shortening of telomeres associated with cell aging, as well as the improvement of immunological functions. It has been reported that meditation reduces inflammatory proteins and pro-inflammatory cytokines such as CRP, IL-6, IL-8, IL-10, TNF-a, and IFN and increases cell-mediated immune response and is associated with inhibition of cellular aging. It has been reported to increase the activity of telomerase.

Conclusion

Psychological mechanisms by which mindfulness meditation has clinical effects include improvement of metacognitive awareness, emotion regulation, reduction of automatic and self-referential thinking, attention regulation, self-compassion, improvement of values clarification and behavioral self-regulation, and exposure, extinction, and reconsolidation. Among them, psychological mechanisms other than self-compassion and value clarification have been reported to be related to neurobiological changes in the brain regions involved. Mindfulness meditation brings mental relaxation as an awake but low-metabolism state, which is different from general relaxation, and the activity of the frontal-limbic system and fronto-parietal neural networks appears to be dependent on the amount of experience of meditation training. Also, recently, there has been a report that meditation affects the activity of telomerase, which can prevent the shortening of telomeres associated with cell aging, as well as the improvement of immunological functions.

Bibliography

Aftanas LI, Golocheikine SA. Human anterior and frontal midline theta and lower alpha reflect emotionally positive state and internalized attention: high-resolution EEG investigation of meditation. Neurosci Lett. 2001;310(1):57–60.

Alda M, Puebla-Guedea M, Rodero B, Demarzo M, Montero-Marin J, Roca M, Garcia-Campayo J. Zen meditation, length of telomeres, and the role of experiential avoidance and compassion. Mindfulness. 2016;7:651–9. https://doi.org/10.1007/s12671-016-0500-5.

Baer RA, Smith GT, Hopkins J, Krietemeyer J, Toney L. Using self-report assessment methods to explore facets of mindfulness. Assessment. 2006;13(1):27–45. https://doi.org/10.1177/1073191105283504.

Barnhofer T, Duggan D, Crane C, Hepburn S, Fennell MJ, Williams JM. Effects of meditation on frontal alpha-asymmetry in previously suicidal individuals. Neuroreport. 2007;18(7):709–12. https://doi.org/10.1097/WNR.0b013e3280d943cd.

Bergen-Cico D, Possemato K, Cheon S. Examining the efficacy of a brief mindfulness-based stress reduction (brief MBSR) program on psychological health. J Am Coll Heal. 2013;61(6):348–60. https://doi.org/10.1080/07448481.2013.813853.
Birnie K, Speca M, Carlson LE. Exploring self-compassion and empathy in the context of mindfulness-based stress reduction (MBSR). Stress Health. 2010;26(5):359–71. https://doi.org/10.1002/smi.1305.
Black DS, O'Reilly GA, Olmstead R, Breen EC, Irwin MR. Mindfulness meditation and improvement in sleep quality and daytime impairment among older adults with sleep disturbances: a randomized clinical trial. JAMA Intern Med. 2015;175(4):494–501. https://doi.org/10.1001/jamainternmed.2014.808.
Brefczynski-Lewis JA, Lutz A, Schaefer HS, Levinson DB, Davidson RJ. Neural correlates of attentional expertise in long-term meditation practitioners. Proc Natl Acad Sci USA. 2007;104(27):11483–8. https://doi.org/10.1073/pnas.0606552104.
Brown KW, Ryan RM. The benefits of being present: mindfulness and its role in psychological well-being. J Pers Soc Psychol. 2003;84(4):822–48.
Cahn BR, Polich J. Meditation states and traits: EEG, ERP, and neuroimaging studies. Psychol Bull. 2006;132(2):180–211. https://doi.org/10.1037/0033-2909.132.2.180.
Carmody J, Baer RA, Lykins ELB, Olendzki N. An empirical study of the mechanisms of mindfulness in a mindfulness-based stress reduction program. J Clin Psychol. 2009;65(6):613–26. https://doi.org/10.1002/jclp.20579.
Chambers R, Gullone E, Allen NB. Mindful emotion regulation: an integrative review. Clin Psychol Rev. 2009;29(6):560–72. https://doi.org/10.1016/j.cpr.2009.06.005.
Chiesa A, Serretti A, Jakobsen JC. Mindfulness: top-down or bottom-up emotion regulation strategy? Clin Psychol Rev. 2013;33(1):82–96. https://doi.org/10.1016/j.cpr.2012.10.006.
Epel E, Daubenmier J, Moskowitz JT, Folkman S, Blackburn E. Can meditation slow rate of cellular aging? Cognitive stress, mindfulness, and telomeres. Ann N Y Acad Sci. 2009;1172:34–53. https://doi.org/10.1111/j.1749-6632.2009.04414.x.
Gu J, Strauss C, Bond R, Cavanagh K. How do mindfulness-based cognitive therapy and mindfulness-based stress reduction improve mental health and wellbeing? A systematic review and meta-analysis of mediation studies. Clin Psychol Rev. 2015;37:1–12. https://doi.org/10.1016/j.cpr.2015.01.006.
Hasenkamp W, Wilson-Mendenhall CD, Duncan E, Barsalou LW. Mind wandering and attention during focused meditation: a fine-grained temporal analysis of fluctuating cognitive states. NeuroImage. 2012;59(1):750–60. https://doi.org/10.1016/j.neuroimage.2011.07.008.
Hollis-Walker L, Colosimo K. Mindfulness, self-compassion, and happiness in non-meditators: a theoretical and empirical examination. Personal Individ Differ. 2011;50(2):222–7. https://doi.org/10.1016/j.paid.2010.09.033.
Keng S-L, Smoski MJ, Robin CJ. Effects of mindfulness on psychological health: a review of empirical studies. Clin Psychol Rev. 2011;31(6):1041–56. https://doi.org/10.1016/j.cpr.2011.04.006.
Kuyken W, Watkins E, Holden E, White K, Taylor RS, Byford S, Evans A, Radford S, Teasdale JD, Dalgleish T. How does mindfulness-based cognitive therapy work? Behav Res Ther. 2010;48(11):1105–12. https://doi.org/10.1016/j.brat.2010.08.003.
Lazar SW, Bush G, Gollub RL, Friccione GL, Khalsa G, Benson H. Functional brain mapping of the relaxation response and meditation. Neuroreport. 2000;11(7):1581–5.
MacCoon DG, MacLean KA, Davidson RJ, Saron CD, Lutz A. No sustained attention differences in a longitudinal randomized trial comparing mindfulness based stress reduction versus active control. PLoS One. 2014;9(6):e97551. https://doi.org/10.1371/journal.pone.0097551.
MacLean KA, Ferrer E, Ailchele SR, Bridwell DA, Zanesco AP, Jacobs TL, King BG, Rosenberg EL, Sahdra BK, Shaver PR, Wallace BA, Mangun GR, Saron CD. Intensive meditation training improves perceptual discrimination and sustained attention. Psychol Sci. 2010;21(6):829–39. https://doi.org/10.1177/0956797610371339.
Marchand WR. Mindfulness-based stress reduction, mindfulness-based cognitive therapy, and Zen meditation for depression, anxiety, pain, and psychological distress. J Psychiatr Pract. 2012;18(4):233–52. https://doi.org/10.1097/01.pra.0000416014.53215.86.
Marchand WR. Neural mechanisms of mindfulness and meditation: evidence from neuroimaging studies. World J Radiol. 2014;6(7):471–9. https://doi.org/10.4329/wjr.v6.i7.471.
Neff K. Self-compassion: an alternative conceptualization of a healthy attitude toward oneself. Self Identity. 2003;2(2):85–101.
Ochsner KN, Gross JJ. The cognitive control of emotion. Trends Cogn Sci. 2005;9(5):242–9. https://doi.org/10.1016/j.tics.2005.03.010.
Phelps EA, Delgado MR, Nearing KI, LeDoux JE. Extinction learning in humans: role of the amygdala and vmPFC. Neuron. 2004;43(6):897–905. https://doi.org/10.1016/j.neuron.2004.08.042.
Rolls ET, Grabenhorst F. The orbitofrontal cortex and beyond: from affect to decision-making. Prog Neurobiol. 2008;86(3):216–44. https://doi.org/10.1016/j.pneurobio.2008.09.001.
Shahar B, Britton W, Sbarra DA, Figueredo A, Bootzin R. Mechanisms of change in mindfulness-based cognitive therapy for depression: preliminary evi-

dence from a randomized controlled trial. Int J Cogn Ther. 2010;3(4):402–18. https://doi.org/10.1521/ijct.2010.3.4.402.

Shapiro SL, Brown KW, Biegel GM. Teaching self-care to caregivers: effects of mindfulness-based stress reduction on the mental health of therapists in training. Train Educ Prof Psychol. 2007;1(2):105–15.

Slagter HA, Lutz A, Greischar LL, Francis AD, Nieuwenhuis S, Davis JM, Davidson RJ. Mental training affects distribution of limited brain resources. PLoS Biol. 2007;5(6):e138. https://doi.org/10.1371/journal.pbio.0050138.

Tang Y-Y, Ma Y, Wang J, Fan Y, Feng S, Lu Q, Yu Q, Sui D, Rothbart MK, Fan M, Posner MI. Short-term meditation training improves attention and self-regulation. Proc Natl Acad Sci USA. 2007;104(43):17152–6. https://doi.org/10.1073/pnas.0707678104.

Van Dam NT, Sheppard SC, Porsyth JP, Earleywine M. Self-compassion is a better predictor than mindfulness of symptom severity and quality of life in mixed anxiety and depression. J Anxiety Disord. 2011;25(1):123–30. https://doi.org/10.1016/j.janxdis.2010.08.011.

8 Research on Brain Imaging of Meditation

Boung Chul Lee

Many researchers are interested in how to scientifically prove the effects of meditation and develop it efficiently. Which areas of the brain function during meditation and how does each method of meditation differ? What parts of the brain change when one first begins practicing meditation, and what is the difference between the brains of masters vs beginners? Much research is being conducted to answer these types of questions, and in this chapter, I will attempt to summarize this research, focusing on recent findings.

In general, the brain is composed of brain cells whose primary components are proteins and carbohydrates, axons whose primary component is fat, and cerebrospinal fluid whose primary component is similar to that of plasma. In MRI brain images, the areas with many brain cells are shown as grayish gray matter, axons are shown as white matter, and cerebrospinal fluid is shown as black ventricles. As MRI started to be used in medicine in the 1980s, research on the brain became popular. MRI is a method of measuring and imaging electromagnetic waves according to changes in the spin of hydrogen atoms in body tissue by applying a magnetic field to the person who enters the test tube, enabling detailed observation of the brain structure without exposure to radiation. Voxel-based morphometry is used to study structural changes in the brain, and it is a method of statistically comparing the difference in size, thickness, shape, etc. between the test group and the control group by taking 3D images of the brain.

As a method of research on functional brain imaging, fMRI is the most popularly used tool to research mindfulness today. fMRI measures changes in hemoglobin, a constituent protein of red blood cells, according to its oxygen-binding state. Neurons use more oxygen when they are active than when they are at rest. In this case, blood flow in microvessels rises to meet the increased demands of oxygen. This change in blood flow is called the BOLD (Blood Oxygen Level-Dependent) effect, and is the basis for fMRI measurement signals. As an indirect method of measuring nerve cell activity by measuring changes in blood flow in a local area, it ultimately measures and compares the state before and after stimulation. Nerve activity results in an increase in blood flow after about 2 s, rising to a maximum in about 4–6 s and lasting about 10 s. This change in blood flow occurs in a range of two to three millimeters of the activated area. Although the temporal and spatial resolution of fMRI is relatively superior to other research methods, the change in the actual BOLD effect is about 0.2%, which is less than the 0.3 to 0.4% attributed to the noise of the fMRI system. Therefore, repeated measurements are needed to

B. C. Lee (✉)
Department of Psychiatry, Hangang Sacred Heart Hospital, Hallym University, Seoul, Republic of Korea

J.-H. Chae, H.-Y. Lee (eds.), *Meditation in Psychiatry and General Medicine*, https://doi.org/10.1007/978-981-95-7147-5_8

	Spatial Resolution	Time Resolution	Cost	Invasion
fMRI	1mm	6~10s	high	none
EEG	1cm	1ms	medium	none
PET	4mm	1 min	very high	radiation
SPECT	8mm	2~8s	high	radiation

Fig. 8.1 Comparison of brain imaging methods on meditation Carter & Shieh (2010)

confirm the response to a single stimulus. In addition, the fact that fMRI scans generate a lot of noise should be taken into account in research on meditation. Of course, there are EEG tests with high temporal resolution and PET (Positron Emission Tomography) tests that can measure individual neurotransmitters. However, for various reasons, fMRI has been the mainstream method for brain imaging studies on meditation so far (Fig. 8.1) Carter & Shieh (2010), Schmidt & Walach (2014).

Brain imaging studies on meditation were conducted with various subjects and regions of the brain of interest according to the practitioner's state (early, middle, late) and the elements of meditation (control of attention, control of emotion, self-awareness). Although MBSR (Mindfulness-Based Stress Reduction) and MBCT (Mindfulness-Based Cognitive Therapy) are the representative programs of the clinical application of meditation, these programs are not just being used for research purposes, but also include a variety of therapeutic aspects such as cognitive-behavioral therapy. In order to study the effects of meditation alone, Tang et al. separated only the elements of meditation to create IBMT (Integrative Body Mind Training) and conducted a study using subjects who went through the program. Tang et al. (2009)

Brain Imaging Research

The first brain structure study on meditation began in 2005. The study reported that when comparing practitioners who had been meditating for about 10 years with ordinary people, there was less cerebral cortical decline due to aging amongst the practitioners and changes in brain structure appeared in the prefrontal cortex and insula Lazar et al. (2006). Another study on Zen meditation found that there was less gray matter loss due to aging in practitioners, particularly in the putamen Pagnoni & Cekic (2007). Yet another study that compared practitioners of Vipassanā meditation with a control group reported a higher density of gray matter regions in the insula (Rt. Ant. Insula), temporal lobe (Inf. Temporal gyrus), and hippocampus (Rt. Hippocampus) amongst practitioners of meditation Hölzel et al. (2008). In a follow-up study, it was confirmed that gray matter density of the left hippocampus increased after participation in an 8-week MBSR program, and it was also found that there was an increase in the posterior cingulate cortex, the temporoparietal junction, and the cerebellum amongst participants compared to the control group. A meta-study (that synthesized and analyzed similar studies) on changes in brain structure reported an enlargement of the inferior temporal gyrus as the most prominent feature. In another study, this area was reported to be directly proportional to the time spent practicing meditation.

A functional study of the brain that primarily used fMRI observed differences in brain activity by comparing meditation practitioners to control groups before and after the start of a meditation program. Speaking of an interesting study, when various noises were heard by meditators and a control group in an fMRI study, activity of the posterior cingulate cortex, one of the parts of the DMN (Default Mode Network), decreased proportionally to the duration of meditation. Additionally, when brain activity was measured after subjects heard a startling noise, it was also found that the activity of the amygdala decreased proportionally to the degree of meditation practice. Inferring based on these results, the more one practices meditation, the less unnecessary activity of the DMN is caused by noise. Additionally, there is a decrease in emotional response proportionate to the duration of practice when negative stimuli are presented.

Currently, several researchers have combined the results of various studies conducted up to this point and separated mindfulness meditation into several elements. I think it will be helpful to understand these elements by connecting them with the corresponding parts of the brain.

Tang saw meditation as being composed of three specific elements, namely attention control, emotion control and self-awareness. He also said that the corresponding areas of the brain are where changes were being observed repeatedly in studies on meditation, and this was consistent with the functional areas of the brain revealed in various brain imaging studies in the past Tang et al. (2015). Looking at the areas of the brain that correspond to each element of meditation, he reported that 'attention control' corresponds to the anterior cingulate cortex, the medial prefrontal cortex, and the striatum, 'emotion control' involves the anterior cingulate cortex, medial prefrontal cortex, and the amygdala, and 'self-awareness' involved the insula, medial prefrontal cortex, and the precuneus (Fig. 8.2) Tang et al. (2015).

On the other hand, Falcone divided the elements of meditation into three networks, namely, the 'alerting network' which alerts us to maintain focused attention on a specific stimulus, the 'orienting network' which selects a specific stimulus from a variety of stimuli, and the 'executing network' that regulates focused attention. If you think about it in terms of meditation practice, the alerting network that focuses one's consciousness on breathing, the orienting network that selects and maintains one's focus on the stimulus of breathing among various senses, and the executing network that returns one's consciousness back to breathing after being distracted by various thoughts are all working together. In terms of each function, it is described that the alerting network involves the right frontal lobe (dorsolateral prefrontal cortex, anterior cingulate cortex) and the right parietal lobe, the orienting network involves the parietal lobe and the temporoparietal junction, and the executing network involves the anterior cingulate cortex, anterior insula, and basal ganglia (Fig. 8.3).

However, a limitation of these studies is that each region of the brain is actually in a variety of studies, making it difficult to determine its function by simply connecting a function to a region of the brain. In addition, when observing active areas of the brain, differences between the two groups may not have been observed due to the

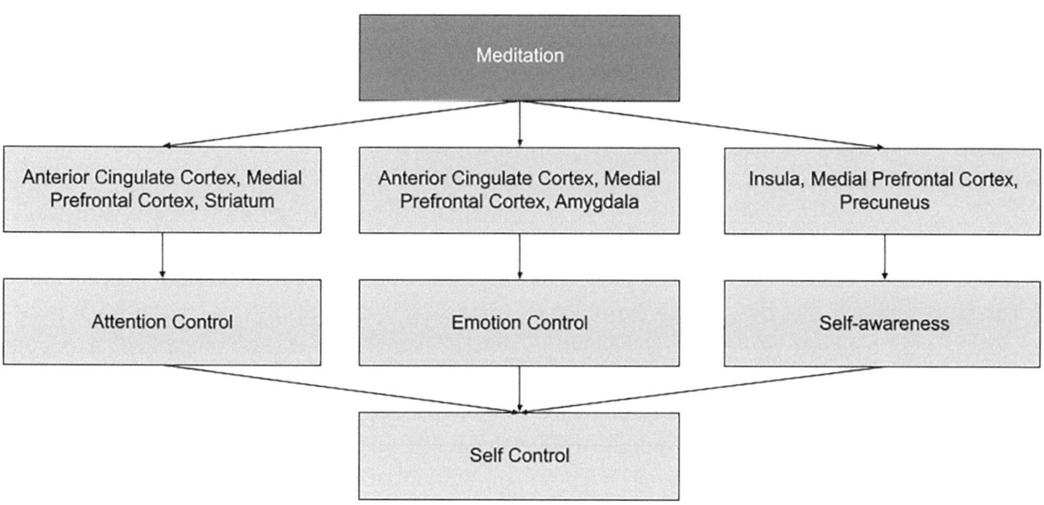

Fig. 8.2 Schematic diagram of the regions of the brain associated with the elements of meditation according to Tang

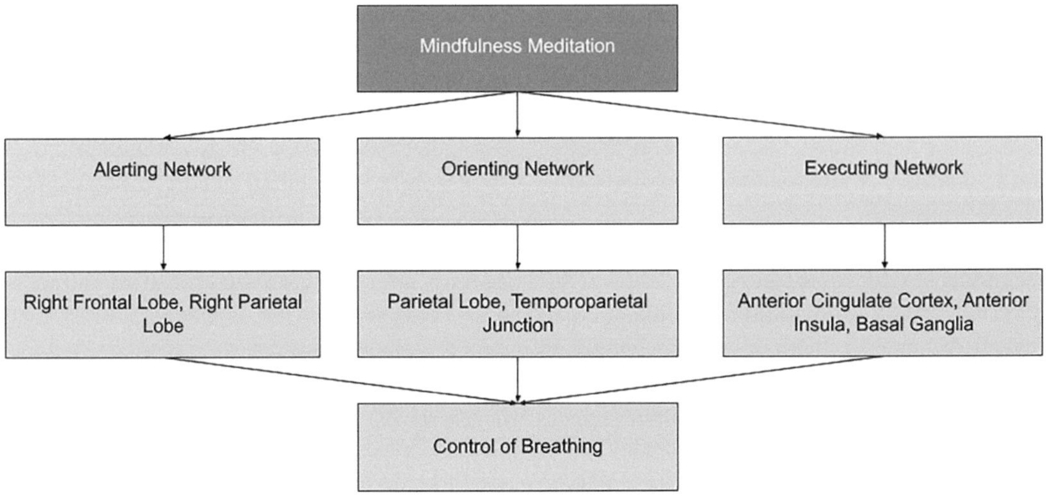

Fig. 8.3 Schematic diagram of the elements of mindfulness meditation and related regions of the brain according to Falcone

ceiling effect or the floor effect. However, when we take into account the temporal and spatial constraints up to this point, a functional evaluation of the brain is considered to be the most powerful way to explain the various aspects of meditation.

In a meta-study of brain functional neuroimaging research, there was a difference in the changes that occurred between beginners and experienced practitioners in the medial frontal gyrus/anterior cingulate cortex and the left insula /inferior frontal gyrus Falcone & Jerram (2018). Furthermore, a meta-analysis that compared beginners to a control group also reported a difference in the right insula.

Regions of the Brain Associated with Meditation

Hippocampus

It has been reported that the size of the hippocampus differs between meditators and control groups. As an area where new brain cells continue to generate even in adulthood, significant changes in the size of the hippocampus were observed even after implementing an 8-week MBSR program. In addition to its commonly known function responsible for memory, the hippocampus is involved in the function for regulating emotions, and it has been reported that there was a decreased density or volume in the hippocampus for patients suffering from psychiatric disorders such as major depressive disorder or PTSD. Although the cause for the decrease in volume has not yet been precisely identified, it is assumed to be due to a loss of nerve cells, a loss of glial cells, and a decrease in neurogenesis. On the other hand, antidepressant treatments increase the volume of the hippocampus (Fig. 8.4).

Default Mode Network

The Default Mode Network (DMN) is a part of the brain that is activated spontaneously during periods of rest, where there is no conscious thought. Although the brain in a resting state, so-called 'zoning out' is like meditation in that they both maintain a relaxed state without being immersed in any specific task, meditation is different in that it is a state of mind that is constantly conscious of thoughts, sensations, and emotions that arise and pass away, and is continuously observing phenomena that occur in an individual's body and mind. In other words, there is a difference between the mind in the

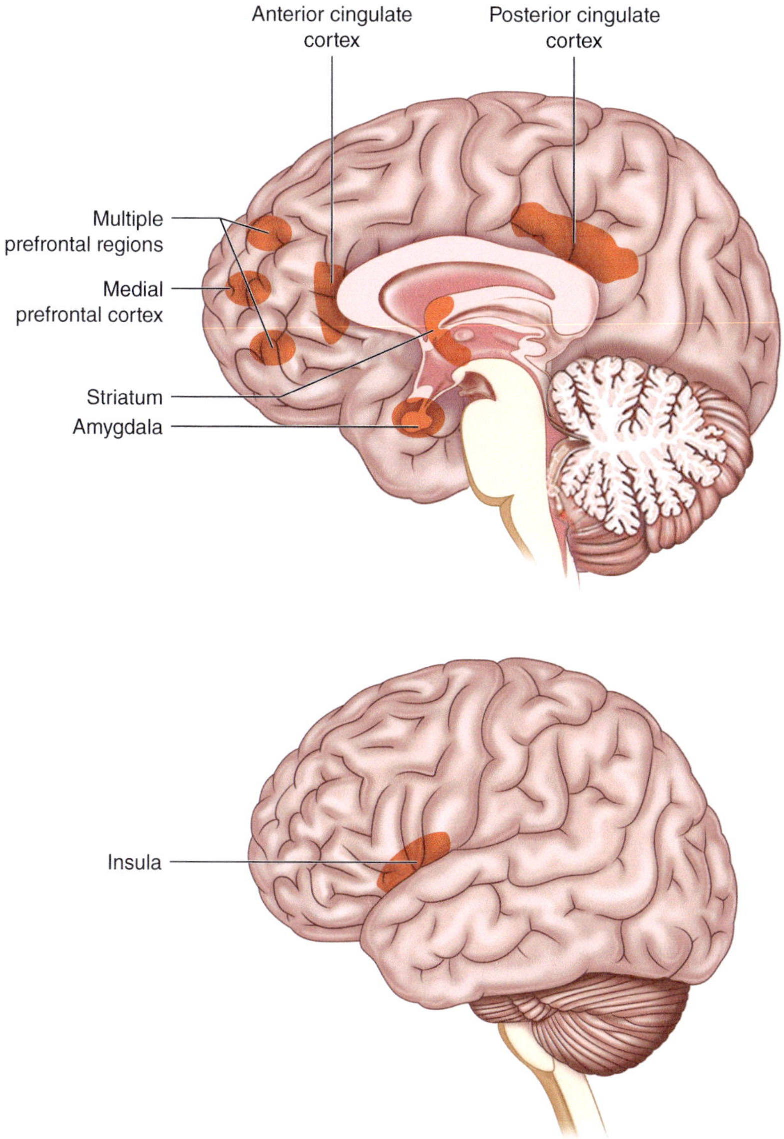

Fig. 8.4 A schematic diagram of the regions of the brain associated with mindfulness meditation

DMN state where it wanders here and there and during meditation where it holds onto the phenomena that occur inside and outside an individual in a state of awareness. This default mode network is associated with activity in the posterior cingulate cortex, precuneus, and the medial prefrontal cortex. While these areas of the brain are activated when it is in a state of not doing anything specific, their activity decreases during meditation.

Posterior Cingulate Cortex

The posterior cingulate cortex and the precuneus are the primary regions of the brain included in the default mode network, and their activity is typically reduced when the activity of the default mode network is reduced through meditation. A decrease in their activity due to meditation has been observed in several studies, particularly fMRI studies. These are areas of the brain that can reflect changes even in short-term practice. Their activity is lower than usual even in the case of beginners who report being in a 'state of quietly paying attention to their breath.'

Amygdala

The amygdala is a region of the brain associated with feelings of fear and anxiety.

In cases of post-traumatic stress disorder or phobias, it is often overactivated in the presence of an anxiety-inducing stimulus. The amygdala is activated by negative stimuli and is inhibited by the prefrontal cortex. Activity of the amygdala is reduced through mindfulness meditation, and this has been shown to occur not only in the meditative state but also in a non-meditating state Desbordes et al. (2012).

Insula

The insula is one of the regions where structural or functional changes are most consistently observed in meditation brain imaging studies. The insula is responsible for interoceptive awareness and visceral awareness such as that of breathing or the heartbeat, and is also involved in empathic response. In other words, it is involved in being aware of the sensations and physiological processes that arise in one's own body. Studies have also reported that there are differences that occur in the insula when you focus on your body posture or when you try to sense and be conscious of your breathing, touch, and body temperature. In cases where you have depression or anxiety disorders, you will have issues being aware of bodily sensations or emotions expressed by bodily sensations. It was confirmed that the size of the insular was reduced in these cases, and it was found that treatment of and recovery from the disease were slower when there was such a structural change.

Anterior Cingulate Cortex

The anterior cingulate cortex is a region of the brain involved in the proper distribution of attention, impulse control, emotion control, and ethical judgment. Like the Stroop test, the anterior cingulate cortex is in charge of the function of detecting errors when receiving various information, and it shows abnormalities in patients with attention deficit disorder or obsessive-compulsive disorder. In meditation, anterior cingulate cortex activity is increased in the act of maintaining attention. However, as with the parietal lobe, the anterior cingulate cortex is less active in skilled meditators due to a reduced need for resources to maintain attention.

Striatum

Along with the anterior cingulate cortex, the striatum is a region of the brain involved in maintaining attention. Abnormalities are found in attention-related disorders such as obsessive-compulsive disorder or autism. The caudate and putamen, which make up the striatum, are known to be related to reward-based learning, and are activated when learned behavior becomes familiar and habitual through conscious effort. During meditation, they are activated in a state where one's attention is focused continuously on a phenomenon without effort. It has also been found that there is an increased level of activity in the striatum even during rest periods after practicing mindfulness. There are reports that practicing meditation increases the secretion of dopamine, a neurotransmitter related to reward, in the striatum.

The Lateral Prefrontal Cortex and the Parietal Lobe

The lateral prefrontal cortex and the parietal lobe are regions of the brain involved in conscious concentration. It functions to keep our attention undistracted when we focus our attention on a specific action, and for beginners practicing meditation, these regions are related to making an effort to try to consciously focus on breathing or bodily sensations. Therefore, they are activated when effort is made during the process of a beginner practicing meditation. However, as the practitioner becomes more adept and does not need to make as much of an effort to maintain their focus, there is a decrease in activity in these regions Brefczynski-Lewis et al. (2007). Therefore, unlike the anterior cingulate cortex or the insula, where activity is continuously strengthened according to the level of meditation practice, activity increases at first in the lateral prefrontal cortex and parietal lobe, but then decreases as the practitioner becomes more skilled and does not need to exert as much effort during meditation.

The prefrontal cortex is involved in self-regulation and adaptive behavior in response to changes in one's environment. Studies have shown that when various changes occur in functionally uncertain situations, the prefrontal cortex functions based on self-control and self-regulation necessary to reach an optimal decision by analyzing a variety of data. During breathing meditation practices, the amygdala and posterolateral prefrontal cortex are considered to be involved in regulating emotion Doll et al. (2016).

Conclusion

There are three elements of meditation, namely attention control, emotion control and self-awareness. Connecting the regions of the brain related to each function is most helpful in confirming the effects of meditation related to brain imaging. During meditation, attention control corresponds to the act of maintaining focus on an object, keeping the mind focused on the breath or sensations, and bringing the mind back from thoughts about the past or future and keeping it in the present moment. The prefrontal cortex, striatum, and anterior cingulate cortex are involved here. Emotion control is the element that regulates negative moods during meditation through non-judgmental acceptance and awareness of the here and now and maintains calmness and positive emotions. The prefrontal cortex and amygdala are involved here. Self-awareness is a metacognition that recognizes the conscious self and includes consciousness about the physical sensations that arise from within the body. The insula is primarily involved here. Additionally, various other regions of the brain are involved such as the default mode network, the temporal lobe, and the parietal lobe. As research progresses, the relationships and roles of all of these regions of the brain and elements of meditation will gradually become clearer.

Bibliography

Brefczynski-Lewis JA, Lutz A, Schaefer HS, Levinson DB, Davidson RJ. Neural correlates of attentional expertise in long-term meditation practitioners. Proc Natl Acad Sci USA. 2007;104(27):11483–8. https://doi.org/10.1073/pnas.0606552104.

Carter M, Shieh JC. Guide to research techniques in neuroscience. Elsevier; 2010. https://doi.org/10.1016/C2009-0-01891-1.

Desbordes G, Negi LT, Pace TWW, Wallace BA, Raison CL, Schwartz EL. Effects of mindful-attention and compassion meditation training on amygdala response to emotional stimuli in an ordinary, non-meditative state. Front Hum Neurosci. 2012;6:292. https://doi.org/10.3389/fnhum.2012.00292.

Doll A, Hölzel BK, Bratec SM, Boucard C, Xie X, Wohlschläger AM, Sorg C. Mindful attention to breath regulates emotions via increased amygdala-prefrontal cortex connectivity. Neuroimage. 2016;134:305–13. https://doi.org/10.1016/j.neuroimage.2016.03.041.

Falcone G, Jerram M. Brain activity in mindfulness depends on experience: a meta- analysis of fMRI studies. Mindfulness (NY). 2018;9:1319–29. https://doi.org/10.1007/s12671-018-0884-5.

Hölzel BK, Ott U, Gard T, Hempel H, Weygandt M, Morgen K, Vaitl D. Investigation of mindfulness meditation practitioners with voxel-based morphometry. Soc Cogn Affect Neurosci. 2008;3(1):55–61. https://doi.org/10.1093/scan/nsm038.

Lazar SW, Kerr CE, Wasserman RH, Gray JR, Greve DN, Treadway MT, McGarvey M, Quinn BT, Dusek JA, Benson H, Rauch SL, Moore CI, Fischl B. Meditation experience is associated with increased cortical thickness. Neuroreport. 2006;16(17):1893–7.

Schmidt S, Walach H. Meditation–neuroscientific approaches and philosophical implications. Spring; 2014. https://doi.org/10.1007/978-3-319-01634-4.

Pagnoni G, Cekic M. Age effects on gray matter volume and attentional performance in Zen meditation. Neurobiol Aging. 2007;28(10):1623–7. https://doi.org/10.1016/j.neurobiolaging.2007.06.008.

Tang YY, Hölzel BK, Posner MI. The neuroscience of mindfulness meditation. Nat Rev Neurosci. 2015;16:213. https://doi.org/10.1038/nrn3916.

Tang YY, Ma Y, Fan Y, Feng H, Wang J, Feng S, Lu Q, Hu B, Lin Y, Li J, Zhang Y, Wang Y, Zhou L, Fan M. Central and autonomic nervous system interaction is altered by short-term meditation. Proc Natl Acad Sci USA. 2009;106(22):8865–70. https://doi.org/10.1073/pnas.0904031106.

Movement-Based Meditation, Somatics

9

Hyu-Jung Huh and Sunje Kim

Somatics is a general term that refers to various fields related to body work or movement that emphasize internal sensory experiences. 'Soma,' a term often used for various types of movement-based treatment, focuses on how one feels one's body from one's own point of view rather than that of others.

The origin of Somatics can be traced to traditional Asian movement practices such as yoga. In the West, somatic movement dates back to the late nineteenth and early twentieth centuries, and popular phenomenology or existential philosophy at this time influenced various techniques of Somatics based on 'experiential learning.' Early Somatic techniques in the West were created by Elsa Gindler and Heinrich Jacoby Gimmler in Germany at the end of the nineteenth century. Based on their work, various figures who are considered the 'pioneers of Somatics' were very active in Europe, including Frederick Matthais Alexander, Moshe Feldenkrais, Mabel Elsworth, Gerda Alexander, Ida Rolf, Milton Trager. These figures developed various techniques to increase physical awareness based on their own experiences going through the process of recovering from various personal difficulties such as physical injury. Since then, various types of techniques of various people were passed down over the course of a century, and in the 1980s, this series of techniques began to be called 'Somatics' thanks to Thomas Hanna, an American philosopher and movement therapist. Currently, various types of techniques in the field of Somatics are used in various fields such as occupational therapy, clinical psychology, and education.

Recently, Laura Schmalz et al. presented a new perspective that views various types of techniques based on Somatics as a kind of mindful movement. From this point of view, various techniques of Somatics were conceptualized as a kind of Movement-Based Contemplative Practice (MBCP). We will briefly review the characteristics of Somatics as Movement-Based Contemporary Practices (MBCP) based on the concepts and descriptions of Laura Schmalz et al.

Characteristics of Somatics from the Perspective of Meditation

Movement Based

Many techniques based on Somatics are based on movements with internally occurring intentions. Most techniques involve the process of adjusting one's movements based on feedback from one's

H.-J. Huh (✉)
Department of Psychiatry, Incheon St. Mary's Hospital, Incheon, Republic of Korea

Department of Psychiatry, College of Medicine, The Catholic University of Korea, Seoul, Republic of Korea

S. Kim
Soma Yoga Movement Center, Seoul, Republic of Korea

J.-H. Chae, H.-Y. Lee (eds.), *Meditation in Psychiatry and General Medicine*, https://doi.org/10.1007/978-981-95-7147-5_9

joints or muscles. In contrast to movement triggered automatically by external influences, intentional active movement is an essential part of recognizing oneself as a subject, and this is further important to the development of self-consciousness. Carefully made intentional movements can contribute to reconstructing an individual's perception as a subject. As a result, it can contribute to exploring and changing various perceptions of self.

On the other hand, there are also techniques based on Somatics related to automatic movements that are not voluntarily controlled. When performing these techniques, one lets themselves be as they are and allows movement to happen. These movements sometimes appear to be similar to those of animals. In other cases, 'movement' is experienced purely as something internal, such as vividly felt warmth, vibration, or flow of energy. In the development process during infancy, involuntary movements precede voluntary ones. In other words, infants experience spontaneous movement before experiencing 'I am moving.' Various movements of Somatic techniques can contribute to reconstructing one's awareness of oneself as the subject by returning to the initial stage of learning to control voluntary muscle movements.

The types of movement that Somatics deals with include not only large movements, but also very fine and small movements, and even imagining movement as a purely internal image. Neurobiologically, actual movement and imagining movement as an internal image are achieved by nearly identical mechanisms.

In this context, all meditation techniques contain elements related to movement. Even in a static form of meditation such as sitting meditation, generally speaking minute movements constantly occur in accordance with the rhythm of breathing. However, what is emphasized in typical meditation practices is different from what is emphasized in Somatic techniques. While Somatic techniques are concerned with paying attention to the process of recognizing and controlling how one moves by clearly understanding the intention of movement, other forms of meditation techniques emphasize simply paying attention to observing the breath.

Embodied Cognition

Over the years, there has been a shift in cognitive neuroscience from a view of the mind as something abstract to a view of the mind as embodied cognition of the various senses that come from the body. The term 'embodied mind' was first coined by Francisco Varela, and he used this concept in contrast to that of the disembodied mind, or in other words a mind as existing with independent properties distinct from the body or the environment. Living organisms are autonomous beings that can actively create and maintain their own physical and psychological identity, and they embody what they perceive through movement and activity. From this point of view, humans exist as embodied subjects. As such, it is difficult to understand mental functions as sensation, cognition, and motivation when they are separated from the body and the environment.

Similarly, according to the 'grounded theory' of cognition, human cognition is not based merely on abstract computations, but on sensorimotor systems in the brain. This perspective has influenced developmental theory, psychoanalysis, and body-based psychotherapy, and it views the body's sensory system as playing a key role in the formation of self-consciousness. If the views of these schools of thought are taken together, they suggest that the experience of self is not simply limited to the activity of neurons in the brain, but is the result of a complex interaction between the body, brain, and environment. Additionally, the experience of self requires a smooth integration of various information about interoception, proprioception of motor sensation and touch, and space.

Observation of sensations in the body and sensory experiences has been considered to be important even in traditional forms of meditation, and many Somatics-based techniques consider this to be their most important element. Most Somatic techniques, such as Yoga, Qigong, Taichi, the Alexander Technique, and the Feldenkrais Method, explicitly emphasize focusing on interoceptive, proprioceptive, and sensorimotor experiences. These techniques utilize the concept of 'one's being as the body' and encourage an embodied experience of self.

A Contemplative Element

The dictionary definition of contemplation is to 'observe a particular object deeply and closely with sustained attention,' and the term is often used primarily in religious or spiritual contexts. The most important theoretical basis in research related to contemplative or meditative practice is neurophenomenology. Neurophenomenology refers to a scientific methodology that explores the 'explanatory gap' between the subjectivity of consciousness and neurobiological phenomena. In other words, neurophenomenology began with an attempt to connect the information obtained through a phenomenological report on the inner world from a first-person perspective in relation to an individual's subjective experience of consciousness with the brain's complex and dynamic activity system. The method of emphasizing the first-person point of view places value on increasing individual awareness of moment-to-moment experiences. Thus, this method provides subjective access to the subtle properties of experience before they are expressed in words or are passed onto thought. The first-person point of view that exists in many forms of contemplative practices and traditions helps to raise self-awareness in a systematic way. Although there are some differences in methods between Somatic techniques, many have systematic methods of training that help one pay attention to experience in a reflective way. Several Somatic techniques help one pay attention to the feedback of bodily sensations and proprioception that occur when performing certain movements or when breathing. Because the various types of movements used in Somatic techniques increase the intensity of various stimuli related to proprioception, it can be more effective than sitting meditation in cultivating awareness of the body and self.

Taken together, the contemplative elements present in various Somatic techniques can cultivate concentration and equanimity, which seems to help reconstruct self-identity. Recently however, some Somatics-based techniques have been used in ways unrelated to psychological factors, such as changing one's self-identity. For example, in the case of Hatha Yoga, there are cases where Somatic techniques are used, like physical therapy or exercise. In these cases, there has been debate as to whether Somatic techniques should be regarded as containing contemplative elements. Therefore, when using a Somatics-based technique in a specific situation, it is necessary to clarify which elements that constitute the technique are emphasized.

Somatics-Based Movement and Neurobiological Mechanisms

Cognitive Factors and Processes Associated with Movement

What has received particular attention in the field of studying cognitive factors related to movement is the methods of paying attention during the process where movement or motion arises.

Automatic Versus Intentionally Controlled Movements

Most movements are highly automated, often not requiring special attention. Even complex actions such as driving do not require externalized attention. Likewise, when one's attention is not focused, the mind wanders. On the other hand, when a specific movement occurs, the mind may switch back and forth between an automated mode and an intentionally controlled mode. For example, in traditional forms of sitting meditation, practitioners are instructed to turn their attention towards observation so that habitual (automated) mental reactions are stopped and new, more healthy reactions can be created. Therefore, in cultivating mindfulness, it is very important to switch back and forth between an automated mode and an intentionally controlled mode through paying attention. These elements are also very important when it comes to movement, and are necessary especially when learning new movement skills.

The shift from an automated mode to a controlled mode can occur in a variety of situations. For example, it may appear in a situation where you want to carefully correct a habitual movement, such as correcting your posture when swinging a golf club. In addition, when you discover something dangerous, you may also need to quickly modify and change your movements. In this case, a change in movement may occur without being conscious of it, only to become aware of it at a later time.

The Cognitive Model of Anticipating/Predicting Movement

The information processing model describes the process of behavioral change in detail. When we perform a certain movement, we anticipate changes in sensation caused by movement through a predictive model, and we consider the dynamics of that specific movement. Corollary discharge is also called efference copy, and this refers to a phenomenon in which a command signal is simultaneously transmitted from the upper center to the lower center as well as to the sensory system when movement occurs. This process contributes to the formation of an internal representation of the results of sensory signals predicted by movement based on one's memory and sensory information accumulated in relation to movement commands.

The visual or proprioceptive sensory information perceived in the process of movement is constantly compared to evaluate if it matches internal representations predicted moment by moment. This process determines whether a movement is actually being performed as intended. If the actually perceived sensory information is consistent with what was predicted, there is no need to pay further attention to the movement. This process maximizes the efficiency of attention and cognitive processing so that the central nervous system can pay attention only to unexpected stimuli without wasting metabolic energy. If there is a discrepancy between the expected sensory information and the sensory information that is actually perceived, an error signal is generated and a process for correcting the movement is initiated. Error signals catalyze a series of processes that cause muscle activity as well as joining direction and speed to be restructured. Additionally, it causes the sequence of movements itself to be reorganized in a top-down fashion.

Taken together, the motor learning model shows how much the process of movement can be automated or how much of a highly conscious task it is. The information processing model explains that we modify our movements in a more flexible way by looking at how much our expected experience differs from our actual experience. These error detection/alarm signals are a necessary part of survival and adaptation. The mechanism of error correction in these movements is mostly based on neurophysiological mechanisms related to the nucleus accumbens/noradrenaline and neuropsychological mechanisms related to working memory.

Movement and Neurophysiological Mechanisms: The Locus Coeruleus/Noradrenaline System

The noradrenaline system is involved in both the motorized and cognitive aspects of movement-related physiology. Movement is usually accompanied by changes in the autonomic nervous system, such as arterial blood pressure or volume, and the activity of the locus coeruleus / noradrenaline nervous system is sensitive to these cardiovascular changes. Additionally, when moving, the input of sensory signals related to touch increases, and these signals are fed back to the auditory nucleus. These input signals are caused by the stretching of skin over the muscle, the sensation of air or clothing on the skin, etc. As such, movement affects the activity of the locus coeruleus / noradrenaline nervous system through coordination of the cardiovascular system and sensory inputs.

Signals from nerve cell output from the locus coeruleus contribute to controlling the speed or efficiency of movement responses to target stimuli. The neuroanatomical and neuropsychological characteristics of the locus coeruleus nucleus are optimized to deliver signals by capturing unexpected changes well, and help one respond quickly to constantly changing environments. The aforementioned error detection signal serves as a key marker for unforeseen changes in the environment, which facilitates regulation of the locus coeruleus/noradrenaline system.

However, many of the detailed and accurate mechanisms for how the locus coeruleus system regulates movement have yet to be identified. On the other hand, judging by the studies so far, the locus coeruleus system is thought to be an important neural regulating factor in movement, and is thought to interact with other neurotransmitters such as dopamine.

Movement and Neuropsychological Mechanisms: Working Memory

The error correction process associated with movement requires temporary processing and storage of external information. A component of external memory, the episodic buffer, is involved in this process. Episodic buffers temporarily store and process expected information and actually observed information simultaneously, and sometimes also deal with multiple types of information related to internal representations retrieved from long-term memory.

Working memory and motor programming are closely related to each other. The increase in working memory is related to thc preparatory process of movement, especially cognitive regulation. Working memory is thought to play a key role when performing movements that require fine-tuned control of timing. Based on the results of several experiments showing that working memory increases in slow and fine-tuned movements rather than continuous and fast movements, it appears that slow movements typically used by Somatics likely require a large amount of working memory.

On the other hand, movements that require working memory and close attention can affect a mindlessly wandering state of mind. According to several experimental studies examining the relationship between working memory and the wandering state of mind, or in other words various forms of wandering thoughts, decreases when something new is being learned. However, once you learn something and become accustomed to it, the activation of your working memory has a diminishing effect on reducing distractions. For example, once you get used to driving, it becomes possible to drive even in a wandering state of mind. Based on this, it is thought that learning new movements with careful attention will reduce the wandering state of mind. In particular, the majority of Somatic movements based on an attitude of mindfulness can reduce the wandering state of mind by directing attention in a new way, even if the movements are already automated and familiar, such as walking or sitting. This is supported by the fact that as working memory increases, the activation of the default mode network, which is related to the wandering state of mind, decreases.

Examples of Somatic Techniques with Meditative Elements

Yoga

Yoga is estimated to have existed about 5000 years ago. As a Sanskrit term, yoga means 'to yoke a horse to a carriage' or 'to unite' or 'to connect.' The body and mind that move according to desire are likened to a rampaging horse and carriage. Just as a rampaging horse is tied to the carriage to be used freely by the owner, the mind and body that move according to sensory desire are controlled through ascetic practices. A more systemized form of yoga was recorded in Patañjali's classic work, the *Yoga Sutra* around the fifth century.

The goal of practicing yoga is the liberation of human beings, and Patañjali outlines eight limbs as the correct method to accomplish this, namely, moral restraint (*yama*), observances (*niyāma*), posture (*āsana*), control of breath (*prāṇāyāma*), withdrawal from senses (*pratyāhāra*), concentration (*dhāraṇā*), absorption (*dhyāna*), and enlightenment (*samādhi*). A rigorous system of practice including precepts, control of food, mind-body training, and sitting meditation has been passed down through the ages up to the present day. One of the most popular mind-body training methods is 'Hatha Yoga.'

Yoga is a practice that regulates and controls bodily sensations through three practices, namely posture (*āsana*), breathing, and sitting meditation, and it improves the power of self-awareness by paying deep attention to the inner senses by helping the body and mind be in a stable state through harmony of movement and breathing. Usually, practicing postures is a general form of practice, and it is very important to practice controlling the breath during this process.

In general, breathing methods that can be practice safely include, (1) how to briefly hold your breath while adjusting the length and speed of inhaling and exhaling, (2) how to alternate opening and closing the left and right nostrils and become aware of both breathing passages, and (3) breathing through the abdominal cavity and diaphragm, where one quickly and powerfully moves the thoracic cavity. As a technique that controls external light and sound, you can control your external senses and focus your attention solely on your inner self through yoga by repeating a mantra or gazing into candlelight. These yoga practices include elements such as sensory control, concentration, meditation, and absorption, and can ultimately help prepare an individual for sitting meditation.

In his book *Light on Yoga: Yoga Dipika,* B. K. S. Iyengar, a teacher of classic Hatha Yoga, introduced more than 200 postures and 15 techniques as practical ways to practice yoga. The book states that the purpose of practice is to stabilize the mind and body as well as functional movements of the musculoskeletal system, and to develop strong and solid physical strength. However, in order to incorporate the classic 'Hatha Yoga' postures from a more modern Somatics point of view, it is necessary to reconstruct and develop movements in an easier and more comfortable way.

In summary, the techniques of practicing yoga are aimed at purifying the body and controlling external stimuli in order to awaken one's inner senses. This process helps one accept the 'self' that is aware of emotions and thoughts, such as being overly distressed or happy, in a stable and balanced manner and helps one experience psychological distance from this self. This process has elements that are shared with mindfulness meditation, which aims to be aware of, decentralize, and distance oneself from one's senses.

The Feldenkrais Method

The Feldenkrais method was created by renowned physicist and Judo master Moshe Feldenkrais. A strong and athletic individual, Feldenkrais went into exile in England before the Nazis invaded Paris in 1940 and had to find work to earn a living. This environment aggravated a knee injury he sustained while playing soccer in his youth. After hearing the opinion of a doctor that he would not be able to completely recover from his knee injuries even with surgery, he read books on neuroscience, having become primarily interested in the relationship between the brain and the nervous system, and he developed the Feldenkrais method based on the process of working and exploring problems with his own pain.

There are two methods of teaching in the Feldenkrais method: Awareness Through Movement (ATM) and Functional Integration (FI). ATM is a group class that guides movements solely through language, and FI is a private class with a hands-on method. Overall, it can be said that both are processes of learning self-awareness with the help of a teacher rather than being a form of treatment.

Feldenkrais recognized the system and connectivity of the body under the premise that 'no body part can move without affecting other parts,' and this is a method of learning that pursues organic and functional integration. The more than 1000 movements are based on learning conditions such as (1) moving slowly and small within an easy and comfortable range, (2) being curious and paying attention to your movements, (3) and being carefully and clearly aware of your movements. Through this process, one's quality of movement improves when one becomes aware of one's inner senses through the coordination of nerves and relaxation of muscle tension through movement. In this way, the process of exploring movement that awakens one's bodily senses leads to the experience of getting to know oneself. Feldenkrais believed that bodily experiences had a mental component, and emphasized changes through neural plasticity of the brain through learning.

The training of the body and mind and meditative experience of the East through Judo can be found in Feldenkrais' books containing his teachings and philosophy as well as in guides on ATM. ATM guides one to perform simple and easy movements that anyone can do as effortlessly as possible. Additionally, unlike other methods, the Feldenkrais method does not suggest breathing specifically according to one's movement. It says to just try and be clearly aware of when you inhale or exhale. It says to pay attention to your current sense of what you are doing and how you are doing it, and to explore your own path of movement rather than following or copying the movements of others or authority figures.

However, despite these guidelines, as soon as most people start a movement, they try to do it better or work harder. They move and breathe by creating tension in or contracting muscles that are not actually needed for a specific movement. Rather than paying attention to the sensations of the body they are using, people are distracted by improving the strength and speed of their movements, sometimes resulting in pain. As the process of repeating movements more comfortably and easily gradually accumulates, involuntary and unconscious muscle tension and contraction decrease, and you will be able to be aware of your own thoughts and emotions that arise. Through this learning process, we come to realize that this is a movement and life pattern that is familiar to us.

The Feldenkrais method aims to enhance self-awareness through movement, which also leads to the experience of being aware of one's 'self' through one's development and exploration. Through learning to repeat the same movements, one understands the possibilities and limitations of the movements one can do oneself, and in this process, one's judgment and evaluation of a standard of right or wrong movement, good or bad movement disappears. By being aware of one's bodily sensations felt here and now, the Feldenkrais method suggests a way to realize oneself through the process of exploring one's own thoughts and emotions.

The Alexander Technique

The Alexander Technique was created by Australian actor Frederick Matthias Alexander. As someone who stood on stage as an actor reciting plays, Matthias suffered from a problem with his vocalization. He began to receive hospital treatment, but medical methods could not find the root cause. Not seeing much improvement, he began the process of closely observing himself to solve his vocalization problem. While observing his posture and reciting habits on stage in front of a mirror and experimenting with them, he discovered that his posture when on stage was different from that in his everyday life. He learned that he had a habit of tilting his head back every time he recited, and this caused the larynx to be pressed down and his spine to bend, leading to problems with breathing and vocalization. Once he found the cause of the problem in his posture and habits, he made up his mind that he himself could make changes. At the end of that process, he was able to treat his voice. Since then, numerous cases of treatment have become known, and eventually his method was established as the Alexander Technique.

The Alexander Technique can be seen as having begun with awareness of how to use one's own body, that is, the insight that Matthias was using his throat, larynx, vocal cords, and respiratory system incorrectly through continuous observation of his posture and habits. As for the teaching method, one-on-one or group classes including hands-on instruction from the teacher are conducted, and there are various techniques dedicated to fine-tuned awareness of daily postures such as sitting, standing, and walking. Although it originated in the process of Matthais treating himself through recognizing his posture and habit, the Alexander Technique is not simply a way to teach correct posture and movement or to treat pain. The Alexander Technique embodies the process of self-awareness and through this it retrains the body and mind so that they can be used effectively. Although this series of processes can be regarded as educating oneself on one's posture and how to use one's body, it is impossible for an individual person to solely use the body in the process of changing one's posture and habits formed throughout one's entire life.

A key element of the Alexander Technique is consciously using the self by embodying the connectedness of the whole body through the use of carefully segmented body parts. Among its core elements, the three elements of 'self-control,' 'non-doing,' and 'non-judgment' are the most important in understanding and learning the Alexander Technique. 'Self-control' refers to the ability to control one's own unconscious behaviors and nervous reactions by stopping habitual reactions, unconscious reactions, and fixed patterns. Our habit of judging right or wrong affects not only our body posture but also our thoughts and relationships in general. Here, 'non-judgment' refers to the ability to stop judging our habits and reactions. 'Non-doing' refers to not doing something that has been done in the past with familiar and learned behaviors and thoughts. Through this, we are able to set aside unnecessary inner tension and effort.

An element of the Alexander Technique is to learn conscious control by observing one's posture and habits and pausing before performing any action or movement. It helps one use and explore the self in one's use of their body. Here, self refers to not only the body, but also one's whole being, including its mental, emotional, and spiritual aspects. In this way, the Alexander Technique can be seen as similar to the awareness, concentration, cultivation of equanimity, and self-inquiry of meditation not only in its main elements, but also in its concept of the self and what it is aimed at in the process of learning the technique.

Application of Somatics-Based Techniques in Psychiatric Clinical Practice

Various techniques based on Somatics contain elements of 'enhancing one's awareness of the body' and 'distancing oneself.' These are the most essential aspects of mindfulness-based meditation, which is already widely used in clinical practice. From this point of view, Somatics-based techniques can be seen as a kind of 'movement based on an attitude of mindfulness.'

Although mindfulness-based meditation methods are well known to be effective in many areas of mental health, including preventing the recurrence of depression, it is still difficult to apply these methods to patients with relatively severe mental illnesses. The traditional form of sitting meditation requires observing and becoming aware of thoughts and bodily sensations that emerge as they are, but this is not an easy task for patients who suffer from negative thoughts and uncomfortable bodily sensations most of the time. They are sometimes overwhelmed by negative thoughts and sensations after practicing sitting meditation. However, a life with a mindful attitude that allows one to stay in the present moment without judgment is a necessary component for the recovery of patients with severe mental illnesses. The various Somatics-based techniques can be an alternative way for these patients to learn mindfulness. Considering that Somatics-based techniques require a considerable amount of working memory and have the effect of reducing the activation of the default network accordingly, we are hopeful that they can be of considerable help to patients with mental illnesses related to a dysfunctional default mode network. Accordingly, we expect that the wandering state of mind and the pain caused by excessive ruminatory reactions can be alleviated.

As such, several Somatics-based techniques have the potential to be used in psychiatric clinical practice. However, they should be reconstructed in a way that is more suitable for patients, and to do this, the following points should be considered.

First, when taking into consideration the characteristics of patients who have a very low tolerance for pain or uncomfortable sensations, it is necessary to reorganize these techniques into easier and more comfortable movements. For example, muscle strength and flexibility are required to attempt specific yoga postures, but patients may not have the ability to recognize and control pain or uncomfortable sensations, which will diminish the technique's therapeutic effects.

Second, how the techniques are guided may be more important than the movements themselves. More non-directive and friendly guidance is needed. Although the Feldenkrais Method and the Alexander Technique teach us to not make judgments about what is right or wrong due to the nature of learning these techniques, this aspect should be emphasized even more in the treatment of patients. In particular, one should also avoid quickly attempting to correct a patient's movements for the sake of cultivating a mindful attitude. In addition, non-directive guidance is an essential element for one to accept one's own experience through movement and to select and adjust one's behavior based on this, which can serve as a basis for recovery.

Third, it is necessary to have a more prudent and cautious attitude with regard to the use of hands-on teaching methods commonly used in Somatic techniques. The hands-on teaching method used in the Alexander Technique and the Feldenkrais Method is one in which the instructor places their hand on the participant's body to help them become aware of it. However, in the case of patients whose ego is not strong enough or who have experienced trauma where the boundaries of their body have been violated, there needs to be much more care in the use of hands-on methods.

Finally, there should be continued efforts to verify the effects and mechanisms of various Somatics-based techniques. Due to the nature of many of these techniques, it is difficult to design a double-blind randomized control, and the relative lack of programs based on standardized protocols can be pointed out as a methodological weakness of effect validation studies. In the future, more quality studies should be conducted to supplement these methodological blind spots.

Conclusion

In recent years, cognitive science has shifted away from the view that the mind is a separate entity from the body to the view that various functions of the mind are inseparably related to the body and its surrounding environment. In accordance with this trend, various Somatic techniques that deal with body work or movement emphasizing sensory experience from a first-person point of view are receiving attention. The various Somatic techniques enhance awareness of bodily sensations, called interoceptive senses, through moving the body, and connect them with one's own thoughts and emotions, helping one see them at a distance. In this respect, Somatic techniques can be seen as a kind of 'movement based on an attitude of mindfulness.' Somatic techniques have the potential to teach mindful attitudes in a more accessible way to patients with severe mental illnesses who have difficulty accessing traditional forms of meditation. In order to be used clinically, Somatic techniques need to be reconstructed according to the characteristics of the patient while taking advantage of their benefits. Based on this, research should be continued on their clinical effects and mechanisms.

Bibliography

Alexander FM. The use of the self. London: Orion Books; 2001.

Brown R. Authorized summaries of F. M. Alexander's Four Books. London: French Connection Press; 1992.

Doidge N. Brain's way of healing. New York: Penguin Group; 2016.

Emerson D. Trauma-sensitive yoga in therapy: bringing the body into treatment. New York: W.W. Norton & Company; 2015.

Feldenkrais M. Awareness through movement: easy-to-do health exercises to improve your posture, vision, imagination. New York: Harper Collins; 1991.

Hanna T. The body of life. New York: Alfred A. Knopf; 1979.

Iyengar BKS. Light on yoga. New York: Schocken Books; 1966.

Jung T-h. Yoga Sutra (요가수트라). Seoul: Tongmunson; 2000.

Russell TA, Arcuri SM. A neurophysiological and neuropsychological consideration of mindful movement: clinical and research implications. Front Hum Neurosci. 2015;9:282. https://doi.org/10.3389/fnhum.2015.00282.

Schmalzl L, Crane-Godreau MA, Payne P. Movement-based embodied contemplative practices: definitions and paradigms. Front Hum Neurosci. 2014;8:205. https://doi.org/10.3389/fnhum.2014.00205.

Traditional Korean (Joseon) Meditation and Taoism

10

Jungkeun Oh

Traditional Korean (Joseon) meditation refers to Korean meditation practices that are said to have originated in the Dangun period (~2333 BC), the Gojoseon period (2333–108 BC), or even earlier. This term is limited to those methods derived in Korea outside foreign religions such as Confucianism and Buddhism. On the other hand, Taoist meditation refers to the methods of meditation practiced in Taoism, which combines Chinese folk beliefs and Taoist ideas of Lao-tzu and Chuang-tzu.

Traditional Korean meditation and Taoist meditation share many aspects, and they speak of similar principles in similar terms. In both methods of meditation, the practitioner meditates while deliberately controlling their breathing. Both methods speak of the lower abdomen (Danjeon), qi (氣), and the three energies (Jing qi shen, 精氣神). Of course, traditional Korean meditation and Taoist meditation have differences in their specific theory and methods, and can be discussed separately from each other. However, in this chapter, we will limit our discussion to the common characteristics of traditional Korean meditation and Taoist meditation.

We can infer that the reason traditional Korean meditation and Taoist meditation have similar aspects is that both practices have the same roots. However, since this book is on medicine, we will omit historical discussions about which practice preceded the other or whether they were developed independently. Instead, we will focus on the practical application of these methods of meditation. In addition, since this book is about the practical field of study in medicine, rather than having a philosophical discussion, I will write in detail about what methods these practices used.

The method of meditation that has been studied the most in the past and is currently the most actively studied is mindfulness meditation, which entered the realm of medicine and science through Jon Kabat-Zinn. Mindfulness is a translation of the Pali word ‘sati,’ which is said to have been used by the Buddha (Siddartha Gautama). This seems to indicate that mindfulness is rooted in Buddhism, especially in Early Buddhist meditation. Although Jon Kabat-Zinn did not exclusively study and experience Early Buddhism, since he named his program Mindfulness-Based Stress Reduction (MBSR), it can be said that the technique of mindfulness (sati) meditation taught directly by the Buddha was taken as the most important element in MBSR.

Since mindfulness meditation is the most familiar method to scientists, at the beginning of this chapter, I will broadly cover the topic of how mindfulness meditation differs from traditional Korean or Taoist meditation (hereinafter referred to as Korean-Taoist meditation).

J. Oh (✉)
Warm Psychiatry Clinic, Sejong, Republic of Korea

J.-H. Chae, H.-Y. Lee (eds.), *Meditation in Psychiatry and General Medicine*,
https://doi.org/10.1007/978-981-95-7147-5_10

The Difference Between Korean-Taoist Meditation and Mindfulness Meditation

Mindfulness entails being present fully here and now, and paying attention uncritically and intentionally. The flow of mindfulness meditation can be briefly schematized as follows.

1. The practitioner chooses an object and turns their attention towards it. This object can be a raisin, a sound that they hear, the breath they take, or a part or all of their body. It can also be their thoughts, emotions, or their own mind. (In Early Buddhism, mindfulness of breathing was particularly emphasized as a basis for meditation).
2. When one focuses the mind on a single object, other thoughts or feelings almost inevitably arise. The practitioner notices that these thoughts or emotions have arisen, lets them go, and returns their attention to the object they were originally focusing on.
3. This process is repeated indefinitely whenever a thought or emotion arises.

By doing this, the practitioner practices turning their full attention to the present. Of course, mindfulness meditation is not merely focused attention on a single object but rather open monitoring. However, to simplify its schematization, I have excluded the technique of open monitoring.

Mindfulness meditation considers the practice of paying attention to the breath and being present (ānāpānasati) to be important. When practicing this method of meditation, it is accompanied by a guiding mental remark, 'Do not try to control your breath. Simply observe it.' Mindfulness meditation encourages the practitioner to not deliberately control their breathing.

Here we can see the biggest difference between Korean-Taoist meditation and mindfulness meditation, where the former recommends that the practitioner deliberately control their breathing during meditation. In Korean-Taoist meditation, deliberately controlling one's breath in an even manner is called 'Jo-sik,' and is an important concept for this practice.

It can be said that Korean-Taoist meditation has had many different schools throughout the long history of Korea and China. When we consider the practices of these schools, taking deliberate, slow, regular, and deep breaths is central to Jo-sik. (Of course, while practitioners deliberately control their breath in traditional Korean meditation, it is not done outside the boundaries of what is natural).

From the point of view of Early Buddhist meditation, in some ways, traditional Korean meditation is closer to walking meditation than sitting meditation. In early Buddhism, if sitting meditation is commonly known as paying attention to one's breath while being seated, walking meditation is a practice that is done while walking. The basic idea of walking meditation is to pay attention to the changing sensations of the feet while one 'performs the action of walking.' In this sense, because traditional Korean meditation is the practice of paying attention to the abdomen where breathing takes place while 'performing the act of breathing,' it is closer to walking meditation, where one meditates while performing the action of walking. Since meditation in yoga also involves controlling the breath, it can also be said that Korean-Taoist meditation is similar to yogic meditation.

Table 10.1 shows the differences between mindfulness meditation and Korean-Taoist medi-

Table 10.1 Mindfulness meditation and Korean-Taoist meditation

	Mindfulness meditation	Korean-Taoist meditation
Status of controlling breathing	Not controlling breathing and just observing it	Control of breathing (Jo-sik)
Area of attention	Paying attention to the nose or abdomen	Paying attention to the lower abdomen (Danjeon)
Religions or philosophical orientation	Ceasing reincarnation (bodily health is not the primary concern)	Longevity without aging (bodily health is important. The belief that one had better cultivate the body to become enlightened)

tation. At a glance, it appears that mindfulness meditation uses the mind more, whereas Korean-Taoist meditation uses the body more. Compared to other methods of meditation, Korean-Taoist meditation recognizes the worldly desire to live a long and healthy life. Since most people do not live their lives while seeking to transcend their desire to live a long and healthy life, Korean-Taoist meditation has aspects that can be motivating to many people. If the reason why medicine exists is to enable people to live long and healthy lives, it can be said that Korean-Taoist meditation is more closely related to medicine.

Korean-Taoist meditation is not without elements of mindfulness. Although it is a meditation practice where one deliberately controls their breathing, Korean-Taoist meditation recommends that the practitioner turn their full attention to the breath itself (and eventually be mindful of the act of breathing). Only then is one properly practicing breathing meditation. Korean-Taoist meditation shares the same approach to Early Buddhist meditation regarding mindfulness while walking. In walking meditation, one performs the 'act' of walking, but does so while paying full attention to the feeling of their feet.

However, mindfulness meditation more strongly applies detailed techniques to be mindful overall from beginning to end. Since sitting meditation in mindfulness meditation involves solely being mindful, it can be said that cultivating the skill of mindfulness itself is strong in mindfulness-based sitting meditation.

Since the religious and philosophical background of mindfulness meditation is aimed at liberation from suffering and desire (Nirvana), training the mind is important and interest in the body itself is relatively small (of course, its religious background is excluded as much as possible in modern mindfulness meditation reinterpreted by the West).

The body is relatively important to Korean-Taoist meditation, which takes the position that the body must be healthy in order for one to be able to practice effectively. Furthermore, Korean-Taoist meditation does not separate the health of the body from that of the mind. Rather, the health of the body and mind is pursued at the same time.

The Relationship Between Relaxation and Breathing

Meditation does not seek any particular state. However, regardless of what type of meditation you practice, as your practice deepens, you consequently experience relaxation. Although meditation is not aimed at relaxation, it comes as a result of meditation.

Patients who come to the Department of Psychiatry often complain of the pain of stress and tension and want to be relaxed. Psychiatrists apply a number of techniques that have a relaxing effect, even incidentally, to patients. Here, meditation and the attitude of acceptance can be used as a way to promote relaxation.

On the other hand, it is easier to meditate when one is in a comfortable and relaxed state than in a stressful situation where one has many miscellaneous thoughts. Meditation results in relaxation, and relaxation helps meditation.

Then how do relaxation and breathing affect each other?

Lower Abdominal (Danjeon) Breathing in Korean-Taoist Meditation

The lower abdomen (danjeon) is a place where energy (qi) gathers. It refers to an imaginary point 5 cm deep located approximately 5 cm below the navel. In other words, it can be said that it is the area of the lower belly. Thus, as a form of breathing through the lower belly, Danjeon breathing can be said to be a special form of lower abdominal breathing.

Lower abdominal breathing, especially regular, deep, and slow abdominal breathing, stabilizes the mind. It causes the parasympathetic nervous system to be dominant, making the mind calm and comfortable while reducing anxiety and tension. Deep, regular abdominal breathing has the effect of causing the vagus nerve (one of the parasympathetic nerves) to become dominant. When a parasympathetic nerve is dominant, we become relaxed. The comfortable and relaxed state achieved by controlling your breathing in this way helps you to easily enter a meditative state. And if you focus your attention on the movement of the lower abdomen while breathing, it produces the same effect as meditating while being mindful of the abdomen.

Mindfulness Meditation

Mindfulness meditation teaches one to focus their mind on their breath, but not to deliberately control it. When practicing mindfulness meditation on the breath, the object of mindfulness can be anywhere within a whole breath, such as the tip of the nose or the abdomen. Here, the practitioner keeps their mind in one place. The practitioner keeps their attention in one place, and if they have a wandering thought, they look at it, let it go, and then return to the place where they had focused their attention.

If one continues to meditate in this way, one will get out of one's own thoughts and the mind will feel at ease. And when the mind is at ease, the body also relaxes. The fact that the body is relaxed means that the parasympathetic nerve has become dominant, which results in breathing becoming deep and slow. Although you do not deliberately control your breath, it naturally deepens and slows down.

Mindfulness meditation seems to determine that controlling the breath creates an 'intention towards doing something,' which hinders deep relaxation. Meditation can also be said to be a form of deep relaxation, and in mindfulness meditation, even the effort to control the breath is seen as a factor that gets in the way of relaxation. Therefore, it encourages the practitioner to let go of even this effort.

In that case, which comes first, relaxation or breathing? It is difficult to conclude which method is superior when it comes to the matter of which method to choose and whether one should achieve relaxation through controlling one's breath or reach a state of relaxation and calm the breath naturally. This may vary from person to person, so I think it should basically depend on individual preference. Even for the same person, sometimes Early Buddhist mindfulness meditation can be more helpful, and other times Korean-Taoist meditation can be more helpful.

Various Methods of Korean-Taoist Meditation

Since one deliberately controls one's breathing when practicing Korean-Taoist meditation, how one breathes becomes an important topic. There are as many methods of Korean-Taoist meditation as there are ways to breathe.

There are a variety of breathing methods and each school asserts its own rules for breathing. Of course, rules asserted by one side are often contradicted by rules asserted by another side. For example, in a school of Kuksundo, one of the traditional Korean meditation methods, the practitioner practices breathing in for 5 s and breathing out for 5 s in the beginning, and as they progress, they practice breathing in and stopping, then breathing out and stopping. When holding their breath, they do not forcefully do it unnaturally, but as their body and mind adapts, the time between breathing in and out and between breathing out and in naturally increases. As the body and mind develops further, inhalation becomes shorter and the pause between inhalation and exhalation increases, exhalation becomes shorter and the pause between exhalation and inhalation decreases, and the time spent after breathing in gradually becomes longer.

Meanwhile, Bongwoo Kwon Tae-hoon's Danhak practice uses a method of gradually increasing the length of breathing. This practice recommends that the practitioner make breathing in and out thin and long in a 1:1 ratio. Additionally, it does not recommend holding one's breath. At first, the practitioner starts by breathing in for 2 s and out for 2 s, then in for 3 s and out for 3 s, and in for 4 s and out for 4 s. When the practitioner is completely used to their current length of breathing, they increase it by 1 s. In this way, the practitioner continuously increases their in- and out-breath by 1 s. (Bong-woo Kwon Tae-hoon says that he increased the length of his breath by breathing in and out for 2 min each.) Other schools simply teach breathing deeply and in a regulated manner through the lower abdomen, and do not consider the specific length of the breath to be important.

On the other hand, according to the Taoist book *Baopuzi*, the period where the breath is stopped in the middle is longer. A translation of the *Baopuzi* reads as follows: Inhale deeply through your nose, hold your breath, and silently count to 120 in your mind. Then exhale quietly from your mouth. Whenever you inhale or exhale, make it so that the sound of breath is not heard by your own ears...(ellipsis)... As you become accustomed to this exercise, the count in your mind will gradually reach one thousand.

When it comes to breathing, it is difficult to say that one method is more correct than another. Each breathing method has its own reasons. Since the makeup of each person's body is different, one should choose the breathing method that best suits them. If it is uncomfortable to meditate while deliberately controlling your breath, it is also ok to practice Early Buddhist mindfulness meditation without controlling your breathing.

Since the methods of breathing are as diverse as the tradition is old, it is not easy to conclude what they all have in common. While there would be exceptions, if we look for the common characteristics of breathing methods adopted in the traditional Korean and Taoist meditation methods, they are as follows:

1. When breathing, only pay attention to the act of breathing itself.
2. Breathe in a deep, regulated, and slow manner.
3. Breathe while paying attention to the lower abdomen.

Research on Meditation Methods That Control Breathing

Korean-Taoist meditation is a representative method of meditation that involves controlling one's breathing. The following are the results of some studies conducted in the scientific field on meditation that involves controlling one's breathing:

- Training to breathe relaxed, deeply, and slowly increases awareness of cold or hot stimuli, and increases the threshold of feeling pain from these stimuli. Additionally, this training reduces negative emotions.
- The learning and retention of motor skills involves complex neuroanatomical structures. These structures are the dorsolateral prefrontal cortex, the posterior parietal cortex, the primary motor cortex, the basal ganglia, and the cerebellum. However, when one voluntarily changes the pattern and length of their breathing, the same parts of the brain are modulated.
- Qigong teaches breathing long, slow, and deep all the way down to the lower abdomen. Practicing Qigong reduces stress and anxiety in healthy adults.
- Breathing exercises reduce symptoms of stress, anxiety, insomnia, post-traumatic stress disorder (PTSD), depression, and attention deficit hyperactivity disorder (ADHD).
- Patients with inflammatory bowel disease who receive mind-body interventions that emphasize voluntarily regulated breathing practices have shown significant gains in inflammatory bowel disease symptoms, anxiety, depression, and quality of life.

Conclusion

Meditation can be divided into two main categories.

1. Meditation that does not deliberately control breathing: meditation that induces relaxation through the mind and consequently stabilizes breathing (the body). Meditation that uses the mind more (e.g., mindfulness meditation, etc.)
2. Meditation that helps one relax by deliberately controlling one's breathing: meditation that relaxes the mind by regulating the body. Meditation that uses both the mind and body (e.g., traditional Korean meditation, Taoist meditation, yoga, etc.)

Korean-Taoist meditation recommends one breathe voluntarily during practice, and they have a concept of qi and the lower abdomen (Danjeon). These practices use the body more and place more importance on bodily health.

The definition of meditation is diverse, and there are also a variety of specific methods. All methods of meditation can be said to have some aspect of mindfulness, but each method of practice is different from the specific practice of mindfulness meditation. Therefore, when using meditation to benefit mental health, it is necessary to consider various meditation methods without limits. It is important to find a method of meditation that works for the individual and to practice it consistently.

Bibliography

Korean Sources

Gal H. Pobakja (포박자). Seoul: Freedom Publishing; 2014.

Heo GM. Kuksundo Ganghae (국선도강해). Seoul: Bright Culture Media; 2017.

Kim WS. Science meditation (과학명상). Seoul: Communication Books; 2016.

Korean Institute of Religion and Culture Research. Introduction to world religions (세계종교사입문). Seoul: Cheongnyeonsa; 2003.

Mo JG. History of Chinese Taoists—stories of people who dreamed of miraculous powers (중국 도교사-신선을 꿈꾼 사람들의 이야기). Seoul: Yaemoon Seowon; 2015.

Oh J. A study on meditation, breathing, and relaxation (명상법, 호흡법, 이완법에 관한 고찰). J Gongju Natl Hosp (국립공주병원 임상연구 논문집). 2014:23–41.

Yi YJ. Tao, the power of imagination (도, 상상하는 힘). Seoul: Yihaksa; 2003.

English Sources

Brown RP, Gerbarg PL, Muench F. Breathing practices for treatment of psychiatric and stress-related medical conditions. Psychiatr Clin. 2013;36(1):121–40.

Busch V, Magerl W, Kern U, Haas J, Hajak G, Eichhammer P. The effect of deep and slow breathing on pain perception, autonomic activity, and mood processing—an experimental study. Pain Med. 2012;13(2):215–28.

Colebatch JG, Adams L, Murphy K, Martin AJ, Lammertsma AA, Tochon-Danguy HJ, Clark JC, Friston KJ, Guz A. Regional cerebral blood flow during volitional breathing in man. J Physiol. 1991;443:91–103.

Deadman P. The transformative power of deep, slow breathing. J Chin Med. 2018;116:62–8.

Floyer-Lea A, Matthews PM. Distinguishable brain activation networks for short- and long-term motor skill learning. J Neurophysiol. 2005;94:512–8.

Gerbarg PL, Jacob VE, Stevens L, Bosworth BP, Chabouni F, DeFilippis EM, Warren R, Trivellas F, Patel PV, Webb CD, Garbus MD, Christos PJ, Brown RP, Scherl EJ. The effect of breathing, movement, and meditation on psychological and physical symptoms and inflammatory biomarkers in inflammatory bowel disease: a randomized controlled trial. Inflamm Bowel Dis. 2015;21:2886–96.

Halsband U, Lange RK. Motor learning in man: a review of functional and clinical studies. J Physiol-Paris. 2006;99(4-6):414–24.

Iyengar BKS. 요가 디피카. 서울: 도서출판 선요가; 2014.

Kabat-Zinn J. 마음챙김 명상과 자기 치유. 서울: 학지사; 2017.

Kastrup A, Li TQ, Glover GH, Moseley ME. Cerebral blood flow-related signal changes during breath-holding. Am J Neuroradiol. 1999;20(7):1233–8.

McKay LC, Evans KC, Frackowiak RSJ, Corfield DR. Neural correlates of voluntary breathing in humans. J Appl Physiol. 2003;95:1170–8.

Wang CW, Chan CHY, Ho RTH, Chan JSM, Ng SM, Chan CLW. Managing stress and anxiety through qigong exercise in healthy adults: a systematic review and meta-analysis of randomized controlled trials. BMC Complement Alternat Med. 2014;14:8.

Yadav G, Mutha P. Deep breathing practice facilitates retention of newly learned motor skills. Sci Rep. 2016;6:1–8.

Buddhism and Meditation

11

Hyunsoo Jeon

To understand the relationship between Buddhism and meditation, we must first understand what Buddhism is. First, let us look at the meaning of the word Buddhism. The Korean word for Buddhism, 'Bulgyo,' comes from the Chinese word fó (佛, KR: Bul), which is a transliteration of the ancient Indian Pāli word Buddha, and the Chinese word jiào (教, KR: Gyo), which means teaching. In other words, Buddhism refers to the teachings of the enlightened. Buddhism is what a man named Gotama Siddhārtha, born in India about 2600 years ago, taught people after he became a Buddha through practicing meditation. The Buddha sought to answer all of the questions that humans could have, including who he was, how the world was composed and by what principles it moves. After much effort, he found the answer. To know what kind of being one is, one needs to know what the body and mind that make up oneself are. The Buddha used a method of observation to understand these things. And he directly saw them as they actually are. When looking at the Pāli scriptures (Nikāyas), which record what the Buddha said, there are many instances of the expression 'knowing and seeing.' This is seeing clearly by creating a state where one can see without trying to think or reason. Herein lies the relationship between Buddhism and meditation. Meditation is concentrating on what is happening in the present moment with a wholesome mind. The object of meditation may differ depending on the type of practice, but the essence of meditation is observing the object as it is. In this respect, meditation is fundamental to Buddhism. Through meditation, the Buddha understood the properties of the body and mind as well as the principles by which the world moves. After the Buddha's death, as time passed, Buddhism spread to various regions and also became very diverse. Broadly speaking, there is Early Buddhism, Mahayāna Buddhism, and Tibetan Buddhism. In this chapter, I will discuss Buddhism from the position of Early Buddhism.

H. Jeon (✉)
Dr. Hyunsoo Jeon's Psychiatry Clinic,
Seoul, South Korea

Buddhist Meditation

Meditation is practiced in various ways according to various religions and cultural traditions. Here, I will discuss Buddhist meditation. It can be said that there are two main types of Buddhist meditation. There is the macroscopic observation of mindfulness meditation and the microscopic observation of Samatha and Vipassanā meditation. Macroscopic observation consists of closely observing moment to moment what is happening in the body and mind as it is with our sense organs of the eye, ear, nose, tongue, body, and consciousness. While walking, one observes what phenomena arise as one walks, and while eating one observes what phenomena arise when eating. When one is angry, one is aware that they have

J.-H. Chae, H.-Y. Lee (eds.), *Meditation in Psychiatry and General Medicine*,
https://doi.org/10.1007/978-981-95-7147-5_11

become angry. This is the macroscopic observation of mindfulness meditation.

On the other hand, the microscopic observation of Samatha and Vipassanā meditation observes what cannot be seen by macroscopic observation. The eye, ear, nose, tongue, body, and consciousness are limited in their ability to observe objects and therefore cannot observe minute phenomena. It is like the naked eye, which can see the hand but not the cells that make up the hand. To see the cells, you need to use a microscope. Similarly, to see the ultimate materiality or mentality that constitutes the body and mind, instead of observing objects with the eye, ear, nose, tongue, mouth, or consciousness, which are limited in their ability to see these ultimate realities, you need tools that are able to see ultimate materiality or mentality. The tool is the eye of wisdom obtained through samādhi (concentration). Here, samādhi is a state where the mind is fully focused on a single object through the practice of gathering the mind. The normal mind focuses on one object and then quickly moves onto another. It flies back and forth from object to object very quickly. Through the practice of developing samādhi, one continuously practices training the mind that has gone away from the object of meditation to another object to let go of that object and return to the original object of meditation. When one practices this consistently enough for the mind to attain samādhi, the mind becomes focused solely on one object. It does not go to another object even for a brief moment and instead remains completely fixated on that one object. This state is samādhi. Here, there are no defilements in the mind.

When one attains samādhi, one develops the eye of wisdom, and through this eye one can see things that they could not see with the naked eye. Through the eye of wisdom one can see ultimate materiality and mentality. The way to attain samādhi is Samatha meditation. Seeing the properties of ultimate materiality and mentality through the eye of wisdom that is developed by attaining samādhi through Samatha meditation is Vipassanā. The properties of materiality and mentality are 'impermanent' (Pāli: anicca), 'unsatisfactory' (Pāli: dukkha), and 'nonself' (Pāli: anattā). Impermanence means that ultimate materiality and mentality arise and disappear at a very rapid rate according to the laws of cause and effect. Unsatisfactory refers to the fact that ultimate materiality and mentality arises and disappears regardless of our will. Nonself means that we have no control over the arising and disappearing of ultimate materiality and mentality.

Although we can also know ourselves through the macroscopic observation of mindfulness, we cannot know exactly what kind of beings we are through that alone. Only when we go all the way to making microscopic observations can we know exactly what kind of beings we are. And then we can live in accordance with our existence. Buddhist meditation is practiced so that we can know who exactly we are and to live our lives accordingly, thereby not doing things that are harmful to us and instead doing things that are helpful to us. Now, we will take a closer look at the macroscopic observation of mindfulness meditation and the microscopic observation of Samatha and Vipassanā meditation. First, we will look at the macroscopic observation of mindfulness meditation.

Macroscopic Observation: Mindfulness Meditation

There are two types of macroscopic observations of mindfulness meditation. There are the structured practices of sitting and walking meditation, and the unstructured practices of observing daily activities (daily life meditation). Each method of meditation has its advantages. Sitting meditation consists of observing the phenomena that occur in the body and mind when sitting still, and here one usually observes the breath. One usually observes the breath coming in and out from the tip of the nose or through the expansion and contraction of the abdomen. When observing, one can even attach labels to the phenomena if necessary. For example, one can use the label 'rising' when the abdomen expands, and 'falling' when the abdomen contracts. Attaching labels is done to facilitate observation. If one attaches labels, one's consciousness can more easily go to the object of observation. Then, as one's power of observation becomes stronger and attaching labels becomes burdensome and interferes with observation, they can be omitted. When practicing sitting meditation, one can observe other objects aside from the breath such as the feeling of the body. The advantage of sitting meditation is that one's observation can become strong since one observes while sitting still. Meanwhile, the mind can become still. When the mind is still, one can observe the phenomena that occur in the body and mind well. In particular, one can observe subtle mental phenomena such as emotions, thoughts, and intentions well. Mental phenomena arise and disappear quickly, making them difficult to observe.

Since we observe the phenomena that arise while walking when we practice walking meditation, we are able to clearly know what happens when we are actually walking. We usually do not clearly know what happens in the body and mind when we walk because we are usually thinking of something or looking at something else. When we see the phenomena that arise when we are walking through walking meditation, they are different from what we think they are. We may think that we walk by simply moving our feet and legs. However, when we actually observe the process of walking, we see that it consists of three stages, namely lifting the foot, moving it forward, and lowering it. And if we look at each of these three stages, we see that there is an intention that triggers these actions. Without intention these actions cannot occur. When we practice walking meditation, we are able to know that our intentions cause the body to move. In other words, we are able to know that the mind moves the body. Through this we can understand the relationship between the body and mind. If intention is the cause, walking is the result. If we expand this observation further, we can see that every phenomenon has a cause; that is, the law of cause and effect applies to all phenomena. This is the advantage of walking meditation. Like other methods of meditation, walking meditation also improves one's concentration and awareness and calms the mind.

The observation of daily activities of daily life meditation also has its own advantages. First, it can greatly expand the time one practices meditation. It is often not easy to set aside time to practice sitting meditation or walking meditation during our busy lives. On the other hand, if we apply meditation to our daily lives, we combine our lives with meditation and can practice at any time. This is because the essence of meditation is focusing on the present moment. If we pay attention to our movements while washing the dishes, we can meditate as long as we are washing the dishes. Since we are aware of what we are doing while living our daily lives, if something wrong occurs, we can easily correct it. We live our daily lives while taking care of our minds moment to moment, allowing us to be aware when negative thoughts or desires arise and to let them go. This allows us to escape from their influence. Even the strongest desires are not strong at first. It is not difficult when we are able to be aware of and let go of the first thought or desire as it arises. It is because we are not able to be aware of and let go of the first thought or desire that it causes the next thought, and the next thought, and the desire to suddenly occur. In addition, when practicing daily life meditation, since we do things while being aware, we are able to know what kinds of phenomena arise. We are also able to experience the phenomena that occur during sitting or walking meditation during our daily lives. Like other forms of meditation, we develop concentration and awareness as well as the wisdom that clearly knows the phenomena that arise. The ideal way to practice mindfulness meditation is to practice sitting or walking meditation in the morning or at night during your own time and to practice daily life meditation during the rest of the day.

Microscopic Observation: Samatha and Vipassanā

Now we will examine the microscopic observation of Samatha and Vipassanā. Since the macroscopic observation of mindfulness meditation is limited in its ability to allow us to clearly know ourselves, we need to practice Samatha and

Vipassanā. Samatha is the practice of cultivating samādhi (concentration). Samādhi refers to the state where the mind is focused on a single object. There are three types of concentration, namely momentary concentration (khan(n밑에 점이 있어요 폰트가 없어서요)ika) samādhi), access concentration (upacāra samādhi), and absorption concentration (appanā samādhi). Among these, absoarkhanikption concentration is known as jhāna, of which there are four stages: the first jhāna, the second jhāna, the third jhāna, and the fourth jhāna. When we cultivate samādhi, we develop the eye of wisdom and are able to see the properties of ultimate materiality and ultimate mentality that cannot be detected by our sense organs or by our ordinary consciousness. With this, we are able to clearly know what kind of beings we are and what phenomena arise when we perform physical or mental actions. We are able to know what kind of phenomena arise when we are walking and what kind of phenomena arise when we perform a mental action. We see the macroscopic observation of mindfulness meditation from a microscopic perspective. Through these two types of observation, we are able to clearly know our existence from both a macroscopic and microscopic perspective.

There are 40 methods of cultivating samādhi, and its specific methods are detailed in the Path of Purification (Visuddhimagga), a commentary on the Buddhist Nikāyas. Of these 40 methods, the most well-known and popular is ānāpānasati, the method of meditation where one focuses their attention on breathing in and out. According to what the Buddha said, the method of cultivating samādhi by focusing on breathing in and out consists of four stages. First, when one breathes in and out long, one knows that they are breathing in and out long. Second, when one breathes in and out short, one knows that they are breathing in and out short. Third, one does not miss a single breath. Fourth, one's breath becomes very subtle. In the first and second stages, one pays attention to any breath that occurs as it is, without any distractions. If you follow the first and second stages well, you naturally enter the third stage, and if you follow the third stage well, you enter the fourth stage. While the Buddha only refers to subtle breathing in the fourth stage, it also includes the formation of a nimitta (a sign of concentration, the union of breath and light) that arises after the subtle breath as well as entering jhāna (absorption).

What Can Be Experienced Through Macroscopic Observation

Now, we will examine in detail what can be experienced through the macroscopic observation of mindfulness meditation practices including sitting meditation, walking meditation, and daily life meditation as well as the microscopic observation of Samatha and Vipassanā. First, we will look at the macroscopic observations of sitting meditation, walking meditation, and daily life meditation.

Through mindfulness meditation we are able to know the properties of the body and mind. The body and mind constantly show their properties, but because we are not aware of them, we do not know them. We will first look at the properties of the body. The body has two types of properties. The first is that the body is actively engaged in life activities according to conditions. Here, life activities have a neutral characteristic. They are neither good nor bad, just like a naturally occurring phenomenon. It is similar to how it rains when the conditions for rain are met, or the wind blows when the conditions for wind are met. The second property of the body is being still. Much like a sack, it does not move itself.

The mind functions on these two properties of the body. The first is reacting to life activities. There are three types of reactions: positive, negative, and neutral. We are affected by these reactions. The life activities of the body do not directly affect us. For example, when a hungry person is annoyed that food is not yet ready, they are having a negative reaction towards the life activity of hunger by thinking 'I'm hungry but why is the food not ready!' and this reaction causes them to be upset. On the other hand, if at this moment the person thinks, 'My digestive system is healthy. Although I'm hungry now, if I wait a bit, the food will be delicious.' They will feel better. Or if they have a neutral reaction, thinking, 'This is the current state of my body,' they will become calm. If we look at it this way, how we react to our life activities affects us.

In addition, it is the mind that moves a still body. We are able to know this in two ways. We are able to know this through the macroscopic observation of practices such as walking meditation discussed earlier, and we are also able to know this through the microscopic observation of samādhi. When practicing walking meditation, we are able to know that intention is always present when we are walking. The body cannot move without intention. The body moves according to the mind. We can also know this through microscopic observation. Samādhi is the mind focused on one object. As discussed previously, when we cultivate samādhi, the eye of wisdom opens and we are able to see ultimate materiality and mentality. For example, when we have the intention to raise our hand, materiality is created by our mind. We are able to see this materiality move to the hand and cause it to be raised. We are able to see that materiality created by the mind moves the body.

If such is the relationship of the body and mind, the mind is important. The mind does not move according to our will, but moves based on certain principles. We are able to see this through meditation. The first principle is that the mind is always turned toward an object. When the mind turns towards an object, it can only be at one object at a time. It cannot be turned towards two objects at the same time. When the mind is turned towards a wholesome object, we are affected in a positive way. Being positively affected means that our mind becomes relaxed, happy, and mentally healthy. When the mind turns towards an unwholesome object, we are affected in a negative way. Being negatively affected means that the mind is suffering, unhappy, and mentally unhealthy. When the mind turns towards a wholesome object, it cannot turn towards an unhealthy object, and vice versa.

The second principle that moves the mind is that when the mind continues to go towards a certain direction, it will create a pathway towards that direction. The reason for this is that the mind does not move according to our will, but rather moves due to conditions. This is because the mind brings up what has been inputted frequently. Inputs occur through six pathways. They occur through the eye, ear, nose, tongue, body and mind, and inputs that occur frequently are brought up in the mind. If we think a lot about the past, thoughts about the past arise. If we think a lot about the future, thoughts about the future arise. If we focus a lot on the present, we will become focused on the present. If we practice meditation consistently for a long time, we will be able to know this. This is the principle by which pathways are formed. Everyone wants to be relaxed, happy, and mentally healthy. It is because we are ignorant that our minds turn towards unwholesome objects despite our desire to be relaxed, healthy, and mentally happy. When we do this, instead of becoming relaxed, healthy, and mentally happy, we will suffer, be unhappy, and become mentally unhealthy. And if we frequently go towards this direction, a pathway will form. Therefore, for our own sake our minds need to go towards wholesome objects and not towards unwholesome objects. To do this, we must clearly know what a wholesome object and an unwholesome object are.

Though there are countless types of wholesome objects, essentially they are the present. Likewise there are also countless unwholesome objects, but essentially they are the past and future. We will examine why the past and future are unwholesome objects while the present is a wholesome object. There are two types of past. There is the positive past such as that of reminiscing, and there is the negative past that causes you to feel regret, anger, injustice, or disappointment. Everyone knows that the negative past is an unwholesome object. Then should reminiscing be seen as a wholesome object? I believe that reminiscing should also be seen as an unwholesome object. There are several reasons to see it that way. Although reminiscing is better than the negative past, it has its own limitations. People who are satisfied in the present moment simply live in the present and do not need to reminisce. It is people who are not satisfied with the present that need to seek comfort through reminiscing.

However, since we cannot just be lost in reminiscence, we will eventually have to return to the present moment, which may not be as satisfactory. If we keep reminiscing, the mind will form a pathway to getting lost in reminiscence. Therefore, it is better to maintain that reminiscing is also an unwholesome object.

There are also two types of future. There is the future of waiting for something good to happen or making plans, and the future of worrying about and being anxious about what is about to happen. The future of worrying and being anxious is an unwholesome object. Then how should we view waiting for something good to happen or making plans? Let us first think through waiting for something good to happen. When a person does something, they choose what is best among various options. They wait because it is better than doing something right now. We must live in the present. When we are waiting for something, we are not able to live in the present. Additionally, if we wait and what happens is different from what we thought, we may become unhappy. Next let us look at making plans. Here making plans refers not to those made by a corporation or by a nation, but rather our simple attempts to draw a picture of the future. When we draw out plans to do something in the future instead of doing something now, thinking that we can do it in the future brings us comfort. However, since we are not doing the thing we are planning to do while planning, it may actually be a waste of time. The benefits of being lost in reminiscence, waiting for something good to happen, or planning are minimal compared to the positive effects that occur when focusing on the present, which we will examine next. In reality, they only come with side effects. Therefore, we can see all types of past and future as being unwholesome objects.

We are able to go to the past or the future in our thoughts. People believe that thinking about the past or the future is simply thoughts and that they have no effect on us. However, when we look at the things that arise which affect us when we think, we are able to know that they are actually much greater than the effects of what actually occurred.

Let us look into the past that actually occurred and our thoughts about the past. When we look at the past that actually occurred, it has four properties. The first is that the past only occurs once. The second is that we cannot control it. The third is that it affects our minds. The fourth is that it leads to chemical changes in the brain. These are the properties of the past that actually occurred. Now let us look into what happens when we think about the past that has occurred. First, it affects our mind. If it were something that made us upset, we would become upset. Second, it leads to chemical changes in the brain. These changes are similar to when the event actually occurred in the past. If we think about this multiple times, we are affected by it multiple times. Although what happened in the past only actually occurs once, we can experience the effects of it multiple times by thinking about it. If we think about it ten times, it is as if it occurred ten times. In this respect, thoughts are greater than reality.

We can control our thoughts by understanding the principles by which our thoughts arise and applying effort. And if we cultivate samādhi and obtain the eye of wisdom, we are able to see what happens when we think of something upsetting that occurred in the past. When something upsetting that occurred in the past arises in the mind, the mentality of mind-door adverting occurs in an instant, followed by seven instances of *javana* (quick action). Mind-door adverting and seven instances of *javana* followed by a subsequent set of mind-door adverting and seven instances of *javana* occur countless times in a single second and affect our minds. This is not something that can be known through our ordinary consciousness, but by cultivating samādhi and obtaining the eye of wisdom, when we have a mental recognition that we are thinking about something, we are able to see this cognitive process arise. The first cognitive process that arises when we think about something is mind-door adverting. This is a cognitive process that occurs when the mind focuses on an object with attention. The type of *javanas* that arise depends on whether the mind is a wholesome or an unwholesome arises. And this cognitive process of mind-door adverting followed by seven *javanas* that occurs repetitively countless times in the brief period of a single second has an incredible effect on us. When we know this, we are able to know that thinking about the past has a much greater effect on us compared to the past that actually occurred. The future has not even occurred once. However, the moment we think about the future, it affects the chemicals in our brain and also has a tremendous effect on our mind.

Let us look at the reason why the present is, in essence, viewed as being a wholesome object. When our mind is present, there are many things that arise that are beneficial to us. First, when the mind is in the present, it is not in the past or the future. This is because by its property the mind can only be in one place at one time. The mind is not affected negatively by the things that can arise when it is in the past or the future that we have examined previously. The majority of our suffering arises when the mind is in the past or the future. When we suffer, it is because we are holding onto an object that causes suffering. If the mind is present and is not holding onto any object that causes suffering, suffering ceases. If the mind goes towards an object in the present all day, it is possible to not suffer at all. Second, when we are present, our focus increases. When the mind is in the past or the present, it does not stay with one object but instead continuously bounces around from one object to another, causing our focus to become weak. However, if we remain with the singular object of the present moment, our focus will become stronger. With this strengthened focus, we are able to break through the nature of objects that we experience. We are able to clearly remember whatever we experience. Third, since our mind is solely focused on what we are doing in the present, we can clearly know what is occurring in the present moment. We can know the properties of the body and mind. When we clearly know a certain object, we will clearly know that we do not know when not knowing a certain object. Therefore, what we know and do not know becomes clear. If we proceed to do something thinking that we know what we are doing, without actually knowing, we will achieve the wrong result. However, if what we know and do not know are clear, we will know what we do not know and stop before something goes wrong. Fourth, by doing things in the present, we will always accomplish more. Fifth, if our mind is in the present, we will not experience suffering and will leave a good impression on others because we are faithfully present. Sixth is that we will be able to sleep well. There are many other benefits aside from these. Therefore, we can consider the present as a wholesome object.

It is necessary for us to look at the properties of mental functions in more detail. We are influenced by what is in our heads, namely our thoughts, emotions, will, and perceptions. However, if we observe these carefully, we can see that it is not we who think, will, or have emotions, but that they arise according to conditions. It is because we do not observe them that we do not know this. However, because their contents are different, we have no choice but to name them distinctly. Depending on their contents, we name them as thought, will, emotion, and perception. The conditions here are not fixed. They can continue to change. The law of cause and effect is continuously applied here. Whether it is a thought, will, or emotion, it is the result of the conditions under which they arise. Our reaction towards them becomes a new condition that brings a new result. This fact has therapeutic implications.

What Can Be Experienced Through Microscopic Observation

Now, we will examine in detail what can be experienced through the microscopic observation of Samatha and Vipassanā. As mentioned above, when one cultivates samādhi through Samatha meditation, they will obtain the eye of wisdom. Through the eye of wisdom we can see the ultimate materiality and mentality that constitute our existence. Everything that exists in the world does so in the form of two aspects, namely conventional reality (sammuti) and ultimate reality (paramattha). Conventional realities are the things that are detected through our sense organs for which we attach agreed-upon names. For example, everyone will see a hand and call it a 'hand,' a foot a 'foot,' and a rock a 'rock.' This is conventional reality. Man-made concepts are also a part of conventional reality. On the other hand, ultimate reality has its own inherent characteristics that cannot be broken down any further. Ultimate reality is therefore the smallest unit and does not change because it has its own inherent properties. It is different from the conventional reality where a hand changes colors or size if the weather gets cold. Of course, this means that the characteristics of ultimate reality do not change during its existence, not that it exists forever. Ultimate reality also arises and disappears depending on conditions. When you obtain samādhi, you are able to see ultimate materiality and mentality.

There are 28 types of ultimate materiality. There are eighteen concrete materialities and ten non-concrete materialities. Concrete materialities are those that actually exist. Non-concrete materialities are materialistic phenomena that are caused by concrete materialities. The eighteen types of concrete materiality are as follows: (1) the earth element, (2) the water element, (3) the fire element, (4) the wind element, (5) color, (6) smell, (7) taste, (8) nutriment, (9) sound, (10) eye sensitivity, (11) ear sensitivity, (12) nose sensitivity, (13) tongue sensitivity, (14) body sensitivity, (15) heart base, (16) masculinity, (17) femininity, and (18) life faculty. The ten types of non-concrete materiality are (1) the element of space, (2) bodily imitation, (3) vocal imitation, (4) lightness, (5) malleability, (6) wieldiness, (7) production, (8) continuity, (9) decay, and (10) impermanence.

When we are able to see ultimate materiality, we can clearly know exactly what kind of things are occurring in us. For example, when you walk, you create an intention to walk, and materiality created in the mind moves from the heart base (mind door) to the leg. And when it touches the leg, the wind element among materiality created by the mind becomes the main factor and causes movement together with the wind element in the leg. When you make up your mind to speak, materiality, including the earth element, created by the mind, moves to the vocal cords, and when it makes contact with the earth element in the vocal cords, you begin speaking. In this way, we are able to see as it is how all movements of the body occur. We are also able to see the regeneration of ultimate reality. Although ultimate materiality forms and disappears very quickly, a cup placed in front of us remains the same. This is because the materiality that constitutes the cup regenerates continuously. Each materiality has a different regenerative force. This is why they exist for different periods of time. Let us take a stone and a loaf of bread as an example. The stone can exist for a long time because its regenerative force is strong. However, a loaf of bread does not exist for as long because its regenerative force is weaker than that of the stone.

When we are able to see ultimate mentality, we are able to know ourselves better. For example, if we are not able to see the ultimate mentality when we become angry, we will not know what actually happens to us when we are angry and how it affects us. The mind as an ultimate reality is composed of consciousness and mental factors. And when the mind perceives an object, the process of mental cognition arises. For example, when you look at ultimate mentality, when you are angry with unwholesome thoughts, mind-door averting arises when your mind is directed at the object of anger, followed by the occurrence of seven *javanas*. This occurs countless times in a second. At this time, there is a consciousness and mental factors that perform the functions of mind-door averting. This is also true for *javanaas*. There is a fundamental consciousness along with mental factors. Regardless of what type of consciousness it is, it is universally accompanied by the following seven mental factors. They are (1) contact, (2) feeling, (3) perception, (4) volition, (5) concentration, (6) life faculty, and (7) attention. The following six mental factors are occasionally present and occasionally absent. They are (1) initial application, (2) sustained application, (3) decision, (4) energy, (5) joy, and (6) desire. Along with these mental factors, there are beautiful mental factors that accompany a wholesome consciousness and unwholesome mental factors that accompany an unwholesome consciousness.

There are 26 types of beautiful mental factors. They are (1) faith, (2) mindfulness, (3) shame of wrongdoing, (4) fear of wrongdoing, (5) non-greed, (6) non-hatred, (7) neutrality of mind, (8) tranquility of the mental body, (9) tranquility of consciousness, (10) lightness of the mental body, (11) lightness of consciousness, (12) malleability of the mental body, (13) malleability of consciousness, (14) wieldiness of the mental body, (15) wieldiness of consciousness, (16) proficiency of the mental body, (17) proficiency of consciousness, (18) rectitude of the mental body, (19) rectitude of consciousness, (20) right speech, (21) right action, (22) right livelihood, (23) compassion, (24) sympathetic joy, and (25) wisdom. There are 14 types of unwholesome mental factors. They are (1) delusion, (2) shamelessness of wrongdoing, (3) fearlessness of wrongdoing, (4) restlessness, (5) greed, (6) wrong view, (7) conceit, (8) hatred, (9) envy, (10) avarice, (11) remorse, (12) sloth, (13) torpor, and (14) doubt.

Beautiful mental factors have a positive effect on the mind, while unwholesome mental factors have a negative effect. A wholesome consciousness is one that is free of two or three among greed, hatred, and ignorance, whereas an unwholesome consciousness is one that is accompanied by greed, hatred, and ignorance. One's mental health suffers when one accumulates the effects of many unwholesome consciousnesses. On the other hand, one's mental health thrives when one accumulates the effects of many wholesome consciousnesses. A consciousness focused on the present is one without greed, hatred, and ignorance. Focusing on the present all day long leads to the accumulation of many positive effects on the mind. If we look closely at what kinds of phenomena arise in our minds moment to moment and deal with the bad phenomena that arise well, we will be able to live our lives with a healthy mind. If we are able to see ultimate mentality, we will be able to clearly know exactly what kinds of phenomena occur in our minds all day and how we are affected by these phenomena.

The Psychotherapeutic Application of Buddhist Meditation

Finally, we will examine how our experiences in Buddhist meditation can be applied to treat mental illnesses. As mentioned above, we are affected by what is in our minds. What is in our minds are mental functions such as will, emotion, and thought. However, if we look at these closely, we learn that these mental functions are the result of the causes or processes that cause them to arise. If we removed the cause or altered the process before they occurred, the mental functions such as thought, will, and emotion would not arise. However, these mental functions arise because we are not able to do this. At this time, your reaction to the mental function that occurred becomes a new cause and brings about a new effect. If we do not know this fact, we will not know that our thoughts and our will arise based on conditions, and will instead believe that we are thinking and we are willing. Rather than creating conditions where good thoughts and will arise, we are swayed by our thoughts and our will that occurred and will continue to react in the wrong way. Will is only something that we bring up. In order to create change we need to establish a system that can lead to change. The same goes for emotions. People believe that they become sad. However, the fact of the matter is that one becomes sad because the conditions for becoming sad have come together. Here, it is important to have a proper response to the emotion. A mistake can make the situation worse. In the case of a panic disorder, panic symptoms arise due to the appropriate conditions. If those conditions are not met, the symptoms do not arise. A therapist helps the patient see the difference between the two conditions.

Often, our physical state impacts our mental state, and at times it can even trigger mental illnesses. The mind has a tendency to be in pain when the body is in pain. If the mind is not in pain when the body is in pain, it can help our mental health. When the mind is in pain, it has the tendency to be in further pain. In this case, if the mind is not in further pain when the mind is in pain, it may not worsen one's mental state. In this case, let us examine how the mind cannot be in pain when the body is in pain. The body is in pain because there is a cause or a process for it to be in pain. If we were to eliminate the cause and take action in the process, the body would not have been in pain. It is because we were not able to do this that the effect of the body in pain occurred. The body in pain is an effect. How we respond to this leads to a new effect. If the mind is in pain when the body is in pain, it negatively affects our body's progress and is harmful to us as our mind is also in pain. Being frustrated or worrying when the body is in pain also means that the mind is in pain. One must know with a calm and wise mind that there is a reason for the body to be in pain in order for the mind to not also be in pain. When this happens, the body will go through the process it must go through while the mind will remain at ease.

We will look at how the mind can avoid being in further pain when it is in pain. When we observe closely, in truth, the mind is in pain because there is a cause for the mind to be in pain and it has gone through that process that led to the effect of the mind being in pain. How we respond to this effect leads to a new effect. If we know this and accept the mind in pain as it is, the mind will not be in further pain. Because the mind arises and passes very quickly, if the mind is not in further pain, we quickly become at ease. Although it can take some time for bodily pain to subside, mental pain can disappear very quickly. For example, when we feel depressed, our mind is in pain. Our response to this depressed state will have an effect on the next mental state. The response, 'How long will this depression last? How will I live in the future? Who caused this to happen?' means that the mind is in further pain. A depressed person may feel unsatisfied with their current life and may not be able to accept it. There is a gap between the situation of their current life and the life they want to live. Their lives are harder the larger the gap is. However, the state of their current life is inevitably as it is due to the law of cause and effect. The current state of their life can change when they do something to change it. Additionally, when they feel depressed, their mind is facing an object that causes them to feel depressed. At this time, they should make an effort to let go of that object and return the wholesome object of the present moment.

Treatment consists of changing our mental conditions (system). We must carefully observe the conditions and change them so that we can bring about the change we want. Additionally, something that must be kept in mind during treatment is that our thoughts are different from reality. The world does not work based on our thoughts, but rather based on reality. The more our thoughts differ from reality, the bigger our problems. When we are not able to deal with our problems well, mental illnesses begin to arise. Although there are varying degrees to which people have mental illnesses, they all have these kinds of problems. In this respect, making an effort to see reality is the true beginning of treatment. For the sake of treatment, and for the sake of living our lives at ease, we must cultivate the wisdom to clearly see reality as it is. With this wisdom we must make an effort to change the conditions that caused our mental illnesses. And through practice, we must learn how to set aside harmful and negative thoughts that are not in accordance with reality.

Conclusion

Meditation is practiced in various ways according to various religions and cultural traditions. Although the object of meditation may vary depending on the type of practice, the essence of meditation is to observe that object as it is. Buddhism, especially Early Buddhism, is an effort to solve all of the questions that humans can have, such as what kind of beings we are, how the world is composed, and by what principles the world moves. Here, we use the method called observation. Observation is at the core of both Buddhism and meditation. It is here that

Buddhism meets meditation. Buddhist meditation can be seen in two ways, namely the macroscopic observation of mindfulness meditation and the microscopic observation of Samatha and Vipassanā. Macroscopic observation is carefully observing moment to moment what arises in our body and mind through our sense organs of the eye, ear, nose, tongue, body and consciousness. The microscopic observation of Samatha and Vipassanā is observing what cannot be seen through macroscopic observation. When we attain samādhi through the practice of Samatha, we will acquire the eye of wisdom. Through the eye of wisdom, we are able to know what our body and mind are made of. I believe that Buddhist meditation includes general meditation. In this chapter, we have looked at what can be experienced through macroscopic observation (mindfulness meditation) and what can be experienced through microscopic observation (Samatha and Vipassanā). And we have looked into how Buddhist meditation can be applied to psychotherapy.

Bibliography

Jeon H. The experience of mindfulness meditation and its psychotherapeutic usefulness (정신과 의사가 경험한 위빠사나 수행: 위빠사나 수행의 정신치료적 유용성). Korean J Psychother. 2006;20(1):30–7.

Jeon H. Stories of healing the mind a psychiatrist learned from the Buddha (정신과 의사가 붓다에게 배운 마음 치료 이야기). Seoul: Bulkwang Publishing Co; 2010.

Jeon H. A psychiatrist's "guidebook for the mind" (정신과 의사가 들려주는 생각 사용 설명서). Seoul: Bulkwang Publishing Co; 2012.

Jeon H. Samatha, Jhāna, and Vipassanā: practice at the Pa-Auk Monastery: a meditator's experience. Somerville: Wisdom Publications; 2018.

Jeon H. Buddhist psychotherapy. New York: Springer; 2021.

Kim J-H, Seunim S, Jeon H. Lessons on the Buddha's emotions (부처님의 감정수업). Seoul: Bulkwang Publishing Co; 2020.

Mon MT. Essence of Buddha Abhidhamma. Yangon: Mya Mon Yadanar Publications; 2010.

Sayadaw P-AT. Knowing and seeing. Scotts Valley: CreateSpace Independent Publishing Platform; 2010.

12 The Third Wave of Cognitive Behavioral Therapy and Meditation

Seunghee Won

Behaviorism emerged as one of the major theories of psychotherapy from the 1920s to the 1950s. Its foundational theories include I.P. Pavlov and J.B. Watson's classical conditioning, B.F. Skinner's operant conditioning, and A. Bandura's social learning theory. Despite the prominence and criticism of psychoanalysis during the 1950s, J. Wolpe, S. Rachman, and H. E. Skinner advanced behavioral therapies based on their respective theories during the same period. In contrast to psychoanalytic theory, which posits that human behavior and thought are influenced by internal mental processes, behaviorism contends that they are shaped by external environmental factors. It considers all human behavior as a result of learning, and in some extreme interpretations, it suggests that free will does not exist.

S. C. Hayes has delineated behavioral therapy into three historical generations. The first generation, emerging in the 1950s, sought to modify behavior through the principles of classical or operant conditioning. This generation concentrated exclusively on overt behaviors, positing that human emotions are learned and predominantly employing techniques such as reinforcement, systematic desensitization, and exposure therapy.

S. Won (✉)
Department of Psychiatry, School of Medicine, Kyungpook National University, Daegu, Republic of Korea
e-mail: wonsh864@knu.ac.kr

The second generation of behavioral therapy introduced cognitive therapy, which is based on A. Beck's cognitive mediating hypothesis. This theory posits that cognition, which influences behavior and emotion, can be altered, thereby enabling desired emotional and behavioral changes through the correction of cognitive errors. The core concepts of cognitive therapy include automatic thoughts, malfunctioning schemas, and cognitive distortions. In the 1970s, cognitive therapy was gradually integrated with behavioral therapies, evolving into Cognitive Behavioral Therapy (CBT). CBT focuses on symptomatic relief, collaborative empiricism, and the improvement of core beliefs. It combines behavioral techniques, such as activity scheduling, contingency management, problem solving, and social skills training, with cognitive techniques. Originally developed as a treatment for depression, CBT's effectiveness was validated and refined through systematic research and clinical practice, leading to its expanded application across a variety of mental disorders and psychological distress situations. Today, CBT is one of the most widely utilized psychotherapies. However, several studies have raised questions about the cognitive mediating hypothesis. While addressing dysfunctional beliefs and automatic thoughts is central to CBT, clinical changes were observed to occur before these cognitive shifts, and changes in negative attitudes were noted solely through medicinal treatment. Some argue that negative

J.-H. Chae, H.-Y. Lee (eds.), *Meditation in Psychiatry and General Medicine*,
https://doi.org/10.1007/978-981-95-7147-5_12

attitudes result from depressive moods. CBT has also faced criticism for being overly rationalistic, lacking integration with basic neuroscience or cognitive psychology, being superficial in its therapeutic relationships, not addressing emotions in depth, and having separate treatment models for each illness. In response to these issues, efforts to overcome the limitations of existing psychotherapies, including CBT, began to emerge in the 1980s and 1990s.

The third generation of behavioral therapy, often referred to as "clinical behavior analysis," is divided into two main branches. The first branch represents a deepening and development of pure behaviorism and includes treatments such as Behavioral Activation, Brief Activation Treatment for Depression, and Integrative Behavioral Couple Therapy. The second branch encompasses methods that integrate various psychological theories and actively incorporate Eastern meditation practices to overcome the limitations of existing psychotherapeutic theories. Unlike the cognitive perspective, the third generation of behavioral therapy is rooted in behavioral theories such as contextualism, functional analysis of behavior, radical behaviorism, and relational frame theory. While it is challenging to identify a single characteristic that encompasses all the emerging methods within this generation, they share a common emphasis on experiences and concepts such as mindfulness, cognitive de-fusion, the dialectic of acceptance and change, commitment, values, spirituality, and relationships. Notable therapies within this generation include the Cognitive Behavioral Analysis System of Psychotherapy, Mindfulness-Based Stress Reduction, Mindfulness-Based Cognitive Therapy, Acceptance and Commitment Therapy, Dialectical Behavior Therapy, and Functional Analytic Psychotherapy. These approaches emphasize experiential processes and aim to foster psychological flexibility and well-being through various innovative techniques.

Although compassion-based interventions (Compassiom-Focused Therapy, Mindful Self-Compassion, Compassion Cultivation Training, Cognitively-Based Compassion Training, Compassionate Mind Training, Attachement-Based Compassion Therapy...) are not formally categorized as third-wave behavioral therapies, they align closely with third-wave principles, especially in their focused on mindfulness, acceptance, and transforming one`s relationship to internal experiences.

Among the treatment modalities gaining attention as third-wave behavioral therapies, behavioral activation and mindfulness-based interventions will be described below.

Modlities of Treatment

Behavioral Activation (BA)

BA is a short-term psychotherapy developed on the foundation of behaviorist theories of depression. Its primary goal is for the therapist and client to collaboratively identify specific behaviors, environmental factors (positive and negative reinforcers), and the interactions between these elements that contribute to the client's current symptoms, mood, and non-functional problem areas. By performing behavioral tasks—such as increasing positive reinforcement, reducing avoidance behavior, planning activities, and graded exposure—BA aims to reduce depressive symptoms and problematic behaviors. Although BA is grounded in a long tradition of behavioral theory and research, it has recently regained attention as an independent method of treatment. C.B. Ferster initially presented behavioral theories based on the functional analysis of depressive behaviors. Building on Ferster's theories, P.M. Lewinsohn developed and advanced appropriate behavioral activation techniques. A. Beck subsequently included Lewinsohn's behavioral activation technique as an essential element of cognitive therapy, utilizing it extensively in his clinical practice. BA emphasizes the functional analysis of behavior to understand the antecedents and consequences that maintain depressive behaviors, thereby providing a structured approach to help clients re-engage with their environment in a positive and meaningful way.

Although the depression behaviorism model and behavioral therapy developed intensively in the 1970s were clinically effective, their decisive inclusion and implementation as part of CBT or Interpersonal Therapy stemmed from a series of studies in which P.M. Lewinsohn himself participated. These studies concluded that behavioral therapy was no more effective than cognitive therapy. However, in 1996, N.S. Jacobson and colleagues published pivotal research that revitalized interest in behavioral therapy. To compare the effectiveness of various treatment methods within CBT, Jacobson et al. randomly assigned 150 depressed patients to three groups. The first group performed only behavioral techniques, the second combined behavioral techniques with cognitive restructuring, and the third received standard CBT. The study's results indicated no significant difference in the effectiveness of treatment among the three groups. Subsequent studies reported that the therapeutic effects lasted up to 2 years even when behavioral techniques alone were used during the acute stages of depression. Jacobson concluded that behavior therapy has a therapeutic effect comparable to that of CBT. He noted that behavioral therapy is much easier to practice and apply clinically than other methods, making it highly applicable for treating depression. Jacobson referred to the collective series of behavioral therapies used to treat depression as BA. This recognition of BA underscored its effectiveness and practicality, reaffirming its value as a standalone treatment for depression.

BA differs from Lewinsohn's earlier behavioral therapy in several key ways:

1. *Individualized approach*: Instead of uniformly applying problem behaviors and target behaviors, BA tailors its approach to individual characteristics through functional behavior analysis, utilizing the ABC model (Antecedent-Behavior-Consequence).
2. *Balance between acceptance and change*: BA seeks to balance acceptance and change rather than attempting to modify all problematic behaviors. This approach recognizes that not all behaviors need to be changed and that acceptance can be a valuable part of therapy.
3. *Acknowledgment of cognition and emotion*: Although BA does not directly address cognition and emotion, it acknowledges their importance in behavioral change, understanding that changes in behavior can influence and be influenced by thoughts and feelings.

A notable distinction between early behaviorist techniques and BA is the latter's acceptance of the importance of negative reinforcement (such as flight and avoidance). BA applies behavioral strategies that address negative emotions and avoidance more centrally. As a behavioral strategy to reduce avoidance behavior, BA helps clients perform ACTIONs (Assess, Choose, Try, Integrate, Observe, Never) to move away from TRAPs (Trigger, Response, Avoidance Pattern) and towards TRACs (Trigger, Response, Alternative Coping). Standard BA typically involves 20 to 24 sessions, with additional maintenance or strengthening sessions potentially added to prevent recurrence. BA has recently regained attention due to its practical effectiveness. Although the number of well-controlled studies on BA is still limited, many positive results have been reported, and research is actively being conducted to expand its application to various illnesses.

Mindfulness-Based Interventions

Mindfulness, a practice with thousands of years of tradition in the East, has garnered significant public attention in the West over the past few decades. Initially introduced to Western society as a mystical religious practice within Buddhist meditation, mindfulness is now recognized for its practical benefits in healing both mind and body. The medical and psychological communities have increasingly embraced clinical applications and scientific research on meditation. The clinical interest in meditation began to rise notably when H. Benson of Harvard University Hospital used it to treat heart disease in the 1970s and 1980s, publishing his findings. Benson focused on the relaxation response induced by concentration (Samatha) meditation, reporting that meditation improved stress-related diseases, alleviated pain from chronic conditions such as heart disease and cancer, restored psychological balance in various mental illnesses, and had positive psychological effects. The attention shifted towards insight meditation (Vipassanā) after the 1990s, largely due to Jon Kabat-Zinn of the University of Massachusetts Hospital. Kabat-Zinn applied Mindfulness-Based Stress Reduction to patients with chronic pain and reported successful outcomes. The application of mindfulness to these patients showed improvements not only in pain regulation but also in anxiety and depression. Currently, various psychotherapeutic techniques based on mindfulness are being actively developed and disseminated. Mindfulness is not merely a passing trend but is becoming a mainstream element in the third wave of CBT. This wave emphasizes experiential and process-oriented approaches, integrating mindfulness to address a range of psychological issues.

Vipassanā is a compound word in Pāli, consisting of "vi" and "passanā." "Vi" has several meanings, but in Buddhism, it particularly refers to the three characteristics of all phenomena: impermanence (anicca), non-self (anattā), and suffering (dukkha). "Passanā" means "to see through." Thus, Vipassanā refers to the effort to clearly understand the nature of mental and physical phenomena that occur in one's own body. The essence of Vipassanā meditation is to be immediately and clearly aware of all phenomena that occur in the body and mind as they are. Being aware of phenomena as they are means applying one's bare attention without intervening through comparison, analysis, judgment, inference, etc. In Pāli, this concept of "being aware as it is" is referred to as "sati." The dictionary definition of sati includes awareness, attention, and remembering. Sati has been translated into English in various ways, including "nothing," "awareness," "attention," and "mindfulness," before settling on "mindfulness." In Korean, its translations encompass a range of meanings, such as mindfulness, being awake, paying bare attention, passive attention, focusing the mind, and keeping the mind. Vipassanā meditation thus emphasizes a direct, non-judgmental observation of the present moment, aiming to cultivate an immediate and clear awareness of the transient nature, lack of inherent self, and the inherent dissatisfaction of all experiences.

Western psychologists have endeavored to operationalize and define mindfulness from a psychological standpoint, leading to various conceptual interpretations. Jon Kabat-Zinn defines mindfulness as the capacity to attentively engage with the present moment, intentionally observing both body and mind, and accepting each experience as it arises. William K. Brown and Richard M. Ryan define it as enhancing attention and awareness of present experiences or reality, while Alan R. Baer defines it as the non-judgmental observation of a continuous stream of internal and external stimuli. Shauna Shapiro defined mindfulness as a process involving three fundamental components—intention, attention, and attitude. In this framework, mindfulness refers to intentionally attending to present-moment experiences while maintaining an attitude of openness, curiosity, and acceptance toward those experiences. These conceptual definitions reflect a range of mindfulness components, including attention regulation, focused awareness, acceptance of experiences, non-judgmental attitude, openness to experience, metacognitive skills, and insight. Through research on operational definitions and its various components, mindfulness has transitioned from being perceived as a mystical concept to a measurable psychological process. It is now understood as a skill that can be cultivated and enhanced through learning and training. This shift in perception has facilitated the integration of mindfulness into mainstream psychology and clinical practice, offering tangible benefits for mental health and well-being.

Most of the time in our daily lives, we operate on autopilot, akin to putting ourselves on automatic navigation without conscious awareness of our actions. In this state, we are oblivious to the events and thoughts around us, merely reacting based on emotions, sensations, and ingrained habits. However, practicing mindfulness enables us to be more attuned to each moment, allowing us to clearly perceive our thoughts, emotions, and bodily sensations in the present. With mindfulness, we gain the freedom to choose more deliberate actions, liberated from past habits. Moreover, mindfulness empowers us to release worries about past pain and future uncertainties. By enhancing our mindfulness, we can make conscious choices in response to each situation, rather than relying on automatic reactions rooted in past conditioning. This heightened awareness enables us to navigate life with greater intentionality and authenticity, fostering a sense of empowerment and fulfillment.

Several psychotherapeutic mechanisms of mindfulness are proposed:

1. *De-centering*: Mindfulness helps individuals recognize that automatic thoughts are not a true reflection of reality but rather mental processes. Strengthening the ability of the observing self-promotes therapeutic separation between the conceptual self (thoughts, beliefs) and the experiencing self (emotions, sensations), leading to greater psychological flexibility and well-being.
2. *De-automatization*: Through meditation, habitual cognitive processes that operate automatically and unconsciously are weakened. This allows for the cultivation of an active and receptive pattern of awareness, where one becomes more conscious of their thoughts and behaviors.
3. *Acceptance*: Rather than avoiding or struggling against negative stimuli or experiences, mindfulness encourages actively accepting them without judgment or selection. This non-judgmental and non-selective acceptance reduces anxiety and promotes emotional regulation.
4. *Exposure effect*: Mindfulness practices involve cultivating a relaxed state through meditation and observing situations that trigger anxiety. This exposure, while in a relaxed state, leads to desensitization to anxiety-inducing stimuli over time.
5. *Reperceiving*: a shift in perspective in which individuals observe their thoughts, emotions, and experiences from a more objective and less identified standpoint.

The principal mindfulness-based interventions are as follows.

Mindfulness-Based Stress Reduction (MBSR)

MBSR is a group program developed in 1979 by Jon Kabat-Zinn at the University of Massachusetts Hospital. Rooted in Buddhist meditation practices, MBSR has become the most widely distributed among mindfulness-based therapies. By 2013, it had been implemented in over 700 university hospitals and general hospitals worldwide, proving particularly beneficial as a complementary treatment for patients in cancer wards or those experiencing chronic pain. Additionally, MBSR has been introduced into various educational institutions in the United States to help manage stress, with similar applications being explored in Korea in clinical and educational settings. At the core of MBSR is mindfulness, defined by Kabat-Zinn as the intentional and non-judgmental attention to the present moment. He expanded the original seven attitudes of mindfulness—non-judging, patience, beginner's mind, trust, non-striving, acceptance, and letting go—by adding gratitude and generosity, forming a nine-attitude model. Through mindfulness, individuals focus on the present moment, heightening sensitivity to surroundings and reducing reflexive responses, thereby enhancing self-regulation and coping with stress. Moreover, mindfulness disrupts the cycle of rumination, freeing individuals from past-focused or future-anxious thoughts. The key components of MBSR include meditation practices aimed at (1) increasing awareness of sensations, emotions, and thoughts; (2) providing self-regulation strategies; and (3) fostering healthy and adaptive responses to stress. These practices empower individuals to cultivate a deeper understanding of themselves and their experiences while developing resilience and coping mechanisms to navigate life's challenges more effectively.

The MBSR program typically spans 8 weeks, though variations may occur. Participants convene once a week for two and a half hours at a designated location and time. Additionally, there is a full-day practice session between the sixth and seventh weeks. Participants are encouraged to dedicate 45 min each day to practicing mindfulness in their daily lives. The meditation practices in MBSR encompass both formal and informal approaches. Formal meditation includes techniques such as breathing meditation, sitting meditation, body scans, and hatha yoga. Informal meditation involves being mindful of everyday activities, such as eating, observing pleasant and unpleasant events, and noticing recurring thoughts, emotions, and bodily sensations. These practices cultivate calmness and insight throughout daily life. Walking meditation can be formal when done deliberately and slowly with attention to breath, or informal when practiced while paying attention to the legs and feet during routine activities. The eight core themes of MBSR include mindfulness and automatic pilot, perception and creative responding, awareness of the body and breath, stress reactivity, working with difficult emotions and thoughts, mindful communication, integrating mindfulness into daily life, and maintaining mindfulness practice The main teachings of MBSR can be summarized as follows: cultivating awareness of mind and body to reduce physical responses to stress or pain, exploring stress experientially to reduce emotional reactions, maintaining equanimity in the face of change and loss, fostering non-judgmental awareness in daily life, promoting calmness and clarity in every moment, and accessing internal resources to enhance life enjoyment and manage stress effectively. Meta-analytic evidence indicates that MBSR leads to moderate improvements in anxiety and depression and small to moderate reductions in pain and psychological distress.

Mindfulness-Based Cognitive Therapy (MBCT)

MBCT was developed in 2002 by John Teasdale, Zindel Segal, and Mark Williams with the aim of preventing relapse in individuals recovering from depression. This eight-week group program integrates elements of Mindfulness-Based Stress Reduction (MBSR) with principles of CBT initially developed by Jon Kabat-Zinn. Similar to MBSR, MBCT consists of two-hour sessions held weekly, with a full-day training session scheduled after the fifth session. Participants are encouraged to engage in daily guided meditation practice at home. The program incorporates both formal and informal meditation practices, including sitting meditation, the three-minute breathing space meditation, body scans, yoga, and walking meditation. Additionally, cognitive-behavioral skills are taught and discussed, participants are educated about depression, action plans are created to prevent relapse, and strategies for detecting early signs of relapse are provided. While MBCT draws on techniques from traditional cognitive therapy, it differs in how it addresses automatic negative thoughts. CBT primarily focuses on modifying the content of maladaptive thoughts through cognitive restructuring, whereas MBCT emphasizes cultivating mindful awareness and changing one's relationship to thoughts through decentering and experiential practices. Through this process, individuals come to recognize that automatic negative thoughts are mental events rather than accurate reflections of reality. By fostering metacognitive insight, MBCT helps participants experientially understand that thoughts are transient and not inherently true, thereby interrupting the cycle of negative thinking and emotional reactivity and supporting more effective management of depressive symptoms. The eight core themes of MBCT include awareness of automatic pilot, dealing with barriers, mindfulness of the breath and body, recognizing aversion, allowing and letting be, understanding that thoughts are not facts, learning how to take care of oneself, and maintaining mindfulness practice. Studies have shown that MBCT can improve residual symptoms of depression, enhance quality of life, reduce reliance on antidepressant medication, and offer effective prevention against relapse, particularly in individuals who have experienced multiple depressive episodes.

Recently, Mindfulness-Based Cognitive Therapy for Life (MBCT-L), developed in the late 2010s and grounded in the principles of mindfulness-based cognitive therapy, has been introduced to support individuals in navigating everyday challenges and cultivating flourishing in daily life. To distinguish it from this adaptation, the original program is often referred to as MBCT-D (Mindfulness-Based Cognitive Therapy for Depression). While MBCT-L retains the eight-week structure of MBCT, sessions are typically shorter and place greater emphasis on applying mindfulness in everyday life, embodied awareness, compassionate self-care, and the cultivation of well-being rather than primarily focusing on depressive relapse prevention. Within the program, activities such as the "vicious flower" and experience record sheets help participants recognize habitual patterns of thoughts, emotions, bodily reactions, and behaviors, thereby illuminating the cyclical processes that maintain psychological distress. MBCT-L also seeks to cultivate key capacities—including awareness of automatic pilot, embodied awareness, decentering, skillful responding, gratitude, and well-being—through mindfulness practices such as the body scan, sitting meditation, mindful movement, the three-step breathing space, the 50:50 practice, the Ten-Finger Gratitude practice, and befriending meditation. The eight core themes of MBCT-L include stepping out of automatic pilot, cultivating embodied awareness, recognizing habitual patterns of mind and body, responding rather than reacting, accepting experience, developing self-care and compassion, integrating mindfulness into everyday life, and fostering well-being and flourishing. Emerging evidence suggests that the program can reduce perceived stress, enhance mindfulness and self-compassion, decrease rumination, and promote psychological well-being.

Acceptance and Commitment Therapy (ACT)

Acceptance and Commitment Therapy (ACT), developed by Steven Hayes in the late 1980s and formally introduced in 1999 and grounded in relational frame theory and functional contextualism, employs acceptance through mindfulness and change through action as its primary treatment strategies. ACT is a versatile approach that can be applied across various problems and disorders. The central focus of ACT lies in addressing psychological inflexibility, which arises from several interconnected factors (Fig. 12.1):

1. *Cognitive fusion*: This refers to becoming entangled or fused with one's thoughts, where thoughts are taken as literal truths rather than transient mental events.
2. *Experiential avoidance*: Individuals may engage in behaviors to avoid or suppress uncomfortable thoughts, emotions, or sensations, leading to short-term relief but long-term psychological distress.
3. *Dominance of the conceptualized past and feared future, weak self-knowledge*: Ruminating about past events or worrying about the future can hinder present-focused

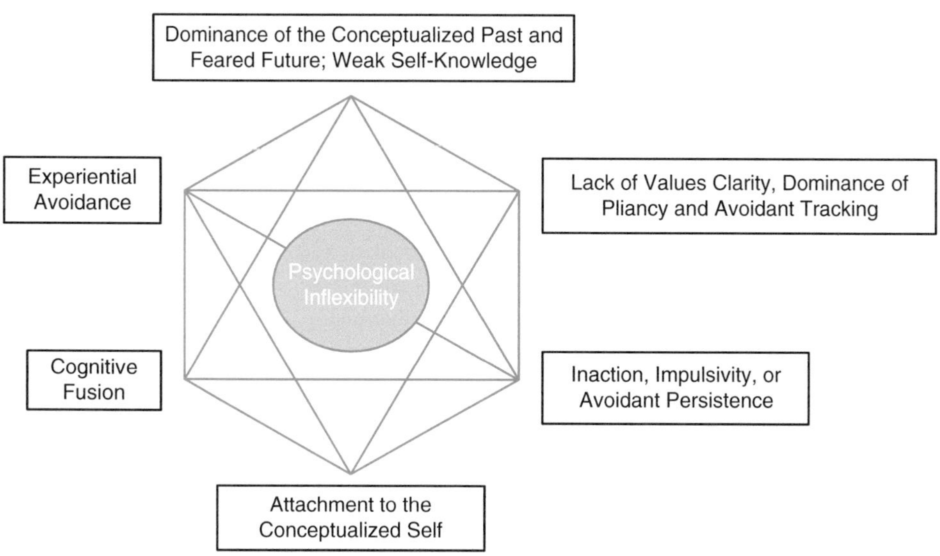

Fig. 12.1 ACT: Psychopathologic hexagon model

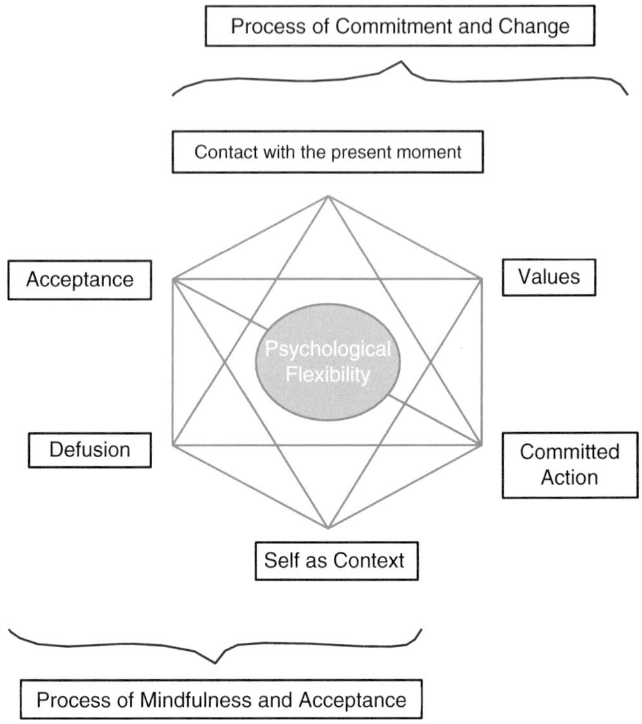

Fig. 12.2 ACT: Mental health hexagon model

engagement and contribute to psychological distress.

4. *Attachment to the conceptualized self*: Holding rigidly to a fixed self-concept can limit one's ability to adapt and respond flexibly to life's challenges.
5. *Lack of values, dominance of pliancy and avoidant tracking*: Failing to clarify and act in accordance with personal values can lead to a sense of emptiness or disconnection.
6. *Inaction, impulsivity, or avoidant persistence*: Behavioral patterns characterized by avoidance, impulsivity, or excessive control can hinder meaningful engagement with life's opportunities and challenges.

ACT aims to foster psychological flexibility, which involves being present in the moment, accepting inner experiences without judgment, and taking action guided by deeply held values. By cultivating mindfulness skills and promoting committed action aligned with values, ACT helps individuals break free from the grip of psychological inflexibility and move toward a more meaningful and fulfilling life.

The mental health state that stands in contrast to psychological inflexibility is psychological flexibility, which can be predominantly attained through two core processes: the "process of mindfulness and acceptance" and the "process of commitment and behavioral change." (Fig. 12.2):

The "process of mindfulness and acceptance" involves (12.2):

1. *De-fusion*: This process aims to help individuals detach from their thoughts and emotions, recognizing them as passing events rather than absolute truths. De-fusion techniques facilitate a more flexible relationship with inner experiences.
2. *Acceptance*: Acceptance involves allowing thoughts, emotions, and sensations to arise without attempting to control or avoid them. It entails acknowledging and embracing experiences as they come, without judgment or resistance.
3. *Self as context*: This process involves developing a perspective that transcends the individual's immediate experiences and identifies with the observing self, which remains stable

and unchanging amidst the flux of thoughts and emotions.

The "process of commitment and behavioral change" includes:

4. *Contact with the present moment*: This process emphasizes being fully engaged and present in the current moment, rather than dwelling on past events or worrying about the future. It encourages active participation in the here and now.
5. *Values*: Identifying and clarifying personal values provides a guiding framework for decision-making and behavior. Values reflect what is deeply meaningful and important to an individual, serving as a compass for actions and choices.
6. *Committed action*: Committed action involves taking intentional steps aligned with one's values, even in the presence of discomfort or uncertainty. It entails making choices and engaging in behaviors that contribute to a valued life direction.

By cultivating these processes, individuals can enhance their psychological flexibility, enabling them to navigate life's challenges with greater resilience, adaptability, and well-being.

ACT focuses on empowering clients to develop a mature perspective on life and psychological well-being by fostering psychological insight and acceptance. Unlike traditional therapeutic approaches that aim to eliminate or change clients' problems directly, ACT emphasizes shifting clients' attitudes toward their problems and seeing them in a different light. It views suffering as a normal and universal aspect of the human experience and treats behaviors aimed at avoiding negative inner experiences (experiential avoidance) as symptoms of dysfunction. ACT recognizes that individuals perceive reality through the lens of language and past experiences, often leading to cognitive fusion, where individuals confuse their thoughts with reality. This fusion can trigger automatic avoidance behaviors in response to negative thoughts or emotions. The disease model of ACT, summarized as FEAR (fusion with thoughts, evaluation of experience, avoidance of experience, reason-giving for behavior), highlights the cycle of dysfunctional behavior driven by cognitive fusion and avoidance. To disrupt this cycle, ACT employs techniques such as cognitive de-fusion, mindfulness, and acceptance. Rather than attempting to change the content of clients' thoughts directly, ACT focuses on accepting the cognitive process itself and helping clients disidentify from their thoughts and emotions. By promoting acceptance and facilitating behavioral changes aligned with clients' values, ACT ultimately aims to transform clients' cognitive content through the accumulation of new experiences. ACT employs therapeutic exercises such as Leaves on a Stream, Thanking Your Mind, the Chessboard metaphor, observing self practices, expansion exercises, mindfulness practices, values clarification, and committed action planning to cultivate psychological flexibility.

The core concepts of ACT are encapsulated in the word "act," which emphasizes accepting thoughts and feelings (A), choosing values to aim for (C), and taking committed action (T). Research, including recent meta-studies, has shown that ACT can be as therapeutically beneficial as CBT. While ACT is applicable to various mental illnesses, it may be particularly effective in treating chronic depression accompanied by dysfunctional behaviors such as substance abuse, addiction, pain, and abnormal eating behaviors.

The ACT Matrix, a recent development in ACT, offers a practical and versatile tool for clinical applications, replacing the traditional hexagonal model. This matrix consists of two intersecting lines, each representing distinct dimensions of human experience and behavior. The vertical axis, known as the line of experience, delineates between two types of experiences: those perceived through the five senses and those arising from mental activity or interoception. This axis helps individuals differentiate between sensory experiences and internal thoughts or emotions. On the other hand, the horizontal axis, termed the line of action, distinguishes between actions aimed at withdrawing from unwanted experiences and actions directed

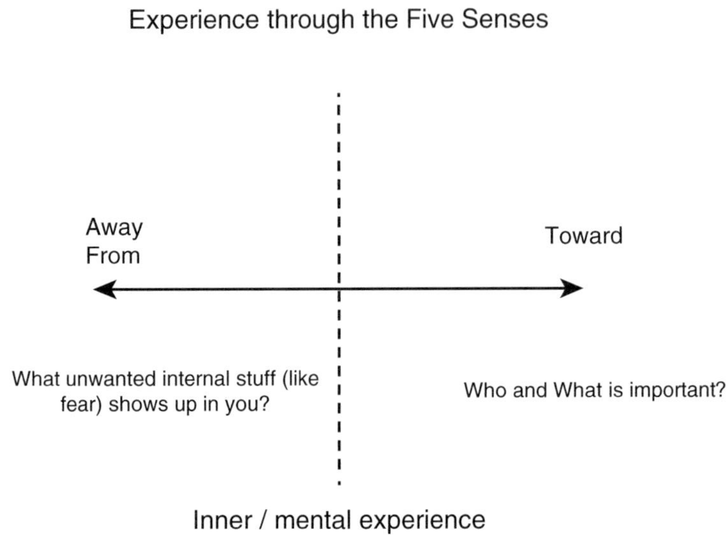

Fig. 12.3 ACT matrix

towards reaching out to someone or something important. This axis facilitates the understanding of behavioral patterns in terms of avoidance versus approach behaviors. By combining these two axes, the ACT Matrix forms four quadrants. Each quadrant represents a unique combination of experiences and actions, offering insights into an individual's current state of psychological flexibility. The matrix serves as a visual aid for clients to become more aware of their behaviors and experiences, ultimately promoting greater psychological flexibility. Overall, the ACT Matrix provides clinicians with a practical tool to guide therapeutic interventions and help clients develop insight and awareness into their patterns of behavior and experience (Fig. 12.3).

Dialectical Behavior Therapy (DBT)

DBT, developed by Marsha M. Linehan in 1994, integrates elements of CBT with mindfulness practices, particularly aimed at treating patients with borderline personality disorder. The foundation of DBT lies in a dialectical worldview, which posits that reality is a synthesis of inherently compatible forces—thesis and antithesis—that integrate to form a new, harmonious force. Central to this worldview is the recognition that opposing properties coexist within reality, emphasizing the importance of acknowledging and reconciling mutual contradictions and unity. From a therapeutic standpoint, DBT acknowledges the tension between three primary opposing characteristics experienced by patients:

1. *Acceptance and change*: Patients grapple with the tension between accepting themselves as they are and striving for personal growth and change.
2. *Gains and losses in recovery*: Patients navigate the tension between the benefits gained through recovery efforts and the losses or sacrifices involved in the process.
3. *Maintaining or changing personal integrity*: Patients face the tension between preserving their sense of self and identity and adapting to new ways of thinking and behaving.

DBT adopts a dialectical perspective in understanding and responding to these tensions. Key principles include:

1. *Multiplicity of perspectives and methods*: Recognizing that there are always multiple viewpoints and approaches to any given situation.
2. *Individual uniqueness*: Acknowledging that each individual possesses unique characteristics and perspectives.

3. *Impermanence of change*: Understanding that change is inevitable and constant.
4. *Validity of opposing viewpoints*: Accepting that contradictory perspectives can both hold validity.
5. *Respect for truth in conflict*: Encouraging the respectful acknowledgment of both sides during conflicts or confrontations.

By embracing these dialectical principles, DBT aims to help patients develop greater self-awareness, emotional regulation, and interpersonal skills, ultimately fostering a more adaptive and balanced approach to life's challenges.

DBT conceptualizes Borderline Personality Disorder (BPD) as a condition characterized by emotional dysregulation, rooted in a combination of heightened emotional sensitivity, intense emotional reactions, and prolonged recovery periods after emotional arousal. This emotional dysregulation is exacerbated by an invalidating environment, which plays a pivotal role in the development and perpetuation of the disorder. DBT identifies BPD as a multifaceted condition involving both motivational issues and deficits in coping skills. Individuals with BPD commonly exhibit deficiencies in self-regulation, interpersonal interactions, and pain tolerance. These deficits manifest as difficulties in managing emotions effectively, establishing and maintaining healthy relationships, and tolerating distressing situations. Furthermore, DBT recognizes the role of maladaptive behavioral patterns and dysfunctional beliefs acquired within the individual's environment. These factors contribute to a motivational context that hinders the utilization of adaptive coping strategies and reinforces maladaptive behaviors. In summary, DBT views BPD as a complex interplay of emotional sensitivity, environmental invalidation, motivational challenges, and skill deficits. By addressing these underlying factors through targeted interventions, DBT aims to empower individuals with BPD to develop effective coping mechanisms, regulate their emotions, and improve their overall quality of life.

DBT adopts a comprehensive approach to treatment that incorporates both acceptance-based strategies and change-oriented techniques. This integrated perspective aims to address the diverse needs of individuals experiencing emotional dysregulation and interpersonal challenges, regardless of the specific problems they face. The acceptance strategy in DBT emphasizes mindfulness practices, which help individuals cultivate present-moment awareness and non-judgmental acceptance of their thoughts, emotions, and experiences. By developing mindfulness skills, clients learn to observe their inner experiences without reacting impulsively or judgmentally, promoting greater emotional regulation and self-awareness. In addition to the acceptance strategy, DBT incorporates change-oriented techniques rooted in CBT. These techniques focus on identifying and challenging maladaptive thoughts and behaviors, developing coping skills, and fostering healthier interpersonal relationships. Through cognitive restructuring, problem-solving, and behavior modification, clients acquire the necessary skills to manage distressing emotions and navigate challenging situations more effectively. Central to the effectiveness of DBT is the therapeutic relationship between clients and their therapist, as well as the broader validating environment in which treatment takes place. This relationship serves as a core mechanism of change, providing clients with validation, support, and guidance as they work towards achieving their treatment goals. By fostering a collaborative and validating therapeutic environment, DBT integrates acceptance-based strategies—such as mindfulness practices and validation techniques—with change-oriented strategies, including behavioral analysis(e.g., chain analysis), problem solving, and skills training in emotion regulation, distress tolerance, and interpersonal effectiveness, thereby promoting lasting improvements in emotional well-being and interpersonal functioning.

Standard DBT is structured to provide comprehensive treatment for individuals with BPD, incorporating various components to address the multifaceted nature of the condition. The key components of standard DBT include:

1. *Group skill training*: Patients participate in weekly group sessions focused on acquiring essential skills to manage their emotions and behaviors. These sessions typically cover four modules: core mindfulness, distress tolerance, emotion regulation, and interpersonal effectiveness. Group training allows participants to learn and practice skills in a supportive and interactive setting.
2. *Individual therapy*: Patients engage in weekly individual therapy sessions with a DBT therapist, during which they apply the skills learned in group training to their specific challenges and receive personalized feedback and guidance. In individual therapy sessions, techniques such as chain analysis, missing link analysis, and diary card review are used to identify problematic behavior patterns and to explore more effective coping strategies.
3. *Phone coaching*: Patients have access to phone coaching between scheduled therapy sessions, allowing them to receive support and guidance from their therapist in real-time during moments of distress or crisis. Phone coaching helps reinforce skill utilization and provides immediate assistance during challenging situations.
4. *Consultation team*: DBT therapists participate in a consultation team, where they receive supervision, support, and guidance from fellow clinicians to prevent burnout and ensure adherence to the treatment model. Consultation teams also facilitate collaboration and ongoing learning among therapists.

Patients participating in standard DBT commit to a one-year treatment program, attending weekly individual therapy sessions, group skills training, and utilizing phone coaching as needed. The structured nature of DBT, along with its emphasis on skill acquisition and application, has been shown to be effective in treating individuals with borderline personality disorder, making it the first psychotherapy recognized as an evidence-based treatment for this population.

Indeed, research findings have highlighted the effectiveness of DBT in treating individuals with BPD, demonstrating moderate to large treatment effects in meta-analyses. However, the application of DBT has expanded beyond BPD to encompass a broader range of mental health conditions characterized by difficulties in emotion regulation and impulse control.

The versatility of DBT lies in its emphasis on teaching practical skills for emotion regulation, distress tolerance, interpersonal effectiveness, and mindfulness, which can be applied across a range of mental health conditions. In recent years, DBT has shown promise in addressing various mental health challenges, including:

1. *Suicidal behavior*: DBT has been effective in reducing suicidal ideation and behaviors by equipping individuals with coping skills to manage emotional distress and develop alternative strategies for responding to crises.
2. *Self-harm*: Individuals engaging in self-harming behaviors, such as cutting or burning, have benefited from DBT by learning healthier ways to cope with overwhelming emotions and regulate impulses.
3. *Substance use disorders*: DBT has been adapted for individuals with substance use disorders, helping them address underlying emotional vulnerabilities and develop skills to cope with triggers and cravings, thereby supporting recovery efforts. DBT for Substance Use Disorders (DBT-SUD) has been introduced.
4. *Post-traumatic stress disorder (PTSD)*: DBT techniques, particularly those focused on mindfulness and distress tolerance, have been integrated into treatments for PTSD to help individuals manage symptoms of hyperarousal, intrusive memories, and avoidance behaviors.
5. *Eating disorders*: DBT has shown promise in treating individuals with eating disorders, such as bulimia nervosa and binge-eating disorder, by addressing emotional dysregulation and promoting healthier coping mechanisms for managing food-related behaviors. DBT for Eating Disorders (DBT-ED) has been introduced.

Many clients with emotional regulation difficulties, such as those diagnosed with BPD, frequently present with co-occurring Post-Traumatic Stress Disorder (PTSD). To address and help them process the distressing memories and emotions associated with trauma, a therapeutic approach of combining DBT with Prolonged Exposure (DBT-PE) has been developed and is being increasingly adopted. For emotionally dysregulated clients with PTSD, it is necessary to discuss a structured and systematic treatment plan integrating DBT and DBT-PE with the client starting from the pre-treatment stage. Even if the client does not initially agree, it is important to discuss this treatment plan again as therapy progresses. Before implementing DBT-PE for PTSD, it is critical that higher-order maladaptive behaviors, such as life-threatening or therapy-interfering behaviors, are effectively regulated through DBT. Depending on the clinical situation, DBT-PE may need to be temporarily suspended in favor of focusing exclusively on DBT.

As research continues to explore the effectiveness of DBT across diverse populations and settings, its potential for addressing complex emotional and behavioral challenges remains a focal point in contemporary mental health care.

Conclusion

The evolution of CBT into its third wave, alongside the rise of mindfulness and meditation, represents a significant shift in therapeutic approaches. These mindfulness-based treatments embody several key characteristics that distinguish them from earlier methods.

Firstly, they embody a synthesis of Eastern acceptance with Western problem-solving approaches, offering a comprehensive model for understanding human beings. By integrating these diverse perspectives, they provide a more holistic framework for addressing psychological issues.

Secondly, mindfulness-based therapies highlight the interconnectedness of mind and body, emphasizing the importance of mind-body healing in promoting overall well-being. This recognition underscores the need to address both mental and physical aspects of health in therapeutic interventions.

Thirdly, these approaches prioritize the cultivation of positive mental states, such as compassion and resilience, rather than solely focusing on eliminating negative elements. By nurturing positive qualities, individuals can develop greater emotional balance and resilience to life's challenges.

Fourthly, mindfulness-based therapies emphasize the role of self-transcendence and expanded consciousness in the healing process. By cultivating awareness and insight, individuals can transcend limited perspectives and tap into deeper sources of wisdom and understanding.

Lastly, these therapies emphasize the importance of changing one's relationship to thoughts, emotions, and experiences, rather than simply solving problems. By fostering acceptance and non-judgmental awareness, individuals can develop healthier ways of relating to themselves and others.

In essence, the third wave of cognitive behavioral therapy, represented by mindfulness-based approaches, stands on the foundation of past methods while integrating new insights and techniques. Rather than discarding previous approaches, it seeks to build upon them, offering a more holistic and integrative approach to mental health and well-being.

Bibliography

Korean Sources

Jeong AJ. Mindfulness based stress relaxation manual (MBSR 마음챙김에 기반한 스트레스감소프로그램 매뉴얼). Jeonju: Jeonbuk National University Press; 2015.

Kim JH. What is mindfulness? Suggestions for clinical and everyday application of mindfulness. (마음챙김이란 무엇인가: 마음챙김의 임상적 및 일상적 적용을 위한 제언). Korean J Psychol Health. 2004;9(2):511–38.

Park SH. Vipassana meditation, mindfulness, and mindfulness-based psychotherapy (위빠사나 명상,

마음챙김, 그리고 마음챙김을 근거로 한 심리치료). Cogn Behav Ther. 2007;7(2):83–105.
Won S. Psychosocial intervention. Korean Society for Affective Disorders (정신사회적 치료. 대한우울조울병학회 편저). In: Textbook of depressive disorders. Seoul: Sigma Press; 2012. p. 218–51.

English Sources

Alessandri M, Heiden L, Dunbar-Welter M. History and overview. In: Heiden L, Herden M, editors. Introduction to clinical psychology. New York: Plenum Press; 1995.
A-Tjak JG, Davis ML, Morina N, Powers MB, Smits JA, Emmelkamp PM. A meta-analysis of the efficacy of acceptance and commitment therapy for clinically relevant mental and physical health problems. Psychother Psychosom. 2015;84:30–6.
Gortner ET, Gollan JK, Dobson KS, Jacobson NS. Cognitive-behavioral treatment for depression: relapse prevention. J Consult Clin Psychol. 1998;66:377–84.
Grossman P, Niemann L, Schmidt S, Walach H. Mindfulness-based stress reduction and health benefits. A meta-analysis. J Psychosom Res. 2004;57(1):35–43.
Hayes SC. Acceptance and commitment therapy, relational frame theory, and the third wave of behavioral and cognitive therapies. Behav Res. 2004;35:639–65.
Hayes SC, Hofmann SG. The third wave of cognitive behavioral therapy and the rise of process-based care. World Psychiatry. 2017;16:245–6.
Hayes SC, Luoma JB, Bond FW, Masuda A, Lillis J. Acceptance and commitment therapy: model, processes and outcomes. Behav Res Ther. 2006;44:1–25.
Hofmann SG, Sawyer AT, Witt AA, Oh D. The effect of mindfulness-based therapy on anxiety and depression: a meta-analytic review. J Consult Clin Psychol. 2010;78(2):169–83.
Hopko DR, Lejuez CW, Ruggiero KJ, Eifert GH. Contemporary behavioral activation treatments for depression: procedures, principles, and progress. Clin Psychol Rev. 2003;23:699–717.
Jacobson NS, Dobson KS, Truax PA, Addis ME, Koerner K, Gollan JK, et al. A component analysis of cognitive-behavioral treatment for depression. J Consult Clin Psychol. 1996;64(2):295–304.
Kabat-Zinn J. Mindfulness for beginners: reclaiming the present moment and your life. Louisville: Sounds True Inc.; 2016.
Kliem S, Kröger C, Kossfelder J. Dialectical behavior therapy for borderline personality disorder: a meta-analysis using mixed-effects modeling. J Consult Clin Psychol. 2010;78(6):936–51.
Kuyken W. Mindfulness for life: How to deal with stress, pain and illness using mindfulness meditation. London: Guilford Press; 2019.
Linehan MM. Skills training manual for treating borderline personality disorder. New York: The Guilford Press; 1993.
Martell CR, Dimidjian S, Hermen-Dunn R. Behavioral activation for depression: a clinician's guide. New York: The Guilford press; 2010.
Polk KL, Schoendorff B, Webster M, Olaz FO. The essential guide to the ACT matrix: a step by step approach to the matrix model in clinical practice. Reno: Context Press; 2016.
Ramnerö J, Törenke N. The ABCs of human behavior: behavioral principles for the practicing clinician. Reno: Context Press; 2011.
Segal ZV, Williams JMG, Teasdale JD. Mindfulness-based cognitive therapy for depression: a new approach to preventing relapse. New York: The Guilford Press; 2006.
Segal ZV, Williams JMG, Teasdale JD. Mindfulness-based cognitive therapy for depression (2nd ed.). New York: Guilford Press; 2013.
Shaw BF. Comparison of cognitive therapy and behavioral therapy in the treatment of depression. J Consult Clin Psychol. 1977;45:543–51.
Zeiss A, Lewinsohn P, Muroz R. Nonspecific improvement effects in depression using interpersonal skill training, pleasant activity schedules, or cognitive training. J Consult Clin Psychol. 2017;47:427–39.

Meditation and Psychoanalysis

13

Bon-Hoon Koo

Throughout history, many theories about the human mind were developed both in the East and in the West to better understand it. Among the representative theories, Buddhism in the East and psychoanalysis in the West have had a great influence on various studies. Rather than merely being theoretical explanations, Buddhist meditation and psychoanalysis have developed into practical ones. Meditation has been used in Buddhism as a way to achieve enlightenment, whereas in psychoanalytic theory, it has been used as a way to solve patients' psychological difficulties.

Meditation has been covered in detail in several chapters of this book, so I have omitted introducing it here. Psychoanalysis is a theory of the mind that began with Sigmund Freud, and is a theoretical system developed primarily through analytic experience through conversations with pathological patients. Psychoanalysis has not only been applied to patients with psychological challenges, but it has also had a great influence on history, culture, and art as a theory that explores human psychology. Freud stated that human drives, primarily sexual and aggressive drives, mature in various ways according to a person's psychosexual stage of development. In this process, there are situations where the individual has to limit their instincts, which causes various internal conflicts. Various methods are utilized to resolve these conflicts, and as the individual's ego and superego develop, various defense mechanisms are utilized and emotions or thoughts that are difficult to handle are suppressed unconsciously. However, if the defense mechanism is underdeveloped and does not cope effectively, or when a neurotic defense mechanism is used, various symptoms such as anxiety, depression, and somatization occur. Psychoanalysis is the process of discovering and understanding this dynamic within the patient through dialogue between the patient and the therapist under the assumption of psychic determinism. During the process of psychoanalysis, it is difficult for the patient to reveal their emotions, thoughts, fantasies, etc., in their unconscious, thereby leading to the appearance of various derivatives of the unconscious. Rather than as words, these derivatives appear indirectly as transference to the therapist through actions, symptoms, thoughts, and language, or as transference to external reality relationships, past memories, and dreams. Through a therapeutic alliance and an uncritical and unrestrained approach based on an empathetic response, the therapist responds to these aspects of the patient, continuously understanding and accepting them in various ways, and experiencing them repeatedly through practice. After Freud's death, psychoanalysis developed into ego psychology, which emphasizes the function of the ego. Gradually, as patients suffering from more severe

B.-H. Koo (✉)
Department of Psychiatry, Yeungnam University College of Medicine, Yeungnam University Medical Center, Daegu, Republic of Korea

J.-H. Chae, H.-Y. Lee (eds.), *Meditation in Psychiatry and General Medicine*,
https://doi.org/10.1007/978-981-95-7147-5_13

disorders were analyzed, the theoretical and clinical domains of psychoanalysis were expanded to include object relation theory and self-psychology, which typically dealt not only with conflict theory, but also with pathologies associated with emotional deficiencies in earlier childhood before the Oedipal period between the ages of three and six. As a result, the therapeutic method of psychoanalysis gradually changed. Recently, not only are a patient's past memories revived to gain insight into current symptoms, but the aspect of getting the patient to experience new relationships, primarily by dealing with transference and countertransference relationships through the patient's interaction with the therapist here and now, is also considered to be important.

This chapter examines the relationship between meditation and psychoanalysis, which are representative theories of the mind in the East and the West, respectively. Since the theoretical aspects of meditation and psychoanalysis are so extensive, this chapter will primarily focus on their practical and clinical aspects. Specifically, the chapter will detail the similarities and differences between the realities of meditation and psychoanalysis through several topics.

The Similarities Between Meditation and Psychoanalysis

Dependent Origination and Psychic Determinism

As the law of conditional arising in Buddhism, dependent origination means non-ontological causality. That is, the term means that since everything in the world arises and disappears according to conditions, all beings are made up of a relationship of relative dependence, that "this arises because that exists." In other words, for mental phenomena in Buddhism, the individual's free will is the cause, and this becomes the next link, where its result becomes the next cause. In this way, mental phenomena are viewed from the perspective of the interrelationships that cause them to occur, and this causal theory is called dependent origination (Pāli: paṭiccasamuppāda; Chinese: 緣起).

The basic hypothesis of psychoanalytic theory is psychic determinism, which is the hypothesis that nothing in the mind is arbitrarily determined, that every action and event has a cause, and that everything is determined by things that precede it. It is a kind of principle of causality that sees human behavior of symptoms as having specific motivations. For example, if someone is angry, it is assumed that there is a reason for being angry such as their friend ignoring them or because they failed to get a promotion. Based on this hypothesis, psychoanalysis searches for the cause of a patient that reveals certain emotions, actions, and thoughts by tracing their causal relationship in reverse. Both Buddhist meditation and psychoanalysis can be seen as having a system of thought based on a causal theory.

Nonjudgment and Analytical Neutrality

When observing thoughts, emotions, and feelings that arise during meditation, it is important to be able to see them as they are without judgment. Jon Kabat-Zinn said the following about mindfulness meditation, "Mindfulness is paying attention intentionally and being nonjudgmental, aware of what is occurring here and now in the present moment."

Even in psychoanalysis, when patients reveal derivatives of their unconscious such as thoughts or emotions that come to mind during analysis, it is important for the therapist to look at the patient without being judgmental or discriminatory from their own point of view. This is referred to as neutrality. In other words, it is the perspective that the therapist can only understand the patient when they follow the patient's associations without imposing their own values or standards onto the patient. Meditation and psychoanalysis can be seen as similar in that both seek to see phenomena as they are while excluding the practitioner's or the therapist's values or subjective perspectives as much as possible when looking into various phenomena that arise in the human mind.

Attention and Free Association

Meditation is known to have two important elements. The first is focusing one's attention on a single object and is called focused attention, or Samatha meditation. The second, being an observational element, is observing and being aware of the various phenomena that arise along with the stream of consciousness and is called open monitoring, or Vipassanā meditation. Among them, focused attention consists of intentionally gathering our attention and focusing on a particular object, such as the breath, the movement of the abdomen, or a mantra such as "Oṃ maṇi padme hūṃ" Depending on how proficient we are at meditation, we go from focusing on one object to becoming aware of feelings, thoughts, and emotions, which arise freely within us. After recognizing and observing these phenomena, we return to the object of concentration. During meditation, we continuously repeat these processes countless times.

In psychoanalysis, free association is considered to be very important in the analysis process, and it refers to allowing the patient to verbalize thoughts, emotions, feelings, wishes, images, memories, and so on that come to mind as they arise without filtering them. Through this process of free association, the therapist gradually understands the patient's associations and shares them with the patient. While the patient reveals their unconscious derivatives through free association, the therapist maintains their focus while following the patient's flow of free association. The therapist's attention, expressed as "evenly hovering attention" or "evenly suspended attention," refers to a state in which attention is evenly focused on what the patient is saying and the therapist's own thoughts and emotions.

Thus, both the concentration of attention during meditation and the flow of concentration of observing things as they are are very similar to the flow of the patient's free association and the therapist's attention in psychoanalysis.

Observation and the Observing Ego

Mindfulness meditation in the West explains the phenomena that humans experience in two ways. The first is the "doing mode," which refers to a way of life that attempts to reduce the discrepancies between how one views one's environment and what one thinks one's environment should be. For example, just like a student may exert a lot of effort to be the best in their class even though they are not doing well in school, this way of life consists of attempting to reduce discrepancies and solve problems in one's life. Through the "doing mode," we can engage in productive activities in our lives and shape our environments to better our lives. However, if we are unable to reduce discrepancies despite our efforts, a state of dissatisfaction persists in us and frustration arises, which increases suffering in our lives. In some ways, this condition can also be seen as a state of neurotic pain according to Freud. In other words, despite our wishes to meet our desires, an unsatisfactory state of suffering persists due to the conditions of our external reality or conflicts between the ego and the superego. The second is the "being mode," which refers to a way of life in which one notices and accepts one's environment in the present moment without attempting to forcefully change it. The "being mode" means accepting things as they are without trying to reduce the discrepancy between the state of reality and the state one desires. In Buddhism, the function of being aware of the entire process of a person's mind is called "sati." By being aware of one's mind through sati, one can effectively manage one's mind by removing the causes of attachment that exist in the mind such as desire, selfishness, anger, resentment, prejudice, preconceptions, and values.

Psychoanalysis also explains the ego from two perspectives. As a state where one is directly experiencing, the experiencing ego refers to experiencing and acting unconsciously through things such as one's feelings or thoughts. In contrast, the observing ego observes and perceives the behavior of the experiencing ego. In other words, while one is in the state of being caught up in the experiencing ego, one gradually develops the observing ego through the process of psychoanalysis, increasing one's insight. In the process of psychoanalysis, the therapist may talk about the patient's non-verbal and verbal states as follows. "You are very angry." "You seem to feel that you are very angry," or "You say that you are very angry." "You said x a moment ago, but now you say y," etc. How the therapist explains the patient's condition may affect the degree to which the patient can view their condition more objectively. By repeating this process, the patient eventually develops the ability to observe their own state of mind, such as, "I did x yesterday, but when I looked into my emotions at that time, I think I did y." Additionally, observation in psychoanalysis is very important not only in the process of recognizing the patient's mind, but also in recognizing the therapist's own thoughts and emotions. In other words, the power of observation is also important for the therapist to be able to recognize transference and countertransference, key elements in the process of psychoanalysis. Observing the patient's verbal and non-verbal derivatives well is necessary to be able to recognize transference to the therapist, and the therapist needs the power of observation to know their own minds and also recognize their own countertransference felt by the patient. Just like the process in meditation of changing from a mode of action to a mode of being, this process refers to gradually escaping from one's obsession with experiencing the ego by developing the ability of the observing ego. In other words, escaping from attachment to oneself through the awareness of sati in meditation can be seen as similar to the process of looking into and objectifying oneself through the observing ego in psychoanalysis. Therefore, both meditation and psychoanalysis can be seen as having a common core of increasing the power of observation to be aware of oneself, such as increasing observation through awareness and the observing ego.

The Mechanism of Meditation and Psychoanalysis: Enlightenment and Insight

Meditation begins with the practice of intentionally focusing on and being aware of our actions, thoughts, and emotions, which we are usually not aware of and are mindless of. Through this process, we become aware of the countless ways we avoid reality, and through this we are able to reduce the distortions we have created and see reality as it is. In other words, enlightenment in Buddhism refers to being fully awake in the present moment through the awareness of meditation by realizing our delusion, shaking off false images, restoring our original mind, and maintaining calmness.

In psychoanalysis, research on the treatment factors that change patients has been conducted for a long time. Although there are many therapeutic factors of psychoanalysis, it can be divided into two major categories. First, through the process of psychoanalysis, the patient gradually understands the unconscious (intra-psychic) part of their own mind. In other words, the patient gains insight through an explanatory method of interpreting what the therapist understands about the patient's unconscious, and as this insight increases, it is also accompanied by behavioral changes. Second, just as interactions occur in the relationship between a mother and a child, as interactions continue to occur between the patient and the therapist in the psychoanalytic process, changes may occur through interpersonal action. In other words, the patient has a new interpersonal relationship experience by interacting with the therapist's empathic attitude and accepting response. The process of psychoanalysis can be seen as a process of going back and forth between the patient's internal self-reflection and external experience of transference. Psychoanalysis consists of exploring one's unconscious through this process and understanding the influence of the unconscious on the individual. We gain insight into the unconscious workings of the mind through free association, and our self-awareness increases accordingly. Unlike before, when our self-awareness increases, we are able to make better choices according to our will rather than being swayed by our unconscious. By saying "make the unconscious conscious," about the treatment mechanism of this kind of psychoanalysis, Freud explained psychoanalysis as "where id is, there shall ego be," from the perspective of ego psychology. Both meditation and psychoanalysis enable us to live according to our own free will without being swayed by the phenomena of the unconscious mind by looking into and being aware of them as they are. In this sense, it can be said that there are similarities between enlightenment in Buddhism and meditation and insight in psychoanalysis. Wilfred Bion said that the goal of psychoanalysis is to develop the ego, similar to the process of enlightenment in Buddhism.

Idealism and Psychic Reality

Buddhism has various philosophical perspectives, one of which is the characteristic of idealism. Just like Wonhyo's saying that "all things are created by the mind alone" (一切唯心造), it is our mind that distorts the external environment or the world, and it corresponds to the basic premise for attaining enlightenment in Buddhism. In other words, all phenomena are nothing more than projections of our own minds like objects being reflected in the mirror; the ultimate reality of the universe is only the mind, and all phenomena appear as the mind changes.

There is a concept of psychic reality in psychoanalysis, which refers to looking at the world from the patient's own unconscious point of view. For example, just as a patient says during the process of analysis that "My mother always criticized and scolded me when I was young," or they say of their therapist that "I think my therapist will scold me or look down on me if I am late for therapy," although the therapist cannot confirm what kind of person the patient's mother actually is, they have an image of the patient's mother as it exists in the patient's mind. In this way, regardless of how the therapist actually feels, the patient has in their mind that the therapist perceives them in a negative way, which feels like reality to them.

Both meditation and psychoanalysis enable us to see our distorted perception of the outside world in our own minds as it is. By having us continuously look at a state in which our thoughts are directed to the past or future rather than remaining in the present, meditation helps us gradually realize that our thoughts are not reality and allows us to see reality as it is. Through the analysis process, psychoanalysis also helps us gradually realize that our thoughts are not the actual reality but rather come from our own unconscious. Through this process, the patient gradually changes and understands more and more the difference between fantasy or mental reality and actual reality as they come to realize, "I do not think my mother could have helped it under the circumstances at that time. And even though she criticized me, when I think about her, I think she cared about me and worried about me a lot," or "You (the therapist) have always just been there, but I think I have assumed that you have seen me that way."

Non-self and Ego

As a key doctrine in Buddhism, non-self (Pāli: anattā) does not mean that one does not exist at all, but rather means that one does not have a fixed and unchanging intrinsic nature. In other words, "we" do not have our own unchanging and eternal nature, but rather our existence is conditional and changes based on the law of dependent origination. However, most people believe that there is a fixed entity called "I" and become attached to "I." By identifying their mental and physical processes with an "I" that is believed to actually exist, people have attachments, possessions, distinctions, etc. and fall into conflict. Therefore, realizing that one does not possess these inherent characteristics is the way that Buddhism heals suffering. In Western mindfulness meditation, being completely centered around oneself causes conflict and pain. On the other hand, by creating "distance" from oneself, that is, by seeing oneself objectively through decentering, one is able to escape from these attachments.

In psychoanalysis, the ego is regarded as a dynamic concept rather than being fixed, and it dynamically changes through constant interaction between the id and the superego. The ego in psychoanalysis refers to an "agent" that explains the psychological functions of human beings. Non-self in Buddhism can be seen as a broader concept than the ego. However, both Buddhism and psychoanalysis can be seen as being the same as each other in that they both resolve pain through therapeutic change by having the individual look at themselves and objects objectively.

Perspective on Pain

In Buddhism and meditation, the goal is not to get rid of pain, but rather to be aware of pain as it is, and to accept it and master it instead of being dragged around by it or resisting it. In other words, rather than wishing for pain to disappear forever, meditation helps one realize that pain is an inevitable part of human life and helps one develop the wisdom to deal with it well.

Even in psychoanalysis, the therapist does not instruct or teach the patient how to resolve pain, but rather helps the patient gradually realize for themselves what pain is and what causes it, and to stop resisting pain and develop insight. Therefore, the goal of psychoanalysis, as Freud said, is "transforming your hysterical misery into common unhappiness." In other words, it is transforming human misery into ordinary, everyday unhappiness. Neither meditation nor psychoanalysis attempts to get rid of pain. Rather, they help us accept and deal with pain by relieving ourselves from resisting it.

Compassion and Empathy

Recently in the West, Buddhist compassion meditation has transformed into Mindful Self-Compassion (MSC), Compassion Cultivation Training (CCT), Compassion Focused Therapy (CFT), Cognitively-Based Compassion Training (CBCT), etc., and is rapidly spreading around the world. As an extreme state of empathy and heart-rending toward the suffering of living beings, compassion wishes that others also attain what one wants and also avoid what one does not want.

Even in psychoanalysis or psychotherapy, empathy is considered to be very important as a basic prerequisite for therapy sessions. As a special focused position that opens the door to the interactions that build trust between patient and therapist, empathy in psychoanalysis is the ability to understand another person's point of view. At times in psychoanalysis, empathy is not only seen as a basic prerequisite, but is also seen in self-psychology as a therapeutic factor that strengthens the patient's deficient emotional aspects and weakened sense of self. Self-compassion and compassion in Buddhism and meditation are acts of projecting a positive self-loving mind. Empathy in psychoanalysis can also be seen as a projection of the therapist's goodwill to help the patient.

The Importance of Experience

Meditation values realization through practical experience more than learning through scriptures or books. As a practice of developing awareness of the world through direct meditative experience, in meditation, how one focuses is more important than what one focuses on. Depending on the method of practice, the object of one's focus can vary, and includes the breath, the movement of the belly, sounds or visual stimuli, mantras, and so on. However, meditation places importance on experiential processes such as how one focuses their attention.

Psychoanalysis also places importance on what the patient experiences together with the therapist during the process of learning through regular and continuous meetings and conversations over a long period of time rather than obtaining insight through a single analysis.

Although both meditation and psychoanalysis value experience, the former values the process of experiencing, whereas the latter values the content of experience rather than the process. In other words, psychoanalysis places importance on looking into one's inner world through language to find and understand the truth.

The Differences Between Meditation and Psychoanalysis

Object and Goals

Psychoanalysis is mainly aimed at patients with pathological symptoms. Of course, one can be the subject of psychoanalysis if one is experiencing psychological difficulties in life without having received a formal psychiatric diagnosis, or if one wants to understand one's own psychological problems. However, psychoanalysis primarily deals with the pathological aspects of our mind as it mostly deals with cases of patients who are suffering from psychiatric disorders such as depression or anxiety. On the other hand, meditation is mainly aimed at ordinary people who are not suffering from mental illness, and its main goal is to deal with more common aspects of human suffering and difficulties, to observe the various phenomena that unfold in one's life, and to look at the perspectives of life. Therefore, it can be said that the goal of meditation is to face the suffering in human life, accept it as it is, and live in the present moment in an awakened state.

Due to these differences in their respective objects, as mentioned earlier, meditation can be seen as placing more importance on the *process* of experience, whereas psychoanalysis can be seen as placing more importance on the *content* rather than the process of experience. In other words, in the case of a mental health patient, the pain caused by various pathological symptoms may be too severe when compared to that of normal people, so they may therefore lack the strength to focus on and observe themselves through practices like meditation. Therefore, in psychoanalysis, it is necessary for the therapist to not only help the patient to look at and observe their own mind, but also to help them understand their unconscious little by little, and to help them develop their own insight through new explanations and reinterpretations of their inner world.

How Memories Are Dealt With

Due to the nature of meditation and psychoanalysis, if you look into the flow of your mind, you can surely also face your own memories. If past memories come up during meditation, one just observes and is aware of them, and afterwards, sets them back down. However, in the case of psychoanalysis, the therapist helps the patient examine the contents of their memories that are raised through free association, and through this analysis, they help the patient adopt a new perspective. In other words, insight in psychoanalysis places emphasis on the contents of our minds, whereas enlightenment in Buddhism places emphasis on the nature of the mind itself.

Relationship with the Teacher or Therapist

Buddhism and meditation emphasize the importance of the teacher. In other words, rather than practicing meditation alone, the teacher plays an important role in guiding the practice. Psychoanalysis, of course, also requires a therapist. It is an extremely exceptional case for one to be able to effectively analyze oneself without a therapist, and so a therapist should always be involved. However, although a teacher is also needed in meditation, they only serve to guide the process of meditation, and do not directly form a relationship between teacher and disciple. On the other hand, in the case of psychoanalysis, dealing with the emotions that emerge in the relationship between the therapist and patient, or in other words transference and countertransference, is the most important part of treatment.

The Ethical Aspect

Psychoanalysis emphasizes conventional ethics that are found in regular society, such as maintaining a boundary between the therapist and patient. In other words, it does not deal with other higher-order ethics aside from the standard social ethics such as not having personal contact with a patient. In addition, psychoanalysis pursues a value-neutral attitude in terms of the contents of treatment without making ethical judgments such as what is right or wrong about the patient's story.

Buddhism and meditation, of course, also deal with ethics that transcend the norms of judgment such as what is right or wrong, and ethics soon become a meditative practice. In other words, ethics in Buddhism is not a judgment of what is right or wrong, but rather is to achieve through direct experience how skillful, good, kind, and generous one is. In Buddhism, a person having unethical or immoral thoughts and actions is due to their mind being overly disturbed, and it states that one cannot be mindful and unethical at the same time. Therefore, ethics in Buddhism is regarded as a practice rather than a simple list of norms.

Conclusion

Meditation and psychoanalysis share similarities in terms of the causal nature of their thought systems, their nonjudgmental approaches, how they use attention, the importance of the power of observing the mind as an object, self-maturity through enlightenment and insight, their systems of perceiving oneself and external objects through the mind, their views of pain, their projections of goodness towards oneself and others, and their emphasis on direct experience by going through the process of meditation or analysis rather than a theoretical understanding. On the other hand, meditation and psychotherapy have different main objects, different ways of dealing with memories, different relationships with the teacher or therapist, and different ethical perspectives. However, since both point in the same direction in terms of trying to address human suffering, putting both meditation and psychoanalysis to good use will be helpful (Fig. 13.1).

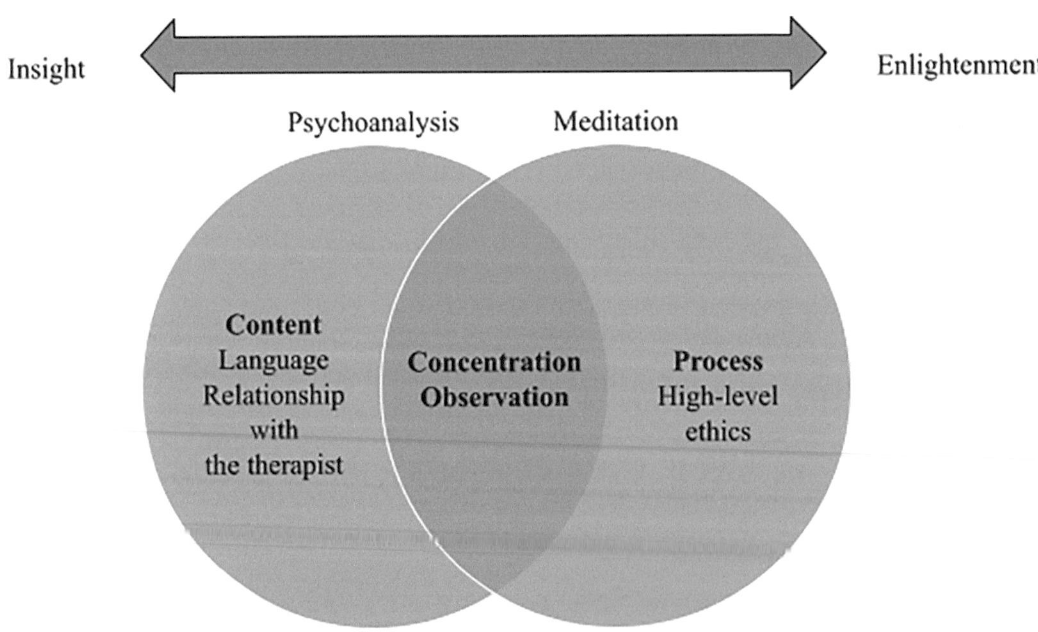

Fig. 13.1 The similarities and differences between meditation and psychoanalysis

Bibliography

Korean Source

Park Y-e. Practical dictionary of Korean-English Buddhist Terms (실용 한-영 불교용어사전). Daegu: Good Connection Press; 2012.

English Sources

Aragno A. The language of empathy: an analysis of its constitution, development, and role in psychoanalytic listening. J Am Psychoanal Assoc. 2008;56:713–40.
Breuer J, Freud S. Studies on hysteria (basic books classics). Reissue ed. New York: Basic Books; 2000.
Buddhapala. Buddha practice. (Korean). Sati Press; 2014.
Choe H-D, Shin S-W. Psychotherapeutic significance of the Buddhist thought of 'not-self' (Anatta). J Korean Neuropsychiatr Assoc. 2005;44:754–62.
Epstein M. Psychotherapy without the self: a Buddhist perspective. New Haven: Yale University Press; 2007.
Gabbard GO. Psychodynamic psychiatry in clinical practice. 5th ed. Washington, DC: Amer Psychiatric Pub; 2014.
Hoffer A. Freud and the Buddha: the couch and the cushion. Boca Raton: Routledge; 2015.
Kabat-Zinn J. Mindfulness for beginners: reclaiming the present moment—and your life. Boulder: Sounds True; 2012.
Kernberg OF. Convergences and divergences in contemporary psychoanalytic technique. Int J Psychoanal. 1993;74:659–73.
Kim S-K. A brief note on psychoanalysis and buddhism. J Korean Psychoanal Soc. 2001;12:30–4.
Kim S-Y. Buddhism and psychotherapy. Psychoanalysis. 2016;27:133–7.
Miller AA, Isaacs KS, Haggard EA. On the nature of the observing function of the ego. Br J Med Psychol. 1965;38:161–9.
Moore B, Fine B. Psychoanalytic terms and concepts. Reprint ed. New Haven: Yale University Press; 1990.
Segal ZV, Williams JMG, Teasdale JD. Mindfulness-based cognitive therapy for depression. 2nd ed. New York: The Guilford Press; 2018.
Wallerstein RS. The concept of psychic reality: its meaning and value. J Am Psychoanal Assoc. 1985;33:555–69.

14 Lacan's Psychoanalysis and Meditation

Kyungchul Shin

It can be said that a groundbreaking change in the ontological perspective began with the rationalist worldview outlined in Descartes' dictum, 'cogito ergo sum' (English: 'I think. Therefore I am'). Through Descartes, we reached a turning point in the seventeenth century where the existing medieval religious worldview was transformed into a worldview centered on human reason.

As another turning point in ontology, Freud argued in 1900 that the unconscious is filled with irrationality and sexual desire in his book *The Interpretation of Dreams*, which caused great antagonism and backlash towards the mainstream view of rationalism. By arguing that the conscious is only the tip of the iceberg and that the unconscious is essential to human thinking and feeling, Freud overturned the worldview of rationalism widely held at that time that emphasized rational thinking and reflection. In other words, he opened the era of the unconscious worldview that transcends reason and consciousness. In this worldview, we can only fully know human existence when we explore the unconscious beneath the conscious. Freud expressed the treatment goals of psychoanalysis as 'replacing neurotic misery with common unhappiness,' 'where id was, there shall ego be,' and 'mental health is the ability to work and to love.' Through the method of the talking cure, it is said that the goal of treatment could be achieved through psychodynamic therapy, which makes the pathological unconscious conscious. Freud refers to health as being able to work and love in society without any pathological symptoms. Therefore, he did not set the goal of therapy beyond the scope of the individual, such as spiritual growth or transcendence of the self.

On the other hand, Jung expanded on Freud's personal unconscious and presented a theory of analytical psychology that includes transcendental concepts such as the 'collective unconscious' and the 'self,' the latter of which is an archetype and the unity of the whole personality. Jung's analytical psychology includes aspects of both personal psychology and transpersonal psychology. The goal of treatment in analytical psychology is individuation and self-actualization, which help one live a life consistent with oneself, with wisdom about the personal and collective unconscious through the expansion of dreams through psychotherapy.

Lacan claims that the human unconscious is structured in language, and he describes human beings as beings of desire and deficiency who are forced to be separated and alienated from 'the Real' due to the emergence of symbolic existence through language. The goal of treatment for Lacan is to pursue *jouissance*(enjoyment) beyond the fantasy given by language and desire, but

K. Shin (✉)
Simwoo Psychiatric Clinic,
Bupyeong-gu, Incheon, Republic of Korea

J.-H. Chae, H.-Y. Lee (eds.), *Meditation in Psychiatry and General Medicine*,
https://doi.org/10.1007/978-981-95-7147-5_14

paradoxically he uses verbal counsel as a means to achieve that goal.

In cognitive behavioral therapy, a 'schema' is a view of oneself and the world, and is a preconceived form of mental structure that functions as a system for perceiving and organizing new information. This preconceived form of schema automatically accepts and organizes new information and modifies itself when encountering exceptional information that is difficult to automatically accept. Cognitive behavioral therapy believes that psychopathologies are caused by cognitive errors such as distorted and automatic thinking, and its goal of treatment is to change cognitive distortion into rational cognition through counseling.

Just as the etymology of both medicine and meditation is derived from the Latin word 'mederi' meaning 'to cure,' meditation fundamentally can be said to have a connotation of healing. Meditation has something in common with the treatment goals of psychotherapy in that it reduces the physical symptoms and psychological problems that negatively affect an individual's life. Meditation, which restores 'being' to human beings, not only improves one's psychological and physical condition through relaxation, but like cognitive therapy, it increases the opportunities for patients to have the experience of approaching their problems from a different perspective or structure through cognitive restructuring.

There are various theories of traditional psychotherapy in the field of psychiatry, but they all have one thing in common: they treat symptoms by helping the patient gain insight into the unconscious or transpersonal aspects that the conscious mind cannot know through 'verbal' counseling with a therapist. On the other hand, meditation can be said to be different from verbal counseling in that it involves directly contemplating one's attachment to mental images, emotions, and thoughts that cause all human suffering and afflictions, cutting them off, and living a life of awareness that leads to healing through 'inner practices' such as concentration meditation or mindfulness meditation.

Here, I have attempted to point out the similarities and differences between Lacan's theory amongst psychotherapeutic theories, and the ontological perspective of meditation within Eastern thought.

The Ontological Perspective of Lacan's Psychoanalysis

Lacan's theory, which originated in France during the twentieth century, is an abstruse theory created using Freud's psychoanalysis, Claud Levi-Strauss' structural social anthropology, and Ferdinand de Saussure's linguistics. Like Freud's theory of psychosexual development, Lacan also describes his own theory of the mental development process.

Newborn infants start out surrounded by what Lacan calls 'The Real,' the natural order of 'real' experiences and objects. Due to undifferentiated neural function, infants perceive the world as identical to themselves and thus have no sense of self-boundaries. Through two significant separations, an infant in 'the Real' emerges as a subject who perceives, thinks, and speaks about the world from a self-centered perspective of subject and object.

The first separation is achieved through the 'mirror stage.' Although newborn infants have a fragmented body under undifferentiated neural functions, by the time they reach 6 months of age, their visual systems are relatively developed and they can recognize their own image despite having less coordinated motor skills. While recognizing the image of themselves reflected in a mirror, they mistake the mirror image, which is the other, for their actual self. At the center of looking at the image of the other (mother) reacting around 'I' (the infant), the integrated mirror image of oneself is placed upon 'I,' and the image of the perceived self and the other are mistakenly identified as reality. Seeing the mental continuity of the newly created ego, the infant feels joy and a narcissistic self is created. The self created in this way is fundamentally the other, obtained at the cost of alienation from the Real, and is the result of identifying oneself with one's own mirror image. In other words, the mirror stage is the stage of imaginary identification, marking the birth of the joyous imaginary self. The infant forms a narcissistic relationship with the image of themselves and their mother. This relationship occurs prior to language, is in the Imaginary, and is a self-other relationship that is a misrecognized dyad (dual relation). This also explains the inevitable misrecognition of reality, which makes the self a form of externality to itself, and which is characterized by paranoid perception. The narcissistic relationship emphasizes the imaginary obsession within which the subject is entrapped. Here, alienation of the real self is the foundation of the essential misrecognition of the mirror stage. Misrecognized attachment acts as a key device that traps the subject in illusion, imaginary desire, or domination.

The second separation takes place as language is built on top of the fundamentally other-like ego, the self-other relationship manifested as an imaginary identification. The subject is castrated through the Oedipus complex within the linguistic cultural sphere, enters the Symbolic of language, and is reborn as a speaking subject. The speaking subject is the result of the second separation, known as the split, which is achieved through the cost of once again being separated from the image of the Imaginary. Castration occurs through the metaphor of the 'name of the father' (French: nom du père) in the Symbolic. The child comes to know their mother's lack of phallus, and their longing to become their mother's phallus is castrated through the 'name of the father' so that they cannot become the mother's phallus. While the Imaginary is characterized by the dyadic relationship, the Symbolic is characterized by a triad. The birth of the subject in the Symbolic through castration signifies the loss of the Real, and creates a fundamental lack in the core of the speaking subject. Due to this lack, the subject becomes that of desire, and thus subjectivity and unconsciousness are linguistically structured in culture, society, and law. Human existence consists of being divided into the imaginary self, that is, the deepest part of the psyche, and the symbolic subject of discourse, action, and culture. The subject is a being that is necessarily separated, that is, alienated and divided, and can never be reverted. There is no possibility of integration. Lacan's theory fundamentally dismantles Descartes' rational self, the 'cogito', which had occupied an important place in Western metaphysics.

According to Lacan, desire is a function of the Symbolic, and desire is a fundamental lack displayed in the speaking subject. Desire is always beyond what can be spoken, and can only ever be dictated by others. It appears as a desire for the desire of the other and is fundamentally intersubjective. In language, the 'signifier', which is the superficial phonetic sign, is not fixed to the 'signified' corresponding to the sign. Instead, signifiers continuously slip in a direction that perpetually replaces fixed meaning. A signifier can speak its meaning only through the mediation of the whole chain of signifiers. Lacan emphasizes the subject as that which fully desires and speaks through the signifier. Lacan's theory of analytic therapy does not cure or eliminate desire, but rather restores the analysis to their latent desires that were hidden due to their symptoms.

The Ontological Perspective of Meditation

Meditation in the East can be divided into Samatha and Vipassanā. As a form of concentration meditation where one focuses their attention on a relatively fixed object, Samatha meditation develops concentration (samādhi) to focus and calm the mind so that it no longer wavers or is agitated and achieves a state of tranquility. On the other hand, Vipassanā meditation, which the Buddha practiced under the Bodhi tree to achieve enlightenment, can be said to be a method of meditation by which one obtains absorption (Pāli: jhāna) through mindfulness (sati).

Although psycho-developmental theory such as that of Freud or Lacan is not advocated from the ontological point of view of Eastern thought that includes Samatha, Vipassanā, jhāna, Buddha-nature (Sanskrit: buddhadhātu, Chinese: 佛性),

just like in cognitive behavior therapy, it has an ontological perspective through a horizontal rather than a developmental mental structure theory. Also similar to Lacan's theory, the ontological point of view of Eastern thought also presents a fundamental critique of the substantial, central, and bounded self.

The five consciousnesses (Sanskrit: pañca-vijñāna-kāya, Chinese: 五識: 色聲香味觸) in which the five senses of sight, sound, smell, taste, and touch are perceived by the mind (Pāli: citta) and the sixth consciousness (Sanskrit: manovijñāna, Chinese: 意識) in which thought is perceived by the mind constitute the six types of consciousnesses within the cognitive process of an ordinary person. The six types of consciousness can be seen as the locus of Lacan's Imaginary and the Symbolic, where the ego, self-consciousness, and the sense of subject and object arise. The seventh consciousness of mentation (Sanskrit: manovijñāna, Chinese 末那識) and the eighth consciousness of storehouse consciousness (Sanskrit: ālayavijñāna, Chinese: 阿賴耶識) are forms of consciousness that are not easily perceived by the average person, and are high cognitive functions that can lead one to absorption (jhāna). One cannot attain a clear view of the indivisible consciousness of absorption that is the fundamental foundation beneath the structure of consciousness in a conditioned state, because ordinary people who do not engage in deep meditative practice are present in the state where the afflictions of self-delusion (Sanskrit: ātma-moha, Chinese: 我癡), self-conceit (Sanskrit: ātma-māna, Chinese: 我慢), and self-attachment (Sanskrit: ātma-sneha, Chinese: 我愛). By strengthening mindfulness (sati) and removing afflictions through the practice of Vipassanā meditation, it is said that the seven consciousnesses will become clear, allowing one to enter the realm of absorption of the emptiness of self (Sanskrit: ātma-śūnyatā, Chinese: 我空).

Only when the fundamental conditioned state of the mind is abandoned, absorption can emerge from below so that the individual subject can manifest the empty present truth and luminous subjectivity. What happens instead is that all beings are encompassed as one indivisible unity. Deepened and expanded awareness leads to the realization that the separate and isolated sense of self-identity is fundamentally fictitious. In Buddhism, human beings are 'non-self' (Pāli: Anattā, Sanskrit: Anātman), not fixed entities that exist in a systematic relationship with the world they experience. Buddhism states that the concept of self and self-image appear as all sensations and feelings (Sanskrit: vedanā, Chinese: 受) become personified as they undergo the process of becoming possessions due to craving (Sanskrit: kāma, tṛṣṇā, Chinese: 愛). Buddhist meditation is the practice of awakening oneself to reach liberation (Sanskrit: Nirvāṇa) by emptying one's mind of wandering thoughts. From the perspective of mindfulness, regardless of any psychological or physical state an individual may be in, one's being exists in and of itself as an undamaged, intact whole from the beginning, and when one connects the wholeness of self and the universe, healing occurs and one obtains the wisdom of bliss.

Despite the differences between the two concerning external phenomena, meditation and Lacan's theory overlap in many areas. Both meditation and Lacanian theory require the denial of the autonomous and substantial self, and imply that traditional rationalism and dualistic thinking in which subject and object are separate, can never lead to the attainment of wisdom beyond reason. Additionally, the state of absorption (jhāna) has conceptual similarities with the Real in Lacanian theory. Although, as Lacan says, the lack at the core of the subject activates the cycle of desire in the subject, the lack of the subject is lacking in the Real. Absorption (jhāna) also means the lack of lacking, pure satisfaction. The goal in Seon (Zen, Chinese: 禅) is the experience of absorption and Nirvāṇa. As absorption is fundamentally empty, it is actually empty in the sense that there is no observing or thinking subject. Everything that is acquired from the five senses, of which the most important is the self or ego, is but a temporary illusion that will decay and collapse with time. Both meditation and Lacanian theory offer critiques of the dualistic way of thinking. It transcends rational debate in a way that questions the methods established according to a dualistic way of thought. The difference is that, for Lacan, healthy existence does not depend on the impossible attainment of the Real, but rather on an understanding of the dynamics that create effort and craving itself. For Lacan, the Real is something that can never be directly understood. Instead, it can only be understood through the Imaginary and the Symbolic. Psychoanalysis does not eliminate desire but restores one to one's original latent desire. As such, it seems that psychoanalysis does not let go of some of its ethical-cultural, that is, its secular goals. While there are methods of transmission for the practice and process of attaining absorption in Buddhism and meditation, it is difficult to clearly find a description of a practical and specific method in Lacan that goes beyond the Symbolic, which is the limitation of the subject. However, in Lacan's later works, he mentions 'Jouissance' and 'beyond the fantasy' which overleap language and desire as the goal of analysis.

Lacan and Ganhwa-Seon

> I am where I do not think, and I think where I do not exist.
> I am there where it was just now, in the place where it was for a moment, still burning in the extinguished, and the real moment of missed birth. I come to be and disappear from what I have stated.
> In the pursuit of the phallus, the subject was the phallus and then came to possess it. Here the final split is inscribed. It is through this final split that the subject projects themselves into the logos.

This example is a random translation of Lacan's text, and here Lacan's writing is notoriously difficult to decipher.

> Disciple's question 1: 'What is the Buddha?'
> Master's answer(hwadu) 1: 'It is a dung stick.'
> Disciple's question 2: 'All dharmas return to one, but where does that one return to?'
> Master's answer(hwadu) 2: 'When I was in Cheongju, I sewed a monk's robe, and it weighed seven pounds.'
> Hwadu(koan) 3: 'Do not think of what is good or what is bad. What is your original form (面目) in this very moment?'
> Hwadu(koan) 4: 'If you have a staff, I will give you a staff. If you do not have a staff, I will take the staff from you.'

These quotes are examples of Hwadu (Chinese: 話頭, Japanese: Watō) or Gong'an (Chinese: 公案, Japanese: Kōan) of Ganhwas-Seon, one of the Buddhist meditation practices. If you read a hwadu passed down from ancient Zen masters, it is a sentence that is impossible to understand logically, similar to Lacan's writing. Samatha meditation or Vipassanā meditation can be seen as a method of reaching absorption by deeply focusing on a single object such as breathing. In contrast, Ganhwa-Seon (Hwaduseon) can be said to be a way to enlighten the real self and absorption by fully immersing oneself in doubt towards the incomprehensible Hwadu.

Because Lacan's style of writing avoids the rational axiomatic account of the unconscious and is a form of omission and oblique imitation of the unconscious, it feels incomprehensible. For Lacan, the only way to understand the unconscious is to directly perceive what is said behind the text through the structure of the text itself. Lacan's unconscious cannot be spoken for itself, and creates a paradox in that we must always rely on the fundamentally alienated linguistic structure to know the structure of desire that is alienated through the Imaginary and the Symbolic. However, simply opposing language itself may fall within the realm of dualistic thinking, which includes the subject-object dichotomy.

This aspect of Lacan is similar to the Seon meditation technique, which uses the paradoxical hwadu to divide the mind and overturn previously held preconceptions. Ganhwa-Seon and Lacan's psychoanalysis are not simply abstract theories, but describe an actual practice and treatment process. The actual experience of Seon (Chinese: 禅, Japanese: Zen) is the achievement of a state of no-self, where the separation between subject and object collapses into a fundamental unity free from attachment to the self and the world. In the context of Lacan's analytic therapy, during the stalemate of treatment where 'the patient is blocked and cannot do anything,' a sudden leap of insight shakes the subject to the core of illusion where the perception of the world was previously considered safe. The subject is then no longer captivated and can observe without clinging. Lacan emphasizes that in the context of analytic therapy, the patient's desire is something that continuously slips away from both their consciousness and the symptoms they experience. By naming and articulating this desire within the therapeutic setting, the patient gives it a conscious form, allowing it to be analyzed.

Conclusion

Eastern thought and Buddhist meditation, due to their nature of transcending human cognitive understanding, may elicit resistance among modern rational individuals towards concepts of self-transcendence. Similarly, Lacan's theories also present challenges for acceptance by contemporary individuals due to the incomprehensibility of the Real and related concepts. While it can be argued that Lacan's theories and meditation practices share implicit similarities in their goals and orientations, there are explicitly more differences than similarities.

Despite being thousands of years apart from each other, Lacan's theory and meditation practice have striking similarities from an ontological point of view. Through the process of practice and treatment, respectively, meditation and Lacan's theory demonstrate that the empirical and fixed notion of self is but a temporary illusion, and both teach a point beyond traditional empiricism, rationalism, and subject-object dualism.

Bibliography

Chew M. Words and emptiness: a comparison between Zen Buddhism and Lacanian psychoanalysis. Scribd; 2012. https://www.scribd.com/doc/60800159/Words-and-Emptiness-Zen-Buddhism-and-Lacanian-Psychoanalysis/.

Choe H-D, Shin S-W. Psychotherapeutic significance of the Buddhist thought of not-self(Anatta). J Korean Neuropsychiatr Assoc. 2005;44(6):754–62.

Evans D. An introductory dictionary of Lacanian psychoanalysis. Routledge; 1998.

Kabat-Zinn J. Mindfulness-based interventions in context: past, present, and future. Clin Psychol. 2003;10(2):144–56.

Kabat-Zinn J, Santorelli S. Mindfulness-based stress reduction in mind-body medicine: a 7-day professional training. Rhinebeck, New York: Omega institute for Holistic Studies; 2008.

Lee J. The implication of the eight noble path in Buddhism and Vipassanā meditation in children education. J Relig Educ Stud. 2010;33:299–323.

Meditation and Analytical Psychology

15

Sang Ick Han

Analytical psychology is a type of depth psychology founded by Swiss psychiatrist Carl G. Jung. Depth psychology refers to a psychology that acknowledges that the human mind has an unconscious. In that sense, meditation as discussed in psychoanalysis refers to the confrontation between the conscious and unconscious. The concept of the unconscious in analytical psychology differs from that in other forms of depth psychology, and consists of a personal unconscious that originates at an individual level and a collective unconscious that is shared at a universal level across humankind. In other words, with such a concept, meditation in analytical psychology can ultimately be seen as the confrontation within the unconscious between the collective unconscious and the individual conscious. Although analytical psychological psychotherapy mainly targets dreams and pictures, and provides treatment through dialectical dialogue based on the process of amplification,[1] once the therapy sufficiently progresses to the extent of experiential recognition of the unconscious, it begins to emphasize treatment through active meditation. Active meditation is a form of meditation in which, after dream analysis or picture analysis has progressed considerably, one actively calls upon the archetype image that arises from one's inner, collective unconscious and has a conversation with one's unconscious. Through this process, it can be said that active meditation, just as in dream analysis or picture analysis, attempts to achieve the integration of the conscious and the unconscious, or in other words, individuation that realizes totality by integrating Self and Ego or self-actualization that is the ultimate goal of analytical psychology.

Active meditation, just as the Chinese characters for meditation 冥想 (Míngxiǎng) means, 'quietly closing your eyes and putting your thoughts (冥, míng) to rest (想, xiǎng),' is closing your eyes, abandoning the passing thoughts from your conscious, holding onto the image that arise

[1] Amplification is psychological work with a practical purpose to understand the symbolic meaning of human dreams, fantasies, or delusions, and is a method of collecting personal and universal associations with a specific image as its focus. It differs from free association, which induces other associations from other images, since other images are evoked by association with one image. The unconscious complex can be expressed through free association, but Jung invented it because it is difficult to see it as the original symbol of the dream image that started free association. (See Yi Booyoung 2011, pp. 213–214).

S. I. Han (✉)
Institute of Analytical Psychology,
Seoul, South Korea
e-mail: hanpsy@catholic.ac.kr

J.-H. Chae, H.-Y. Lee (eds.), *Meditation in Psychiatry and General Medicine*,
https://doi.org/10.1007/978-981-95-7147-5_15

from your unconscious, and continuing to converse with the symbolic images that come to your mind. Meanwhile, it may be to 'realize with the mind's eye rather than the physical eye, the part that the discerning consciousness of daily life cannot capture, the salvation of phenomena that add new meaning, the understanding that there is nothing but everything in the world, that it is one with animals and plants, the whole nature and the whole universe, with a mind that has gone down to the depths and removed the conscious elements at the surface level,' which is generally what meditation seeks to achieve. Perhaps, once you reach that level, it is not different from achieving individuation as described in analytical psychology.

Meditation in Medieval Western Traditions

Through an analytic psychological research on alchemy, Jung attempted to reveal that the absurd explanations and assertions of alchemists are internal mental processes of humans, and to prove that they are universal primitive symbols of humankind which transcend era-specific and cultural characteristics. Although alchemists attempted to create the best materials through material changes in nature, they unknowingly projected their unconsciousness from the beginning to the end of the process of material change. In order to explain the secrets of matter, they projected another secret, their own unconscious. Projections are not made but rather occur. Alchemists understood their own projections as characteristics of matter, but what they actually experienced was their own unconscious. The material transformations, which are said to have occurred externally, symbolically expressed the process of transformation towards individuation that occurred in most alchemists' unconscious.

Alchemists have hallucinations or fantastical perceptual experiences while their actual work is being performed. Just as astrology creates images of constellations and imagines the figures of various animals including reptiles as well as the strange shapes of trees in fire, when alchemy is at work, one sees various colors or images appear that ordinary people cannot see with spiritual eyes, eyes of foresight, and eyes of the imagination in the most sincere attitude of contemplation. The saying in the book of alchemy, 'look with spiritual eyes at the process of growth of a small grain of wheat. Then you can see the Philosopher's Tree.' implies that the process of alchemy is a kind of active meditation. Additionally, by stressing that psychological conditions are absolutely necessary for this process, the words, 'true imagination, not phantasy, must be performed.' in *The Wise Man's Rose Garden* emphasize that the essential secret of alchemy is hidden in the human spirit, or in modern terms, the unconscious. Based on this, Jung said that the true meaning of imagination in the book of alchemy is meditation. Explaining the posture of meditation in the sense of analytical psychology, 'the human mind agrees with the work of alchemy, which surpasses all else, and in order to acquire the "golden understanding" one must keep the eyes of the spirit and the soul open and must observe and recognize the inner light that has kindled one's heart.' Regarding this, Jung explains the parallel relationship between the work of alchemy and the philosophical-psychological process, wherein if one is a practical and chemical experiment in a laboratory, the other is a psychological process, sometimes a conscious mental process, or sometimes a material projected unconsciously in the process of projection. Jung therefore emphasized that one should start with a free and empty mind.

According to *The Complete Master's Manual*, in alchemy, the psychological and personality conditions that alchemists must possess include having a delicate mind and sufficient knowledge of metals and materials. An alchemist should not have a rough and rigid mind, or be greedy, have material greed, indecision, or capriciousness, nor should they be in a hurry or have hasty imaginations. Instead, they should have firm determination, perseverance, patience, gentleness, relaxedness, and moderation. Additionally, *The Wise Man's Rose Garden* mentions conditions of being pious, upright, considerate, kind, having a bright facial expression, and a cheerful heart.

This suggests that a considerable degree of personal maturity is first required to become an alchemist.

If you look at the dictionary definition of meditation in alchemy in *Ruland's Lexicon Alchemie*, it is defined as 'an inner dialogue with someone unseen.' The 'someone unseen,' appearing as a deity or an angel, suggests that Western alchemists place a higher spiritual value on god-like beings than their Eastern counterparts. In this practice, alchemy is not merely physical; it is a process of infusing spirit into matter through a creative dialogue with the Divine. Consequently, the stone becomes spiritualized, while the alchemist achieves a state of volatility and sublimation—freeing themselves from external manipulation and humbling themselves through an act of free will. Alchemy involves infusing more spirit into the stones alchemists work with, especially through creative dialogue between themselves and God. In other words, this means that the stones become more spiritualized and that one becomes more volatile and sublimating by freeing oneself from all manipulation and lowering oneself with free will.

Alchemists' imagination gives special meaning to their proper work and is actually the key to opening the 'door of work.' 'Imagination is either the start within a human being, heaven, or a body that transcends heaven.' The illusory process was never regarded as a substanceless illusion, but rather as a 'subtle body' of something physical, a half-mental nature. It can be said that such concrete theory inevitably became dominant in an era where there is no empirical psychology. The unconscious mind that is activated while an alchemist works is projected onto material objects. In other words, it can be said that the unconscious comes from the outside in that it is activated by material stimuli that come from the outside during alchemy work. The unconscious, which originates from matter, is to some extent a spiritual-material-anti-yin-yang being. The 'imagination' or the act of imagining is a physical activity that intervenes in the cyclical process of material change, which both acts and is also acted upon. Alchemists not only establish a relationship with the unconscious, but also a direct relationship with the substances they hope to transform through their imagination. In this sense, imagination is a deep extract derived from life-giving physical power and soul power.

In alchemy, the transformation of substances first went through a four-stage process. Afterwards, it came down to transformation into the best substance, and eventually changed into three stages. The transformation of the mind that occurs during the projection of the unconscious can be seen to reach the highest levels in the third and fourth stages. The first stage is that of blackening (nigredo, melanosis) and is a state of the original matter (prima materia), a mass of 'chaos' (massa confusa). The second stage is that of whitening (albedo, leukosis), and is a state of dawn, of silver, or of the moon. The third stage was that of turning into gold (citrinitas, xanthosis), but it disappeared in the fifteenth and sixteenth centuries. The final stage is that of reddening (rubedo, iosis), which symbolizes the state of the sun. The four-stage composition of alchemy is consistent with the four-stage unity of the elements, symbolized by the four elements (earth, water, air, fire), or four qualities (hot, cold, wet, dry). It was eventually reduced to three stages, symbolized by three primary colors (black, white, red). It can be seen as related to the internal and spiritual reason why Christian dogma is a Trinity rather than a Quadrinity that includes femininity or the devil, opposite of God. The third or fourth stages of conversion, which are achieved through the projection of the unconscious during the process of alchemy, are ultimately a mental transformation process that occurs through the imaginary process which alchemists perform during their work. In an analytical psychological sense, they are eventually singled out.

Among other meditation practices in the Western tradition, Jung also explained his active meditation in the light of the spiritual exercises of St. Ignatius of Loyola. Spiritual practice is a retreat generally conducted over a period of 30 days and is a personal process between the instructor and the retreatant. The process consists of progression from the first week (sin and reflection, mainly Christian meditation), to the second week (the incarnation and life of Jesus Christ, mainly contemplation), the third week (participation in the process of Christ's passion), and the fourth week (renewal with the resurrected Christ). Specific methods of spiritual training include Christian meditation and the subsequent step of contemplation, which involves continuously contemplating God using one's imagination. It involves drawing a contemplative scene in your mind and remaining within it, seeing people, listening to them, and observing how they behave with your imagination. In addition, prayer using the application of the five senses is also practiced along with spiritual discourse (colloquy), which is a personal inner conversation with divine images such as that of Christ, the Virgin Mary, the Holy Trinity, and so on. Jung viewed the spiritual training of Christian meditation as a petition (petito) rather than a prayer (oratio), and as a reflection of typical Western extroversion rather than the practice of Eastern meditation, which focuses entirely on introverted inner facts. However, although it is true that the experience of God during spiritual training is an object of awe and worship, ultimately, it is about emptying one's mind and sinking into immersion for inner unity with God. Since an internal transformation is achieved through the introverted result of discovering the Christ that exists in one's heart, it is an introverted result that uses an extroverted framework, and can therefore be seen as introversion. What Jung's active meditation and Saint Ignatious's spiritual exercises have in common is that both use imagination. On the other hand, the difference between the two is that active meditation is a method for the conscious ego to reach the unconscious, and is for individuation, where the ego achieves wholeness with the self. It is extremely personal and has no set framework. On the other hand, spiritual training is a religious way to reach God, and it provides a framework for those to practice it to meet Christ.

Meditation in Analytical Psychology

Techniques of analytical psychological psychotherapy include dream analysis, picture analysis, and active meditation. The purpose of Jungian psychotherapy is to achieve individuation by integrating the conscious and unconscious through their encounter with each other. Active meditation is a method of self-reflection that transfers the contents of the unconscious into consciousness through fantasy and builds a bridge to enable the mental transformation process. It is an attempt to improve treatment outcomes by promoting self-realization (individuation) by focusing on meditation, and is in line with monasticism and self-reflection.

As a psychiatrist, Jung discovered through a series of early association experiments a key element in understanding the unconscious in 'the complex,' a mental element that emphasizes emotions that are not controlled by consciousness. Afterwards, although he tried Freud's psychoanalytic dream interpretation, he could not fully understand the patient's unconscious and could not expect to achieve the goal of wholeness, which in turn was the goal of treatment. Additionally, during the period of introversion (1913–1919) after breaking off from Freud, Jung was in a difficult state internally. While trying to overcome the difficulties he was facing as a therapist who treats patients, he discovered active meditation through his experiences. Active meditation is one of Jung's greatest accomplishments aside from dream analysis. By thoroughly focusing one's consciousness on mental images that arise naturally from the unconscious and controlling the emotions, fantasies, obsessions, daydreams, etc. that arise in the unconscious, one actively brings content to their consciousness without any sense of caution or criticism, and has a dialogue with it as if it were an object external to oneself. By paying attention to the internal image, the mental energy (libido) that was available in the conscious mind is transferred to the unconscious mind. During this process, the unconscious libido increases, allowing a series of stimulated images to meaningfully appear in the inner eye. During active meditation, the conscious self actively participates in the unconscious. As the conscious and unconscious gradually accept each other's positions and responsibilities, a confrontation between the two takes place. Active meditation is a method of investigating the self, and although it is more empirical and scientific, it is not a new method. There have been many examples in the past of people discovering similar methods to establish a relationship with forces stronger and more eternal than themselves. Contacting 'the Lord' or trying to hear the invisible word of the Lord as laid out in the Old Testament, an African tribe chieftain having a big dream to solve their difficult problems, shamans communicating with spirits, Christian meditation or contemplative prayer, the Catholic spiritual training of St. Ignatius, medieval alchemy, yoga, Tibetan esoteric meditation, Eastern Taoist health regimen (道家 養生術), and Zen in Buddhism can all be seen as similar attempts. If there is a difference between active meditation and religious meditation, the former is personal, lacks a given plan, and traces the just-so-story in the unconscious. Although it can be said to be most similar to the practices of Zen Buddhism, it differs in its perspective on dreams.

There are two types of fantasies that appear during active meditation. One is an active fantasy and the other is a passive fantasy. An active fantasy is one seen in active meditation and is a posture that seeks to intuitively recognize the unconscious. This means that there is a high degree of clarity as the libido immediately captures all elements that occur in the unconscious and associates all relevant data. Here, there is the possibility of recognition, the conscious and the unconscious show a positive attitude of participation rather than an antagonistic relationship, and the process of the unconscious is characterized by a complementary rather than an antagonistic relationship with the conscious. This can be seen as the highest human mental activity. A passive fantasy is a passive, non-intuitive state, and is a fantasy that is seen when a dissociative state tends to be in opposition to consciousness. On the other hand, as a meaningless phantasm, a fantasy has a temporary meaning, is created by the person themselves, and is based on conscious expectations on the surface of personal matters. In this sense, the word meditation (imagination) is a more appropriate term than fantasy. Active meditation is not useful for everyone. While some will benefit from trying it, forcing it will not be beneficial to others. Typically done at the end of analysis, active meditation objectifies the image so that the image replaces the dream, and so that all mental data is acquired in a creative form, even without a dream. Since all data is generated from the conscious mind, interpretation or judgment may be impossible in some cases. Nonetheless, it is more complete than the language of dreams and contains more than what dreams imply. Thus, it can be considered to be much more beneficial than dream data.

The Process of Active Meditation

Active meditation begins with emptying one's self-consciousness. Liberating oneself from egoic thinking is applicable to most Eastern methods of meditation, and is also a central goal of Zen Buddhist practice. Through active meditation, fantasies that arise from the unconscious are allowed and turned into objects of internal contemplation. This differs from Eastern methods of meditation, which ignore dreams and illusions. However, we must not be so obsessed with fantasy that we block it from flowing out, nor must we not be so careful that our inner good changes endlessly. We can communicate with images by giving them form to internally perceived fantasies such as writing, sculpture, painting, or dance, and for psychosomatic physical symptoms, we can also internally communicate with the affected organs. However, one should not focus too much on aesthetic work, nor should one leave the form to its own devices and think about its meaning first. Finally, at the critical stage, we must face moral questions as our real selves, not as the illusions and virtual selves that have emerged. [Example: mistakes such as hiding the fact that a person is married when a female image (anima) appears in a man].

There are some cases where active meditation is difficult to apply. In cases of latent psychosis or borderline personality disorder, it can be difficult to face the fantasies that arise from the unconscious as the strength of one's ego is weak. Overly intelligent people may also find it difficult to succeed because their intellectual abilities tend to be deceptive and can hinder moral confrontation. A certain level of innocence where there is no true awe towards fantasy is necessary. When something irrational or incomprehensible happens, we must be in a position to solely accept the fact that it happened. Mobilizing the critical abilities of one's thorough consciousness to select only what the consciousness accepts is a valuable attitude. It is taboo to engage in active meditation while being obsessed with the principle of power that seeks to exert supernatural abilities to dominate others. The image of a living person should not be adopted as the object of meditation. One must seriously pursue the totality of the unknown and carry out one's practice with as scientific of an attitude as possible, and those who lack a mature function of their ego must practice active meditation through a solid human relationship that can understand and sympathize with them.

The following are situations where practicing active meditation is helpful. It can be tried first to (1) reduce the amount of excessive dreams (in particular dreams that end with a question mark or illusions during hypothesis are much closer to consciousness and therefore simpler) for those whose unconscious mind is overflowing with lucid fantasies, especially those who are very rational and intelligent, (2) when conversely there is an excessive lack of dreams, (3) when emotional disorders (anger, depression, despair) are the starting point of a problem, (4) when there is a vague feeling of discomfort, weariness, nausea, pain, or something that cannot be defined, (5) when there is a problem with adapting to one's life (this is one of the most frequent reasons for analysis), (6) when one's disability is severe, or (7) when the same mistakes are being made repeatedly.

If, during active meditation, the shadow archetypes of the collective unconscious appear as images in meditation or dreams or are arranged in one's external reality, one may encounter unexpected misfortune or hardship. If one experiences a crisis both within and outside of oneself, one experiences negative emotions such as depression, or one feels that evil is rampant around them, one must be vigilant and exercise caution.

When practicing active meditation, one must have an awe towards one's consciousness and expectations around its creativity, an ethical duty of self-reflection to seek out everything with humility, and a sincere and devout religious attitude.

Conclusion

Currently, active meditation is not actively applied in clinical practice. Perhaps there is a reason why Jung's analytical psychological methods of psychotherapy are not yet well known. The mental world of human beings has transcendental elements that are difficult to accept solely through a logical and rational brain. Although mystical and intuitive judgments based on Eastern thought or meditation are asked for at times, it may be difficult to accept them in situations where the rationality of modern and contemporary natural science is prioritized.

While explaining the sixteen-step process of meditation that appears in the Amitabha Zen Meditation Sutra (阿彌陀禪經), a Chinese Buddhist scripture on yogic meditation translated from Sanskrit, Jung spoke of concentrating on flashy and complex images in the path of yogic meditation just like active meditation, and he also pointed out the similarities between the psychotherapy of analytical psychology and Zen (禪) meditation in Buddhism. Jung also mentioned the differences between Easterners and Westerners regarding religious attitudes. Westerners build high altars to elevate their spirit and try to overcome their external reality and the world, while Easterners build deep altars to enter the depths of their minds and seek inner devotion and a return to nature. For example, Jung stated that while Western churches have high altars and their religious practices include prayer, worship, and song, altars of religious practitioners in India are located two to three meters below the basement of the temple, and yoga is their foundational practice in order to enter the world of absorption (dhyāna), meditation, and the depths of their minds.

In Christianity, one never says during meditation, 'I am Jesus Christ.' Paul says, 'I no longer live as myself, but Jesus Christ lives in me' (Galatians, 2:20). However, in Buddhism, it is said that 'I will attain enlightenment that I am the Buddha.' Christianity achieves its goal within Jesus Christ, whereas in Buddhism one realizes that they are the Buddha. Christianity is about leaving the impermanent and self-obsessed world of consciousness. On the other hand, Buddhists differ in that they believe one's inner nature is divine and one with the essence of the universe based on the eternal foundation of one's inner nature.

The appearance of flashy and complex images in the process of yogic meditation is similar to active meditation in that the practice of meditation for the latter continues while one looks at similar circular images. These extroverted West and introverted East are both one-sided. While at first glance, there may be some resistance among Asians who have become enlightened by the words Zen Buddhism and Confucius, but when looking at it again, there may be another way to express 'one path' or the state of unity. The East underestimates consciousness, while the West downplays one mind, one heart. The West is passionate about objectivity, while the East promotes wisdom, peace, liberation, and steadfastness of spirit. Such one-sidedness is not completely bad, and the human spirit cannot distinguish or develop without this one-sidedness. Through introversion in the West and extroversion in the East, we may be able to achieve harmony between introversion and extroversion, between material and spirit, and unity between consciousness and unconsciousness without following each other's footsteps. Yoga, Zen, Tao Te Ching, the Tibetan Book of the Dead, I Chin, Oriental Lao-tzu philosophy, Confucianism, and Buddhist thought have surprising similarities with the individuation process of analytical psychology. They are in line with the introverted spirit of the West, which has been hidden in the extroverted history of the West from ancient Greece through the Middle Ages to modern times. It is pointless to overemphasize the differences between Eastern and Western thought or to consider which is better or worse. Instead, it is important to understand their mutual differences while at the same time respecting their common human foundations.

At a time when medical meditation and meditation science are gradually emerging, it can be said that the time has come to move forward to develop a new, more practical and scientific method of meditation that integrates consciousness and unconsciousness, rationality and irrationality.

Bibliography

Chang-in Y, Boo-yeong Y. Active meditation (적극적 명상). Bull Psychiatr. 1981;5:303–8.

Han J-G. The philosophical foundations of meditation (명상의 철학적 기초). Seoul: Ewha Womans University Press and Culture Center; 2007.

Jung CG. Psychology and alchemy. 2nd ed. London: Routledge and Kegan Paul Ltd.; 1968.

Jung CG. Psychology and religion, east and *west*. 2nd ed. London: Routledge and Kegan Paul Ltd.; 1969.

Jung CG. The idea of salvation seen in alchemy (연금술에서 본 구원의 관념) (Erloesungsvorstellungen in der Alchemie). Trans. Korea Finance Research Institute. Seoul, Sol Publishing; 2004.

Kim J-T. Analytical psychological considerations on the 'spiritual exercises' of saint Inatius of Loyola (로욜라의 이나시오 성인의 '영신 수련'에 대한 분석심리학적 고찰). Mental Res. 2010;25:27–64.

Shin Y-w. Analytical psychological meaning of the refinement technique in Yongho's secret (용호비결에 나타난 연단술의 분석심리학적 의미). Mental Res. 2018;33:141–94.

Yi B-Y. Analytical psychology: C. G. Jung's Theory of the human mind (3rd edition) (분석심리학: C. G. 융의 인간심성론(3판)). Seoul: One Piece Publishing; 2011.

Yi S-I. Research on transference in analytical psychology (분석심리학에서의 전이에 관한 연구). Mental Res. 2018;33:99–140.

16 Loving-Kindness, Compassion, and Self-Compassion Meditation

Kyoung-Uk Lee

The term mindfulness began to spread in American psychology and psychiatry when Jon Kabat-Zinn began distributing the mindfulness-based stress reduction (MBSR) program after establishing the Stress Reduction Clinic at the University of Massachusetts Medical School in 1979. Clinical application and research on mindfulness-based interventions became prevalent in the late 1970s and 1980s with the pioneering work of Jon Kabat-Zinn. Subsequently, other researchers and clinicians began developing additional mindfulness-based approaches, including dialectical behavior therapy by Marsha Linehan in the late 1980s and mindfulness-based cognitive therapy by Teasdale, Segal, and Williams in the late 1990s. These developments contributed to the growing interest in and application of mindfulness-based interventions in various therapeutic contexts.

Meanwhile, political, social, and environmental issues such as conflict, competition, violence, and war prevalent in modern society naturally aroused interest in human coexistence and cooperation. Consequently, Western academia turned its attention to the development and cultivation of positive attributes such as altruism, empathy, communication, and compassion as potential solutions to these problems. In particular, the emergence of compassion, often referred to as the second stage of the mindfulness revolution, was triggered when the Dalai Lama founded the Mind and Life Institute in 1987. Through this institute, he promoted a multidisciplinary approach to alleviate human suffering by integrating Buddhist practice and wisdom with modern science. Afterward, various compassion training programs have been developed and scientifically evaluated at numerous universities and institutions, including Emory University, the Center for Compassion and Altruism Research and Education at Stanford University, the Max Planck Institute for Human Cognitive and Brain Sciences, and the Center for Healthy Minds at the University of Wisconsin-Madison. It is noteworthy that these programs are expanding their scope of application by minimizing religious elements and are accumulating scientific evidence for compassion meditation by employing scientific methods such as neuropsychology and brain imaging. Additionally, self-compassion meditation, a form of compassion meditation focused on the self, has been introduced and is rapidly gaining popularity as an effective approach to overcome the self-critical and isolated psychological states experienced by individuals in modern society, which is dominated by achievement-oriented values. This practice emphasizes cultivating kindness and understanding towards oneself, par-

K.-U. Lee (✉)
Department of Psychiatry, Uijeongbu St. Mary's Hospital, College of Medicine, The Catholic University of Korea, Seoul, Republic of Korea

J.-H. Chae, H.-Y. Lee (eds.), *Meditation in Psychiatry and General Medicine*,
https://doi.org/10.1007/978-981-95-7147-5_16

ticularly in response to self-criticism and feelings of isolation.

In this chapter, I will first introduce the concepts of loving-kindness, compassion, and self-compassion, and will subsequently examine each of their respective meditation practices.

Loving-Kindness and Compassion in Buddhism

Loving-kindness was introduced in the Metta Sutta in the Suttanipata of early Indian Buddhism. The word "metta" is translated from Pali to English to mean benevolence, loving-kindness, friendliness, amity and goodwill. Compassion was introduced alongside two other sublime qualities that should be cultivated. Altogether, there are four "immeasurables": loving-kindness (metta), compassion (karuna), appreciative joy (mudita) and equanimity (upekkha). They appear in the Early Buddhist Pali Canon in the Tevijja Sutta (the Threefold Knowledge) and Subha Sutta. Loving-kindness refers to a state of the mind that wishes for the happiness and well-being of all sentient beings, including oneself. In Buddhism, compassion is distinguished from loving-kindness in that compassion refers to the wish for all beings to be free from suffering. It is known that practicing loving-kindness can overcome anger, ill will and hatred, whereas the cultivation of compassion serves as an antidote to cruelty.

In Mahayana Buddhism, the aim is to realize Buddhahood, not for oneself alone, but to help all sentient beings achieve enlightenment. Thus, the great compassion (Mahākaruṇā) is considered the prerequisite for wisdom (prajñā) and arises from the recognition of emptiness (sunyata) and non-self (anatman). Understanding the interdependent nature of all phenomena allows for the expression of unconditional, limitless loving-kindness and compassion towards all beings. This perspective marks a clear distinction from Western psychology. In Western psychology, compassion is often viewed as an act of one individual showing mercy to another, based on a sense of separate selves. However, in Buddhism, the distinction between those who show compassion and those who receive it dissolves in the light of nondiscrimination (non-duality) and the realization of non-self.

Tibetan Buddhism has long recognized compassion as a fundamental human potential, studied methods to enhance it, and views it as the key to happiness and profound spiritual transformation. In this tradition, the cultivation and practice of great compassion (Mahākaruṇā) is emphasized and considered as the stepping-stone to bodhicitta (the awakening mind). This approach is well-established in Lamrim (Tibetan: "the stages of the path to enlightenment"), a systematic set of textual instructions. Atisha laid out this step-by-step approach, based on an individual's spiritual capacity, in his book, "Lamp for the Path of Awakening," which became the foundation for the Lamrim tradition. Tsongkhapa, one of Tibet's most influential figures, expanded on this in his celebrated treatise "Lam Rim Chenmo" (The Great Exposition on the Stages of the Path to Enlightenment). Later, Geshe Chekawa arranged and summarized Atishas' teachings into a collection of fifty-nine mind-training (Tibetan, lojong) slogans. Lojong, a core practice in the Tibetan tradition, aims to transform the mind by turning away from self-centeredness and cultivating mental habits that generate bodhicitta. Tonglen, one of these lojong practices, involves the practitioner cultivating compassion by imaginatively taking in others' suffering while giving out happiness to all sentient beings during the breathing process.

Loving-Kindness and Compassion in Psychology

The definition of compassion in psychology aligns closely with Buddhist perspectives, as both emphasize the importance of engaging with suffering and acting to alleviate it. Kanov defined compassion as consisting of three processes that occur in the interaction between oneself and others during suffering: attention to or noticing another's suffering, experiencing an emotional reaction to the suffering, and acting to lessen or relieve pain. Paul Gilbert defined compassion as a "sensitivity to the pain in oneself and others with a commitment to try to alleviate and prevent it." Gilbert introduced an evolutionary perspective, linking compassion to the development of caring behavior, altruism and prosocial behavior in general. Paul Ekman viewed compassion as a response to the suffering of another person, categorizing it into four types based on the focus of one's response: empathetic, action-oriented, concerned, and aspirational compassion. Ekman later proposed the concept of "global compassion," emphasizing the need to alleviate suffering regardless of nationality, language, culture, or religion and insisted that human society should move towards global compassion. Goetz conceptualized compassion as a distinct emotion with specific appraisal processes, signaling behavior, and response profiles. He described compassion as an affective state attuned to suffering, which elicits caring behaviors (e.g., touch, posture and vocalization) and physiological responses that orient the individual toward social approach.

Self-Compassion

In 2003, Kritsin Neff introduced the concept of self-compassion, drawing from Buddhist psychology, as an alternative to self-esteem in measuring psychological health. Self-compassion is extending compassion to oneself in instances of perceived inadequacy, failure, or general suffering. It involves being kind and understanding toward oneself rather than harshly self-critical.

Neff distinguishes self-compassion from self-esteem: while self-esteem involves a positive evaluation of self-worth, self-compassion does not stem from judgments or evaluations. Instead, self-compassion acknowledges the imperfect human condition and relates to oneself with kindness and acceptance in the face of failure. This distinction is crucial, as an excessive focus on improving self-esteem in modern Western society may contribute to negative outcomes such as narcissism, self-centeredness, and a lack of concern for others. Moreover, the comparative nature of self-esteem can increase vulnerability to negative emotions when individuals perceive themselves as falling short.

Research has shown that self-criticism is strongly associated with various psychiatric disorders, including depression, anxiety, and suicide. Self-compassion appears to be a crucial attribute for individuals exposed to mental health threats in highly competitive modern society. It offers a beneficial alternative to self-esteem and, importantly, serves as an antidote to self-criticism. This makes self-compassion particularly relevant in the treatment of psychiatric disorders where self-criticism plays a significant role, such as depression, anxiety, and suicide.

Neff addressed common misconceptions about self-compassion in Western culture, such as the belief that it is weak, self-indulgent, or undermines motivation. She provided empirical evidence countering these misunderstandings. Numerous studies have since investigated self-compassion using self-report measures, examined the effects of self-compassion training on psychosocial outcomes, and explored how experimentally induced self-compassionate states affect behavior.

The Western emphasis on independence and individuation in psychology tends to focus on maintaining and strengthening the self. However, this approach may exacerbate feelings of separation from others and personal suffering through isolation. In contrast, Buddhism views the concept of "self" as a source of human suffering, advocating for minimizing the self and experiencing non-self to achieve authentic happiness. Recent criticisms have been raised regarding the artificial distinction between compassion and self-compassion, leading to further exploration of the role of self in self-compassion.

In conclusion, self-compassion offers a promising approach to improving mental health, particularly in addressing the harmful effects of self-criticism. Its application in the treatment of psychiatric patients could provide a valuable tool in managing depression, anxiety, and suicidal tendencies, making it an important area for continued research and clinical practice.

Mindfulness, Compassion, and Compassion Fatigue

Mindfulness training is a form of insight meditation that develops the ability to regulate cognition and emotion by cultivating non-judgmental attention to present-moment experiences of body sensations, emotions, and thoughts. In contrast, loving-kindness and compassion meditation are often considered forms of concentrative meditation that focus on specific objects or individuals while cultivating positive emotions of benevolence and compassion. While mindfulness primarily targets current experiences that occur in the body and mind, loving-kindness meditation often employs visualization techniques.

The relationship between mindfulness and compassion has been debated. Some argue that mindfulness practice naturally fosters compassion, while others contend that compassion should be cultivated directly, independent of mindfulness. When practicing compassion, mindfulness of one's own reactions to others' suffering is crucial, as it allows for empathy without becoming overwhelmed. This mindful approach also helps prevent compassion fatigue.

Compassion fatigue is generally defined as the emotional and physical exhaustion that can affect helping professionals and caregivers over time. It results from prolonged exposure to the suffering of others and the stress of caring. Some researchers argue that "compassion fatigue" is a misnomer, as true compassion does not lead to fatigue or negative outcomes. According to Buddhist traditions, compassion is associated with the intention for others to be free from suffering, potentially evoking positive or even joyful states of mind rather than negative states of mind or sadness. Moreover, recent neuroscientific research supports the idea that compassion training can increase positive affect and prosocial behavior. Due to these concerns, some researchers have suggested alternative terms such as "empathy fatigue," "secondary traumatic stress."

Loving-Kindness and Compassion Meditation

Traditional Buddhist Compassion Meditation

In Theravada Buddhism, meditation practices are prescribed to develop the four sublime states of mind (Brahma-vihara, divine states of mind, divine abidings). These four immeasurables are loving-kindness, compassion, sympathetic joy, and equanimity, which are states of mind that regard all living beings as infinitely dear and precious. Loving-kindness (metta) is the wish for all beings to be healthy and happy, without discrimination or attachment. Compassion (karuna) is the wish for all beings to be free from suffering and the causes of suffering. Sympathetic joy (mudita) is the ability to rejoice in others' happiness, serving as an antidote to envy. Equanimity (upekkha) is a balanced mind, free from discrimination and rooted in insight.

Buddhaghosa's "The Path of Purification" (Vissudhimagga) outlines a method of loving-kindness meditation using phrases. The practitioner begins by reflecting on the dangers of hatred and the benefits of patience. Then, one repeats phrases such as:

May I be happy and free from suffering
May I be free from enmity
May I be free from afflictions
May I be free from anxiety
May I live happily

After beginning by focusing on oneself, the practitioner gradually extends the practice to include loved ones such as friends, neutral individuals, and even those they dislike or are hostile towards. It is not directed towards the opposite sex or the deceased.

For compassion meditation, Buddhaghosa suggests first contemplating the disadvantages of lacking compassion and the advantages of cultivating it. The practitioner begins with a suffering person, thinking: "This being has indeed been reduced to misery; if only they could be freed from this suffering!" This compassionate mindset is then extended to loved ones, neutral people, and hostile persons successively. Likewise with loving-kindness, one should not direct compassion towards dear people of the opposite sex or towards the deceased at first. These practices aim to cultivate a mind that regards all beings with equal care and concern, fostering a state of universal compassion.

Tibetan Buddhist Practice

Tibetan Buddhism, a form of Mahayana Buddhism, emphasizes the development of bodhicitta (awakening mind), which is the altruistic intention to attain enlightenment for the benefit of all sentient beings. Tsongkhapa, known as the founder of Tibetan Buddhism, suggested two main methods for cultivating bodhicitta: the sevenfold cause-and-effect instruction and the method of exchanging self and others. The sevenfold cause-and-effect instruction includes the following steps: (1) recognizing all beings as having been one's mothers in previous lives, (2) recollecting their kindness, (3) wishes to repay that kindness, (4) cultivating loving-kindness, (5) developing great compassion, (6) generating the extraordinary intention to take responsibility for their welfare, and (7) generating bodhicitta itself. The method of exchanging self and other, combined with the practice of tonglen (giving and taking), is known as lojong (mind training). This practice involves: (1) equalizing self and others, (2) contemplating the disadvantage of self-centeredness, (3) reflecting on the benefits of cherishing others, (4) the actual exchange of self and others, and (5) the meditation on giving and taking (tonglen). In tonglen meditation, practitioners imaginatively take on the sufferings of others and then their own happiness. This process aims to reduce self-centeredness and foster a deeper connection with others and the nature of existence. Tonglen has been adopted and incorporated into various modern psychological and contemplative practices.

Tibetan Buddhist approaches to compassion often emphasize both the emotional (affective) and intellectual (cognitive) aspects of compassion, influencing how modern interventions conceptualize and teach compassion. Tibetan Buddhist compassion practices have inspired several contemporary secular compassion training programs, such as Cognitively-Based Compassion Training (CBCT) developed at Emory University, Compassion Cultivation Training (CCT) developed at Stanford University.

Domestic and International Programs

While Buddhism traditionally distinguishes between loving-kindness (metta) and compassion (karuna), many contemporary meditation programs often combine or use these practices interchangeably. This integration is common in secular mindfulness-based interventions, where loving-kindness and compassion meditations are frequently taught together or as part of a broader program. In Korea, various loving-kindness and compassion programs have been developed, drawing from multiple sources including Buddhism tradition, Gilbert's Compassion-Focused Therapy (CFT) or Compassionate Mind Training (CMT), and Germer & Neff's Mindful Self-Compassion (MSC) program. These adaptations reflect a growing interest in compassion-based interventions within Korean mental health contexts.

It's important to note that due to the limitations of the literature review and space constraints, this overview may not encompass all existing programs, both internationally and within Korea. The field of compassion-based interventions is rapidly evolving, with new programs and adaptations continually emerging.

Loving-Kindness Meditation (LKM)

Loving-kindness meditation (LKM) is a type of concentration meditation aimed at developing cognitive, motivational, and emotional changes through the cultivation of benevolence, kindness, and warmth towards oneself and others. LKM has social characteristics as it extends the object of meditation from oneself to others, fostering feelings of social connection even towards unknown individuals. Sharon Salzberg, a prominent LKM teacher, introduced a practice that involves repeating phrases such as “May I be safe, be happy, be healthy, live with ease.” Recognizing that Western practitioners often struggle with self-directed LKM, Salzberg suggested beginning by thinking about someone who has helped you.

In Korea, Ven. Misan Sunim developed the Heart-Smile Training (HST) based on Mahayana Buddhist philosophy and Zen Buddhism, which teach that we are all naturally endowed with boundless wisdom and compassion. The HST aims to awaken innate loving-kindness through various practices, ultimately leading to an experience of wholeness in the present moment. It consists of a main meditation practice and four auxiliary meditation practices. The main practice provides a full experience of wholeness by filling the body and mind with a feeling of warmth produced from a gentle and warm smile. Auxiliary meditation practices consist of (1) Heart-Smile Gratitude and Acceptance, (2) Heart-Smile Movement 33, (3) Heart-Smile Body Scan and (4) Sound Meditation. The HST is characterized by practices that directly evoke loving-kindness through the body and mind, providing an experiential understanding of oneself and the world as it is.

Jae-Sung Kim developed a loving-kindness-based insight meditation program drawing from Buddhagosa's The Path of Purification and Mahasi tradition. This program aims to realize nirvana through vipassana meditation, supported by the deep concentration attained through loving-kindness meditation. The preparation stage involves asking for and giving forgiveness, a practice influenced by Sayadaw U Janaka of the Mahasi tradition. The LKM practice then progresses from oneself to various categories of individuals: those who are grateful to or respect, loved ones, neutral persons, and finally, those we dislike. The insight meditation (Vipassana) component of Kim's program fosters self-awareness of the body, thoughts, feelings, and emotions through sitting and walking meditation, as well as mindfulness in daily activities.

Compassion Meditation (CM)

In the Korean Buddhist tradition, notable compassion meditation practices have been developed by Venerable Maga Sunim and Jiwoon Sunim. Maga Sunim's program, rooted in Buddhist principles, includes meditations on gratitude for rice, self-acceptance, and positive regard for spouses, family members, and colleagues, and a concluding meditation (prostrations, shared meditation, praising meditation). This program has been adapted for various demographics, including couples, families, office workers, children, teenagers, college students, and the elderly. Jiwoon Sunim's compassion meditation program incorporates compassionate hand contemplation, compassionate tea meditation, and compassionate walking meditation. The compassionate hand contemplation involves visualizing a compassionate hand delivering love and compassion to one's body, while reflecting on the Buddhist concepts of the four elements and emptiness through observing the three characteristics of impermanence, suffering and non-self.

In Western countries, several evidence-based compassion cultivation programs have been developed within academic settings. Cognitively-Based Compassion Training (CBCT), developed by Geshe Lobsang Tenzin Negi at Emory University in 2004, is based on the Indo-Tibetan Buddhist lojong tradition. This eight-week program aims to cultivate empathy, prosocial skills, and social connectivity through six modules: attention stability and clarity, insight into the nature of mental experience, self-compassion/self-acceptance, cultivating impartiality/inclusiveness, gratitude and affection, and empathetic concern and engaged compassion. These modules represent the two primary categories of skill development including resilience and compassion. CBCT employs analytical meditation to shift one's perspective from self-centeredness to altruism, emphasizing interconnectedness. A number of research projects have been conducted on various groups such as those with PTSD, parents with children with autism, depressed patients, and people who have attempted suicide.

Compassion Cultivation Training (CCT) was developed in 2012 by Thupten Jinpa in collaboration with a team of psychologists, neuroscientists, and contemplative scholars at the Center for Compassion and Altruism Research and Education (CCARE) at Stanford University. Jinpa, who is the Founder and Chairman of Compassion Institute, served as the principal author of CCT. The program was designed as a secular, eight-week course to cultivate compassion, empathy, and kindness for others and oneself. Like CBCT, CCT draws inspiration from Indo-Tibetan Buddhist traditions but has been adapted into a non-religious format applicable to various groups and individuals. This program consists of weekly 2-h sessions that include group discussion, lectures, in-class practices, and homework assignments. Through this cohort-based experience, participants develop skills in mindfulness, self-compassion, and compassion for others. CCT comprises six progressive steps: (1) settling the mind, (2) cultivating loving-kindness and compassion for loved ones, (3) self-directed compassion and kindness, (4) embracing shared common humanity, (5) cultivating compassion for others, and (6) active compassion training. The effectiveness of CCT is dose-dependent and does not treat psychopathology or replace psychotherapy. Research has shown CCT to improve compassion across multiple domains, enhance emotion and cognitive regulation, and decrease worrying and suppression of emotions.

Paul Gilbert developed Compassion Focused Therapy (CFT) to address shame and self-criticism by integrating concepts from evolutionary psychology, social psychology, Bolby's attachment theory, Buddhist psychology, and neuroscience. CFT posits that humans have evolved with three primary emotion regulation systems: the threat system, the drive system, and the affiliative/soothing. According to CFT, the human capacity for reasoning, reflection, and mentalization, which evolved later, is easily influenced by these emotional control systems. When faced with negative events, cognitive processes such as reflection, negative bias, and self-criticism can activate negative emotions, potentially leading to mental health problems. Conversely, self-compassion is theorized to activate the soothing system, which can deactivate the threat protection system. In CFT, compassion is conceptualized as emerging from a social motivational system that enables engagement with distress and promotes caring and kind responses to the needs of self and others. The primary therapeutic technique of CFT is compassionate mind training (CMT), which includes strategies to help individuals develop experiences of inner warmth, safety, and soothing. These strategies include appreciation exercises, mindfulness practices, and compassion-focused imagery exercises. A significant focus of CFT is addressing fear towards compassion and resistance to self-compassion, as many clients struggle to access the soothing and social safety system. Research has shown that CFT can be effective in reducing anxiety, depression, self-criticism, shame, and inferiority. Effectiveness studies have been conducted with various populations, including those with psychosis, personality disorders, and eating disorders.

Mindful Self-Compassion Meditation (MSC)

Mindful Self-Compassion (MSC) was developed by Christopher Germer and Kristin Neff, integrating Buddhist philosophy, neuroscience, and psychotherapy principles. MSC's rapid global spread may be attributed to its relevance in addressing self-criticism and shame, which are prevalent in competitive, achievement-oriented modern societies. The Center for MSC continually adapts programs for specific groups, including educators, healthcare professionals, and adolescents. Unlike previous mindfulness interventions, MSC explicitly teaches self-compassion, although compassion has been considered an implicit aspect of mindfulness training. MSC helps individuals respond to difficulties with:

1. Mindfulness: being aware of the present-moment experiences as it is rather than resisting or avoiding inner discomfort or distress
2. Common humanity: recognizing that suffering and imperfection are parts of a universal human condition rather than being separate from others
3. Self-kindness: responding with warmth, kindness and compassion rather than self-criticism

MSC is primarily a resource-building program designed to cultivate our capacity for self-compassion. A typical MSC group consists of eight 2.5–3 h sessions and a half-day silent retreat, with 10–25 participants. It includes three core meditations (affectionate breathing, loving-kindness for ourselves, and giving and receiving compassion), four additional meditations, and 18 informal practices for daily life. Meta-analyses have shown that self-compassion interventions increase self-compassion, compassion for others, mindfulness, and well-being, while decreasing depression, anxiety, and psychological distress across diverse populations. MSC training may be particularly beneficial for mental health professionals at risk of burnout or compassion fatigue. Additionally, it has been shown to improve emotion regulation in medical students and clinical psychologists.

Conclusion

The widespread adoption of mindfulness practices in psychology, education, medicine, and business has paved the way for what can be termed a "second mindfulness revolution," focusing on loving-kindness, compassion, and self-compassion. This trend is evidenced by leading universities worldwide developing and disseminating compassion-based meditation programs. Notably, self-compassion interventions have gained particular traction among individuals in competitive societies who struggle with self-criticism. These programs offer a potential antidote to the harsh self-judgment often cultivated in achievement-oriented cultures. To ensure the ethical implementation of compassion interventions, it is crucial to address concerns similar to those raised about mindfulness practices, such as commercialization, spiritual materialism, and the risk of reducing complex traditions to mere techniques devoid of moral context. Simultaneously, there is a need for a multidisciplinary approach that integrates the original Buddhist philosophy of compassion with clinical and scientific frameworks. This integration can provide a robust empirical foundation for compassion-based interventions while preserving their philosophical integrity. Such an approach would facilitate the expansion of these practices into clinical settings, supported by a strong evidence base.

Bibliography

Aguilar-Raab C, Jarczok MN, Warth M, Stoffel M, Winter F, Tieck M, Gulewitsch MD, Raab K, Bhasin MK, Herpertz SC, Friederich HC. Enhancing social interaction in depression (SIDE study): protocol of a randomized controlled trial on the effects of a cognitively based compassion training (CBCT) for couples. BMJ Open. 2018;8(9):e020448.

Analayo B. Compassion and emptiness in early Buddhist meditation. Windhorse Publications; 2015.

Cho SK. Buddhist mind training and the cultivation of compassion: a Korean perspective. In: Seppälä EM, Simon-Thomas E, Brown SL, Worline MC, Cameron CD, Doty JR, editors. The Oxford handbook of compassion science. Oxford University Press; 2014.

Cho S, Lee H, Oh KJ, Soto JA. Mindful attention predicts greater recovery from negative emotions, but not reduced reactivity. Cognit Emot. 2018;32(3):600–13.

Choi Y, Cho E. The influence of heart-smile meditation on the self-esteem and happiness of nursing students. J Korean Acad Psychiatr Ment Health Nurs. 2019;28(4):321–30.

Crego A, Yela JR, Riesco-Matías P, Gómez-Martínez M, Vicente-Arruebarrena A. The benefits of self-compassion in mental health professionals: a systematic review of empirical research. Psychol Res Behav Manag. 2022;15:2599–620.

Dahl CJ, Lutz A, Davidson RJ. Reconstructing and deconstructing the self: cognitive mechanisms in meditation practice. Trends Cogn Sci. 2015;19(9):515–23.

Dalai Lama. The power of compassion. HarperOne; 1995.

Dalai Lama. Transforming the mind: teachings on generating compassion. Thorsons; 2000.

Desbordes G, Negi LT, Pace TW, Wallace BA, Raison CL, Schwartz EL. Effects of mindful-attention and compassion meditation training on amygdala response to emotional stimuli in an ordinary, non-meditative state. Front Hum Neurosci. 2012;6:292.

Ekman P. Darwin's compassionate view of human nature. JAMA. 2010;303(6):557–8.

Ekman P. Moving toward global compassion. Paul Ekman Group; 2014.

Ferrari M, Hunt C, Harrysunker A, Abbott MJ, Beath AP, Einstein DA. Self-compassion interventions and psychosocial outcomes: a meta-analysis of RCTs. Mindfulness. 2019;10(8):1455–73.

Figley CR. Compassion fatigue: coping with secondary traumatic stress disorder in those who treat the traumatized. Brunner/Mazel; 1995.

Galante J, Galante I, Bekkers MJ, Gallacher J. Effect of kindness-based meditation on health and well-being: a systematic review and meta-analysis. J Consult Clin Psychol. 2014;82(6):1101–14.

Germer CK. The mindful path to self-compassion. Guilford Press; 2009.

Germer CK, Neff KD. Teaching the mindful self-compassion program: a guide for professionals. Mindfulness. 2019a;10(6):1088–100.

Germer C, Neff KD. Mindful self-compassion (MSC). In: Itvzan I, editor. The handbook of mindfulness-based programs: every established intervention, from medicine to education. Routledge; 2019b. p. 357–67.

Germer CK, Neff KD. Teaching the mindful self-compassion program: a guide for professionals. Guilford Publications; 2019c.

Gilbert P. Introducing compassion-focused therapy. Adv Psychiatr Treat. 2009;15(3):199–208.

Gilbert P. The origins and nature of compassion focused therapy. Br J Clin Psychol. 2014;53(1):6–41.

Gilbert P. Compassion: from its evolution to psychotherapy. Front Psychol. 2020;11:586161.

Gilbert P, Procter S. Compassionate mind training for people with high shame and self-criticism: overview and pilot study of a group therapy approach. Clin Psychol Psychother. 2006;13(6):353–79.

Gilbert P, McEwan K, Matos M, Rivis A. Fears of compassion: development of three self-report measures. Psychol Psychother Theory Res Pract. 2011;84(3):239–55.

Goetz JL, Keltner D, Simon-Thomas E. Compassion: an evolutionary analysis and empirical review. Psychol Bull. 2010;136(3):351–74.

Gwon S. Research on modern secular compassion meditation in the west-in relation to Tibetan Lojong practice and its application [Doctoral dissertation]. Graduate School of Dongguk University; 2018.

Halifax J. Being with dying: cultivating compassion and fearlessness in the presence of death. Shambhala Publications; 2008.

Hofmann SG, Grossman P, Hinton DE. Loving-kindness and compassion meditation: potential for psychological interventions. Clin Psychol Rev. 2011;31(7):1126–32.

Hutcherson CA, Seppala EM, Gross JJ. Loving-kindness meditation increases social connectedness. Emotion. 2008;8(5):720–4.

Jazaieri H, McGonigal K, Jinpa T, Gross JJ, Goldin PR. A randomized controlled trial of compassion cultivation training: effects on mindfulness, affect, and emotion regulation. Motiv Emot. 2013;38(1):23–35.

Jinpa T. Mind training: the great collection. Wisdom Publications; 2006.

Kanov JM, Maitlis S, Worline MC, Dutton JE, Frost PJ, Lilius JM. Compassion in organizational life. Am Behav Sci. 2004;47(6):808–27.

Kim JS. The effects of a loving-kindness and compassion meditation program on the self-regulation of anger and forgiveness. Korean J Counsel. 2014;15(3):1185–202.

Kim JB. A study on meditative utilization of loving-kindness and compassion: focused on compassion practice in early Buddhism and Tibetan Buddhism [Doctoral dissertation]. Wonkwang University; 2019.

Kim JJ, Parker SL, Doty JR, Cunnington R, Gilbert P, Kirby JN. Neurophysiological and behavioural markers of compassion. Sci Rep. 2020;10(1):1–9.

Kim S, Song Y, Lee KU. Effect of mindful self-compassion training on anxiety, depression and emotion regulation. Mood Anxiety. 2022;18(1):10–6.

Kirby JN, Tellegen CL, Steindl SR. A meta-analysis of compassion-based interventions: current state of knowledge and future directions. Behav Ther. 2017;48(6):778–92.

Klimecki OM, Leiberg S, Lamm C, Singer T. Functional neural plasticity and associated changes in positive affect after compassion training. Cereb Cortex. 2013;23(7):1552–61.

Klimecki OM, Leiberg S, Ricard M, Singer T. Differential pattern of functional brain plasticity after compassion and empathy training. Soc Cogn Affect Neurosci. 2014;9(6):873–9.

Kreplin U, Farias M, Brazil IA. The limited prosocial effects of meditation: a systematic review and meta-analysis. Sci Rep. 2018;8(1):2403.

Lang AJ, Casmar P, Hurst S, Harrison T, Golshan S, Good R, Essex M, Negi L. Compassion meditation for veterans with posttraumatic stress disorder (PTSD): a non-randomized study. Mindfulness. 2020;11(1):63–74.

Leary MR, Tate EB, Adams CE, Allen AB, Hancock J. Self-compassion and reactions to unpleasant self-relevant events: the implications of treating oneself kindly. J Pers Soc Psychol. 2007;92(5):887–904.

Leaviss J, Uttley L. Psychotherapeutic benefits of compassion-focused therapy: an early systematic review. Psychol Med. 2015;45(5):927–45.

Ledoux K. Understanding compassion fatigue: understanding compassion. J Adv Nurs. 2015;71(9):2041–50.

Lutz A, Slagter HA, Dunne JD, Davidson RJ. Attention regulation and monitoring in meditation. Trends Cogn Sci. 2008;12(4):163–9.

McIntyre R, Smith P, Rimes KA. The role of self-criticism in common mental health difficulties in students: a systematic review of prospective studies. Ment Health Prev. 2018;10:13–27.

Ñāṇamoli B. The path of purification: Visuddhimagga. Buddhist Publication Society; 2010.

Neff K. Self-compassion: an alternative conceptualization of a healthy attitude toward oneself. Self Identity. 2003a;2(2):85–101.

Neff KD. The development and validation of a scale to measure self-compassion. Self Identity. 2003b;2(3):223–50.
Neff KD. Self-compassion, self-esteem, and well-being. Soc Personal Psychol Compass. 2011;5(1):1–12.
Neff KD. Self-compassion: theory, method, research, and intervention. Annu Rev Psychol. 2022;73:553–77.
Powers J. Introduction to Tibetan Buddhism. Snow Lion Publications; 2007.
Purser RE, Loy D. Beyond McMindfulness. HuffPo. 2013;1(7):13.
Salzberg S. Real happiness: the power of meditation. Workman Publishing; 2011.
Sayadaw UJ. Vipassana meditation: the path to enlightenment. Pariyatti Publishing; 2003.
Shonin E, Van Gordon W, Compare A, Zangeneh M, Griffiths MD. Buddhist-derived loving-kindness and compassion meditation for the treatment of psychopathology: a systematic review. Mindfulness. 2015;6(5):1161–80.
Sun S, Pickover AM, Goldberg SB, Bhimji J, Nguyen JK, Evans AE, Patterson B, Kaslow NJ. For whom does Cognitively Based Compassion Training (CBCT) work? An analysis of predictors and moderators among African American suicide attempters. Mindfulness. 2019;10(11):2327–40.
Thomason S, Moghaddam N. Compassion-focused therapies for self-esteem: a systematic review and meta-analysis. Psychol Psychother Theory Res Pract. 2021;94(3):737–59.
Ubeysekara A. Four divine abodes (Brahma Viharas) in Theravada Buddhism. Ari's World. https://drarisworld.wordpress.com/2020/02/23/four-divine-abodes-brahma-viharas-in-theravada-buddhism/; 2020, February 23.
Wallace BA. Buddhism with an attitude: the Tibetan seven-point mind-training. Snow Lion Publications; 2001.
Werner AM, Tibubos AN, Rohrmann S, Reiss N. The clinical trait self-criticism and its relation to psychopathology: a systematic review - update. J Affect Disord. 2019;246:530–47.
Wilson AC, Mackintosh K, Power K, Chan SWY. Effectiveness of self-compassion related therapies: a systematic review and meta-analysis. Mindfulness. 2019;10(6):979–95.

Mindfulness-Based Intervention for Depression

17

Ji-Ae Yun

Mindfulness-Based Cognitive Therapy (MBCT) for Depression has been developed as an 8-week course group therapy to educate patients on how they can escape the maladaptive cognitive process through the integration of mindfulness meditation training and cognitive behavior skills. Unlike previous depression treatments, which focused on treating acute episodes and alleviating painful depressive symptoms, MBCT focuses on ensuring that people get along well after the depressive episode is over to reduce the risk of recurrence. The ultimate purpose of MBCT is not just to improve symptoms, but to fundamentally improve the relationship between thoughts, emotions, and bodily sensations that cause a deeper level of understanding in patients, preventing depression from recurring.

Understanding of Psychological Factors Associated with the Recurrence of Depression and the Mechanisms of Treatment

In order to understand the principle of MBCT, a theoretical understanding of recurrent depression is required. In the process of establishing MBCT, attention was focused on why people who recovered from depressive episodes suffer from depression again.

The mechanism of MBCT is achieved through changes in psychological factors related to the risk of relapse of depression. The MBCT developers built their interventions on the assumption that people who have suffered from depression may react differently to sad mood states than people who have never been depressed.

MBCT improves clinical outcomes through alterations in mindfulness, rumination, worry, compassion, cognitive reactivity, aversion, attention regulation skills, metacognition, and positive affect. The effect of mindfulness-based interventions on basic biobehavioral processes is also based on attention and emotion regulation. These processes are key targets in depressive relapse because both biased attention and impairments in emotion regulation are two core psychological processes that are implicated in vulnerability to depressive relapse.

Rumination is repetitive, automatic, and negative thinking about oneself and is an established predictor of the onset, severity, and maintenance of depression. When engaged in these past or future-based ruminations, people may often experience these thoughts as if they were actually occurring and demand attention as immediate threats, which causes activation of the amygdala. Many studies have found that greater levels of mindfulness have been shown to reduce rumination. Additionally, rumination was found to sig-

J.-A. Yun (✉)
Department of Neuropsychiatry, Daejeon Eulji Medical Center, Daejeon, Republic of Korea

J.-H. Chae, H.-Y. Lee (eds.), *Meditation in Psychiatry and General Medicine*,
https://doi.org/10.1007/978-981-95-7147-5_17

nificantly mediate the relationship between global mindfulness and depressive symptoms. In Particular, certain facets of mindfulness, which are acting with awareness, non-judging, and non-reacting, played a role in the reduction of rumination and subsequent depressive symptoms. Non-judging present-moment awareness may interrupt the cycle of rumination about past regrets or future fears, breaking the link between cognitive reactivity (the process in which a slight deterioration in mood reactivates the cognitive patterns seen in past depressive episodes hidden behind recovery) and depressive symptoms. Furthermore, regardless of the number of past depressive episodes, a significant reduction in ruminative thoughts in individuals with current or past depressive episodes was found after mindfulness intervention.

Another important mechanism of action in MBCT is to improve the ability to intentionally shift patients' attention, enabling more flexible cognitive and behavioral responses, and attention control and emotional control by improving working memory capacity. Intentional attention can be the resource to help people behave under cognitive or emotional demands, not impulsively or automatically. MBCT increases attention-regulating ability, so that the promotion of attention to negative information is reduced and the inhibition of attention to positive information can be reduced.

Although there is still insufficient evidence, there is a mechanism that is thought to be responsible for the effectiveness of MBCT. Hypergeneralized autobiographical memory is known as a cognitive modality associated with depression and suicidal behavior. Although MBCT did not have a statistically significant moderating effect on the outcome of depressive symptoms, MBCT can reduce hyper-generalized autobiographical memory and increase memory specificity. They also reported much more specific life goals after MBCT and expressed higher achievability. Self-discrepancy refers to the distance between the current actual self-concept and ideal self-guides, and a high level of self-discrepancy is associated with depressed mood. The MBCT group did not show this increase, although this was not directly explained by the change in depressive symptoms. Emotional reactivity is used as an indicator of vulnerability to depression and treatment response, and it was observed that emotional reactivity decreased overall in the MBCT group. Also, the therapeutic effect of MBCT was related to reporting that they experienced an increase in momentary positive emotions.

Mindfulness becomes a means of recognizing distressing thoughts and emotions, actively accepting such experiences, destroying networks related to recurrence through self-compassion, and offsetting the risk of recurrence. The factors of mindfulness that accompany facing painful thoughts and emotions with kindness, empathy, and patience are thought to be crucial to the process of change.

MBCT as an Alternative to Conventional Depression Treatment

According to the National Institute for Health and Care Excellence (NICE) guidelines, people with a history of relapse of depression should continue to take antidepressants for at least 2 years. Antidepressant maintenance treatment must be taken to show a protective effect, and the effect does not last beyond the period of taking it. However, the rate of drug maintenance is low, and it may not be available to some subjects. In addition, antidepressants suppress symptoms but do not target the cause of the depressive episode itself. The important point is that patients usually do not try to take antidepressants indefinitely. Patients with high risk of recurrence have less antidepressant retention than patients with low risk, and many patients prefer psychosocial interventions that provide long-term protection against recurrence or relapse.

MBCT shows the potential to greatly contribute to reducing the prevalence of depression in the primary care environment as an alternative to the limitations of conventional depression treatment. In addition, MBCT can be an approach to meet the needs of many patients. In fact, more than 30 people can participate in MBSR classes at a time. This is different from the existing treatment methods that try to deal with the specific thoughts of an individual. Therefore, MBCT has been fully developed with empirical support, is available to many patients, and is a very effective treatment in terms of cost.

The Composition of MBCT

MBCT is a group-based skill training that has been manualized for a total of eight sessions once a week, 2 h per session. The class consists of a variety of formal and informal meditation exercises. Initial sessions include more guided meditation that pays attention to breathing or body sensation. Later, it focuses more on developing independent and individual exercises and expanding conscious awareness of mental events, including previously avoided thoughts and emotions. Homework is an essential element of treatment, and patients practice mindfulness training for 45 min every day using guide meditation recordings.

MBCT includes elements of cognitive therapy and psychological education for depression. People learn that trying to resist or avoid unwanted thoughts or emotions can actually add to the pain and perpetuate depression rather than help solve it. It also supports participants to engage in activities that promote well-being, such as taking a bath, listening to music, and taking a walk. Cognitive therapeutic factors include establishing behavioral plans to help patients recognize the initial warnings that appear when symptoms worsen and developing actions to be taken at that time.

The therapeutic perspective of MBCT and cognitive behavioral therapy (CBT) shows a clear difference. MBCT aims to improve metacognition by focusing on recognizing the relationship between thoughts and feelings, not on changing the content of thoughts. In other words, the purpose is to experience thoughts, feelings, and beliefs as a mental event without thinking of them as a reflection of one aspect or truth about oneself. One of the big differences between existing CBT and MBCT is the attitude of the therapist. When participants practice new ways of thinking and emotion, it is essential to practice the therapist's own mindfulness so that they can provide real resources to participants. In doing so, the therapist can directly implement an instantaneous attitude of mindfulness to negative emotions that may occur within the group. Also, the therapist does not try to give or fix any solutions to the participants' problems.

Research Results on MBCT Efficacy and Treatment Guidelines

Several randomized controlled trials (RCTs) found that MBCT lowered the risk of recurrence in patients with a history of 3 or more relapses of depression. Therefore, treatment guidelines of the American Psychiatric Association 2010 recommended MBCT as an augmentation therapy of medication treatment in the 'continuation phase,' which is the period of maintaining treatment to prevent recurrence of depression.

Subsequent studies have also reported a lot of evidence on the effect of MBCT on the prevention of relapse in depression. Results from six RCTs, showed that MBCT reduced the risk of relapse of depression by 34% compared to conventional treatment in patients with a history of 3 or more depressive episodes. In two RCTs of this study, MBCT showed similar effects to maintenance administration of antidepressants. In a UK study, 212 adults with recurrent depression were randomly assigned to either MBCT or antidepressant maintenance treatment. As a result, MBCT showed a similar risk of relapse to antidepressant maintenance treatment. This study suggested that MBCT could be an alternative option instead of repetitive pharmacological treatment for patients with recurrent depressive episodes.

A meta-analysis study published in 2016 analyzed 1258 patients from nine RCTs. The results of this study showed that MBCT reduced the risk of recurrence of depression during 60 weeks of maintenance treatment compared to other active treatments and antidepressant treatments. These results showed similar results regardless of gender, age, educational level, and therapist, and it was most effective for patients with higher severity of depressive symptoms before treatment. Furthermore, MBCT is found to be delivered safely and effectively in real-world healthcare settings, not research clinics. The rate of reliable deterioration (3%) was comparable to other psychotherapeutic interventions delivered in similar settings.

Acceptability of MBCT and rates of session attendance were generally high, and rates of drop out from treatment were relatively low and very similar to those observed in other studies.

Recently, many studies have reported that MBCT is helpful in acute depressive episodes. In a meta-analysis of 8 studies in which MBCT was applied to acute depressive episodes, MBCT showed a significantly higher effect size. The meta-analysis, which inspected moderators of effect size and estimated MBCT treatment effects over time across 31 studies, yielded mean effect sizes of large and medium effects for no treatment and alternative treatment comparisons, respectively.

As the evidence for MBCT increases, recently updated guidelines not only prevent recurrence of depression but also gradually expand the scope of MBCT application. According to the 2023 CANMAT guidelines, MBCT is recommended as a second-line treatment for acute depression (level 2 evidence) and as a first-line maintenance treatment for relapse prevention (level 1 evidence). According to the 2022 VA/DoD Clinical Practice guidelines, MBCT is suggested as a first-line treatment for uncomplicated MDD patients (weak for). Additionally, for initiation of treatment in pregnant or breastfeeding women or older adults (≥65 years) with mild to moderate MDD, Va/DOD recommended offering MBCT as a first-line treatment. The 2022 NICE guidelines stated that MBCT can be used as a first-line treatment for people with a new episode of less severe depression. In addition, since 2018, a recommendation has been newly added to administer MBCT alone to people who have remitted from depression while being treated solely with antidepressant medication and who have been assessed as being at higher risk of relapse, but who do not wish to continue taking antidepressants. The 2019 American Psychological Association's treatment guidelines recommended MBCT instead of antidepressants as an initial treatment for the general adult population with depression. MBCT was also recommended as a treatment to prevent relapse.

MBCT was found not only to be effective as a treatment, but also to those who needed a psychosocial approach for well-being, MBCT was found to be accessible, well-received, and cost-effective. In one study that calculated the actual cost-effectiveness, MBCT was cheaper than antidepressant maintenance treatment for the last 3 months of the 15-month total treatment period, and MBCT showed more favorable cost-effectiveness in the long run. From a structural point of view, MBCT is also an economical psychological intervention tool, as it can be delivered in groups with up to 15 participants. Thus, NICE guideline 2018 and 2022 recommend that in people at high risk of relapse who have remitted following acute pharmacological treatment and who are expected to experience more severe depression if they relapse, the combination of MBCT with clinical management (antidepressant drug tapering) appears to be the most cost-effective option.

MBCT's Future Focus and Key Questions

Which Patients Are More Effective with MBCT?

Studies on which patients will benefit more from MBCT and which factors are important for the treatment effect are still insufficient. Current reports indicate that MBCT currently shows significant benefits in patients with 3 or more depressive episodes. On the other hand, patients with recurrent depression were also highly likely to drop out of MBCT. In addition, patients with a history of suicide attempts were also highly likely to drop out of MBCT. It has been shown that people with high cognitive reactivity and severe rumination are very difficult to apply to MBCT, but they may be the ones who can benefit the most if they can finish the MBCT. Evidence is accumulating that MBCT may provide the greatest benefit to patients reporting childhood trauma. A study of police officers found that mindfulness-based interventions were also effective in men-centered occupations. Among them, the participants who had high neuroticism, high openness, and recognized social norms favorable for mindfulness had more effects.

Is It Applicable to Patients at Risk of Suicide?

The application of MBCT to patients at risk of suicide is challenging, but it can be an active approach. Several attempts are being made to apply MBCT with Safety Planning Intervention to patients at high risk of suicide. The findings reported in the studies were mostly favorable to mindfulness-based intervention as an effective strategy for suicidal behavior.

A study of the effectiveness of adjunct MBCT in outpatients who are at elevated suicide risk found significant reductions in suicidal ideation and depressive symptoms, but not hopelessness, with MBCT treatment. The treatment was also feasible, acceptable, and safe for these participants. A qualitative study found that patients reported that improved emotion regulation and group treatment modality were helpful in improving clinical symptoms. A small percentage of patients reported that aspects of the treatment increased emotional distress and triggered suicidal thinking; however, this was temporary or not directly related to suicidal behavior.

Adverse Events in Meditation Practices and Meditation-Based Therapies

As the popularity of mindfulness meditation increases, the safety of mindfulness meditation needs to be further evaluated. In a systematic review of 83 mindfulness-based intervention studies, the most common adverse events were anxiety (33%, 18), depression (27%, 15) and cognitive anomalies (25%, 14); gastrointestinal problems and suicidal behaviors (both 11%, 6) were the least frequent. The overall prevalence of meditation adverse events (8.3%) is similar to those reported for psychotherapy practice in general.

However, there has not been a consistent, systematic way to define and report adverse events of mindfulness. It could be difficult to differentiate adverse events from distressing experiences, which can be understood as integral to meditation practice or actually expected reactions involved in the process of achieving the true benefits of mindfulness. Defining adverse events and standard assessment of adverse events is critical. Future studies are needed to show how treatment outcomes are affected by context and individual differences, including their medical and psychological state.

Conclusion

Mindfulness-based cognitive therapy (MBCT) shows its effectiveness through changes in negative thinking patterns in depressive disorder. In particular, it was confirmed that it was effective in preventing recurrence after recovery from depression in patients who had experienced recurrent depressive episodes, and it was also found to be effective in acute depressive episodes. Therefore, MBCT can be another therapeutic alternative that can overcome the limitations of existing medication treatment. In addition, the advantage of MBCT as a group-based treatment that can be administered to a large number of subjects is excellent in cost-effectiveness, showing the potential to greatly contribute to reducing the high prevalence of depression.

Bibliography

Baer R, Walsh E. Treating acute depression with mindfulness-based cognitive therapy. In: Treating depression: MCT, CBT and third wave therapies. John Wiley & Sons Inc; 2016. p. 344–68.

Bangor University. Implementation of mindfulness-based cognitive therapy into the UK National Health Service in 2012 | Centre for Mindfulness Research and Practice | Bangor University; n.d. Retrieved 16 Apr 2019, from https://www.bangor.ac.uk/mindfulness/nhs.php.en.

Barnhofer T, Crane C, Brennan K, Duggan DS, Crane RS, Eames C, Radford S, Silverton S, Fennell MJV, Williams JMG. Mindfulness-based cognitive therapy (MBCT) reduces the association between depressive symptoms and suicidal cognitions in patients with a history of suicidal depression. J Consult Clin Psychol. 2015;83(6):1013–20.

Batink T, Peeters F, Geschwind N, van Os J, Wichers M. How does MBCT for depression work? Studying cognitive and affective mediation pathways. PLoS One. 2013;8(8):e72778.

Britton WB, Shahar B, Szepsenwol O, Jacobs WJ. Mindfulness-based cognitive therapy improves emotional reactivity to social stress: results from a randomized controlled trial. Behav Ther. 2012;43(2):365–80.

Chesin MS, Sonmez CC, Benjamin-Phillips CA, Beeler B, Brodsky BS, Stanley B. Preliminary effectiveness of adjunct mindfulness-based cognitive therapy to prevent suicidal behavior in outpatients who are at elevated suicide risk. Mindfulness. 2015;6(6):1345–55.

Chesin MS, Brodsky BS, Beeler B, Benjamin-Phillips CA, Taghavi I, Stanley B. Perceptions of adjunctive mindfulness-based cognitive therapy to prevent suicidal behavior among high suicide-risk outpatient participants. Crisis. 2018;39(6):451–60.

Crane C, Williams JMG. Factors associated with attrition from mindfulness-based cognitive therapy in patients with a history of suicidal depression. Mindfulness. 2010;1(1):10–20.

Crane C, Barnhofer T, Duggan DS, Hepburn S, Fennell MV, Williams JMG. Mindfulness-based cognitive therapy and self-discrepancy in recovered depressed patients with a history of depression and suicidality. Cogn Ther Res. 2008;32(6):775.

Crane C, Winder R, Hargus E, Amarasinghe M, Barnhofer T. Effects of mindfulness-based cognitive therapy on specificity of life goals. Cogn Ther Res. 2012;36(3):182–9.

Davidson RJ. Mindfulness-based cognitive therapy and the prevention of depressive relapse: measures, mechanisms, and mediators [review of mindfulness-based cognitive therapy and the prevention of depressive relapse: measures, mechanisms, and mediators]. JAMA Psychiatry. 2016;73(6):547–8.

Deen S, Sipe W, Eisendrath SJ. Mindfulness-based cognitive therapy for treatment-resistant depression. In: Eisendrath SJ, editor. Mindfulness-based cognitive therapy: innovative applications. Springer International Publishing; 2016. p. 133–44.

Disorders, G. D. P. F. T. T. of D., & Guideline Development Panel for the Treatment of Depressive Disorders. APA clinical practice guideline for the treatment of depression across three age cohorts. PsycEXTRA Dataset. 2019. https://doi.org/10.1037/e505892019-001.

Eisendrath SJ, Gillung E, Delucchi KL, Segal ZV, Nelson JC, McInnes LA, Mathalon DH, Feldman MD. A randomized controlled trial of mindfulness-based cognitive therapy for treatment-resistant depression. Psychother Psychosom. 2016;85(2):99–110.

Farias M, Maraldi E, Wallenkampf KC, Lucchetti G. Adverse events in meditation practices and meditation-based therapies: a systematic review. Acta Psychiatr Scand. 2020;142(5):374–93.

Gilmartin H, Goyal A, Hamati MC, Mann J, Saint S, Chopra V. Brief mindfulness practices for healthcare providers - a systematic literature review. Am J Med. 2017;130(10):1219.e1–e1219.e17.

Jury TK, Jose PE. Does rumination function as a longitudinal mediator between mindfulness and depression? Mindfulness. 2019;10(6):1091–104.

Krick A, Felfe J. Who benefits from mindfulness? The moderating role of personality and social norms for the effectiveness on psychological and physiological outcomes among police officers. J Occup Health Psychol. 2020;25(2):99–112.

Kuyken W, Hayes R, Barrett B, Byng R, Dalgleish T, Kessler D, Lewis G, Watkins E, Brejcha C, Cardy J, Causley A, Cowderoy S, Evans A, Gradinger F, Kaur S, Lanham P, Morant N, Richards J, Shah P, et al. Effectiveness and cost-effectiveness of mindfulness-based cognitive therapy compared with maintenance antidepressant treatment in the prevention of depressive relapse or recurrence (PREVENT): a randomised controlled trial. Lancet. 2015a;386(9988):63–73.

Kuyken W, Hayes R, Barrett B, Byng R, Dalgleish T, Kessler D, Lewis G, Watkins E, Morant N, Taylor RS, Byford S. The effectiveness and cost-effectiveness of mindfulness-based cognitive therapy compared with maintenance antidepressant treatment in the prevention of depressive relapse/recurrence: results of a randomised controlled trial (the PREVENT study). Health Technol Assess. 2015b;19(73):1–124.

Kuyken W, Warren FC, Taylor RS, Whalley B, Crane C, Bondolfi G, Hayes R, Huijbers M, Ma H, Schweizer S, Segal Z, Speckens A, Teasdale JD, Van Heeringen K, Williams M, Byford S, Byng R, Dalgleish T. Efficacy of mindfulness-based cognitive therapy in prevention of depressive relapse: an individual patient data meta-analysis from randomized trials. JAMA Psychiatry. 2016;73(6):565–74.

Lambert D, van den Berg NH, Mendrek A. Adverse effects of meditation: a review of observational, experimental and case studies. Curr Psychol. 2021. https://doi.org/10.1007/s12144-021-01503-2.

Lee S-H. Effects of mindfulness-based therapy on depressive disorder. J Korean Neuropsychiatr Assoc. 2018;57(2):133–8.

Lenz AS, Hall J, Bailey Smith L. Meta-analysis of group mindfulness-based cognitive therapy for decreasing symptoms of acute depression. J Spec Group Work. 2016;41(1):44–70.

Ma SH, Teasdale JD. Mindfulness-based cognitive therapy for depression: replication and exploration of differential relapse prevention effects. J Consult Clin Psychol. 2004;72(1):31–40.

Maddock A, Blair C. How do mindfulness-based programmes improve anxiety, depression and psychological distress? A systematic review. Curr Psychol. 2021. https://doi.org/10.1007/s12144-021-02082-y.

Mayor S. Mindfulness based therapy is as effective as antidepressants in preventing depression relapse, study shows. BMJ. 2015;350:h2107.

Parikh SV, Quilty LC, Ravitz P, Rosenbluth M, Pavlova B, Grigoriadis S, Velyvis V, Kennedy SH, Lam RW, MacQueen GM, Milev RV, Ravindran AV, Uher R, CANMAT Depression Work Group. Canadian network for mood and anxiety treatments (CANMAT) 2016 clinical guidelines for the Management of Adults with major depressive disorder: section 2. Psychological treatments. Can J Psychiatry. 2016;61(9):524–39.

Perestelo-Perez L, Barraca J, Peñate W, Rivero-Santana A, Alvarez-Perez Y. Mindfulness-based interventions for the treatment of depressive rumination: systematic review and meta-analysis. Int J Clin Health Psychol. 2017;17(3):282–95.

Raj S, Ghosh D, Verma SK, Singh T. The mindfulness trajectories of addressing suicidal behaviour: a systematic review. Int J Soc Psychiatry. 2021;67(5):507–19.

Riemann D, Hertenstein E, Schramm E. Mindfulness-based cognitive therapy for depression [review of mindfulness-based cognitive therapy for depression]. Lancet. 2016;387(10023):1054.

Segal ZV, Teasdale J. Mindfulness-based cognitive therapy for depression, Second Edition. Guilford Publications; 2018.

Sipe WEB, Eisendrath SJ. Mindfulness-based cognitive therapy: theory and practice. Can J Psychiatry. 2012;57(2):63–9.

Teasdale JD, Segal ZV, Williams JM, Ridgeway VA, Soulsby JM, Lau MA. Prevention of relapse/recurrence in major depression by mindfulness-based cognitive therapy. J Consult Clin Psychol. 2000;68(4):615–23.

Tickell A, Ball S, Bernard P, Kuyken W, Marx R, Pack S, Strauss C, Sweeney T, Crane C. The effectiveness of mindfulness-based cognitive therapy (MBCT) in real-world healthcare services. Mindfulness. 2020;11(2):279–90.

Toscano AL. Efficacy of mindfulness based cognitive therapy in the treatment of symptoms of active depression: a meta-analysis. Towson University Institutional Repository; 2015. https://mdsoar.org/handle/11603/2047.

van der Velden AM, Kuyken W, Wattar U, Crane C, Pallesen KJ, Dahlgaard J, Fjorback LO, Piet J. A systematic review of mechanisms of change in mindfulness-based cognitive therapy in the treatment of recurrent major depressive disorder. Clin Psychol Rev. 2015;37:26–39.

Williams JMG, Crane C, Barnhofer T, Brennan K, Duggan DS, Fennell MJV, Hackmann A, Krusche A, Muse K, Von Rohr IR, Shah D, Crane RS, Eames C, Jones M, Radford S, Silverton S, Sun Y, Weatherley-Jones E, Whitaker CJ, et al. Mindfulness-based cognitive therapy for preventing relapse in recurrent depression: a randomized dismantling trial. J Consult Clin Psychol. 2014;82(2):275–86.

18 Mindfulness-Based Interventions for Psychosis

Young-Chul Chung and Ling Li

Psychosis includes schizophrenia, delusional disorder, and brief psychotic disorder, as well as non-affective psychosis, which consists of non-classified psychosis, and affective psychosis, which consists of mania and depression accompanied by psychotic features. These various psychoses are classified as serious mental illnesses not only because of the severity of the symptoms themselves but also because they harm a person's ability to function in daily life. To optimally treat a severe mental illness, it is essential to not only provide treatment via medication, but also to provide in parallel psychosocial interventions that serve to identify and approach various environmental factors including various traumas a patient experienced while growing up, their parents' personalities and family atmosphere, and economic challenges. Research on schizophrenia/psychosis in the past few decades, including genetic and brain imaging studies, has focused on identifying its biological causes. However, the results of a recent large-scale genome-wide association study showed that 128 single-nucleotide polymorphisms (SNPs) could only explain around 3.4% of the risk of schizophrenia. On the other hand, 53–68% of first-episode psychosis patients have experienced psychological trauma in childhood, and it has been reported that childhood trauma increases the risk of developing psychosis by 33%. Therefore, an effort must be made now to understand the patient's environmental factors that have been previously neglected, strengthen psychosocial interventions that work together to solve those problems, and establish a system to provide such mental health services.

Currently, according to the guidelines published by the UK's National Institute for Health and Care Excellence (NICE) and the American Psychiatric Association (APA), the standard psychosocial intervention for psychosis/schizophrenia is cognitive behavioral therapy (CBT). The NICE guidelines recommend that at least 16 sessions of CBT be provided over a period of 6 months. Although the 1997 edition of the APA guidelines stated that there was insufficient evidence to recommend cognitive behavioral therapy, the guidelines changed their position in the 2004 edition, stating that there was considerable evidence for CBT. However, despite evidence that cognitive behavioral therapy is effective in improving positive symptoms, it is still very limited in improving negative symptoms. Recently, various Mindfulness-Based Interventions (MBI) are being applied in various fields. Although the application of meditation in the field of psychosis

Y.-C. Chung (✉)
Department of Psychiatry, Jeonbuk National University Hospital, Jeonju, Republic of Korea
e-mail: chungyc@jbnu.ac.kr

L. Li
Department of Psychiatry, Jeonbuk National University Medical School, Jeonju, Republic of Korea

J.-H. Chae, H.-Y. Lee (eds.), *Meditation in Psychiatry and General Medicine*,
https://doi.org/10.1007/978-981-95-7147-5_18

was delayed compared to other approaches due to concerns about the side effects caused by meditation, several good randomized controlled trials have been consistently published. Therefore, in this chapter, we will provide a brief clinical description of psychosis/schizophrenia, introduce recently announced MBI results and considerations, and discuss cases where side effects were reported due to meditation. Through this, we will attempt to show the new prospects of applying MBI for treating psychosis and the specific treatment protocols that need to be carefully considered.

Epidemiology

When examining the occurrence of diseases according to age, illnesses such as cancer, cardiovascular diseases, and neurological diseases increase as people age. However, most mental illnesses, including psychosis, are found to occur at the highest rates in people in their 20s and 30s. According to the Ministry of Health and Welfare survey conducted in Korea, the annual occurrence of disorders on the schizophrenia spectrum disorder is 0.2%. When adjusting for the number of people hospitalized, it was estimated to be about 115,000. The annual occurrence of psychosis is 0.03% or 30 per 100,000 people, meaning that there are about 16,000 new cases occurring every year. In 2013, the number of schizophrenia patients who received medical services was reported to be 182,146 (Korea National Health Service).

Clinical Features

There are various symptoms of schizophrenia. They can be broadly divided into positive symptoms such as relational thoughts, delusions, and auditory hallucinations, and negative symptoms such as blunted affect, illogic, and apathy. Rather than describing each symptom in detail, it is important to understand why ideas of reference or persecutory ideas, which are the representative positive symptoms, occur. Psychoanalytically, schizophrenia is interpreted as the result of the projection of inner fear or feelings of dislike. In modern psychology, threat perception is explained as an important cause of schizophrenia. Projection involves taking it out externally and blaming others because you are in a situation that is too difficult or you are angry. As such, it can first and foremost be a great help in understanding the patient's difficult feelings. However, having hateful thoughts or an aggressive attitude towards others does not automatically cause harm like when others threaten to harm you. For this to happen, one must experience threats to one's existence and self-esteem while growing up, from being subtly ignored by others to being constantly rejected and hurt in big and small ways (Fig. 18.1).

In other words, when a chronically accumulated threat is combined with a weak internal (covert) projection (Fig. 18.2), ideas of reference or persecutory ideas occur. Negative symptoms include a lack of change in emotion, monotonous expression, and decreased speech or behavioral function. These symptoms can be understood as the result of avoidant behavior where one completely blocks out and isolates oneself in order to avoid painful perceptions. Wilfred Bion said that psychotic patients feel bombarded by stimuli welling up from within and destroy their mental devices (quote "attack on linking") in order to get rid of these experiences. Negative symptoms can be understood as everything disappearing as a result of the destruction of the patient's mental devices. Therefore, positive symptoms are mainly problematic in the acute stage, but negative symptoms are prominent in the prodromal and chronic residual stages.

Although the trauma that the patient experiences before the onset of psychosis and during the treatment process is not a clinical symptom, it is an important factor that must be understood for the patient's psychological treatment. The first trauma is one received from people while growing up (parental abuse or neglect, bullying, physical assault, sexual assault). It is said that patients who experience two types of trauma are five times more likely to be diagnosed with psychosis, and 30 times more likely when there are three

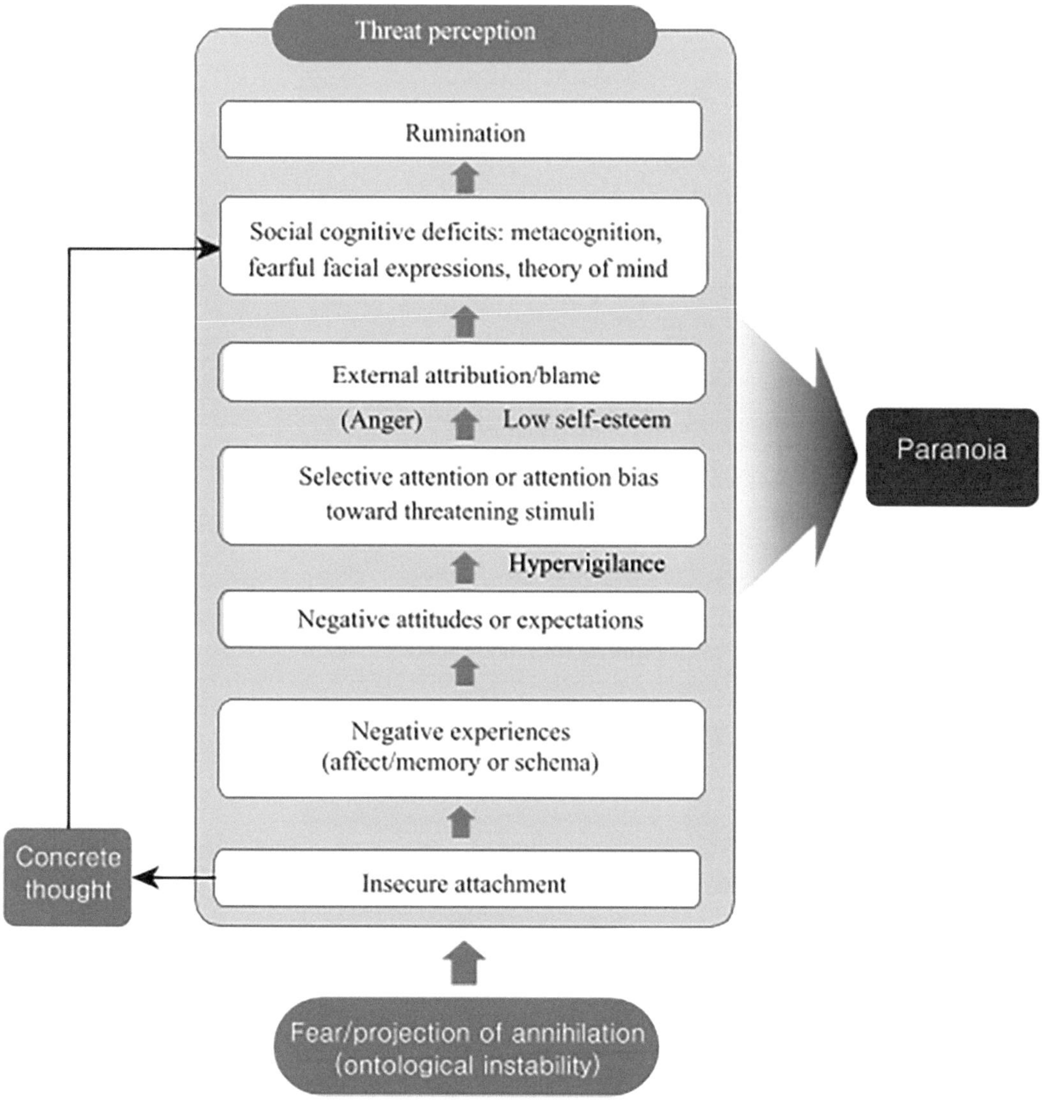

Fig. 18.1 Theory on the development of paranoia: based on the threat anticipation model

types of trauma. The second trauma is caused by experiencing the psychotic symptom itself for the first time. Persecutory delusions or auditory hallucinations can themselves be traumatic because it is often difficult to acknowledge or accept those symptoms given that they can be very scary, frightening, or confusing experiences. The third is the trauma experienced during the treatment process. It is trauma that comes from the shame or humiliation felt by being hospitalized against one's will and being forced to receive treatment because one is confused and cannot distinguish reality when first experiencing symptoms of psychosis. The fourth is the trauma of having to deal with social discrimination and surveillance while receiving maintenance treatment. Because patients are usually vulnerable and do not know how to defend themselves or attack others, in some respects they are actually victims of socioeconomic factors. When their symptoms worsen as a result of discontinuing treatment, these patients have to endure the trauma of being socially ostracized due to incidents of aggression towards unspecified people.

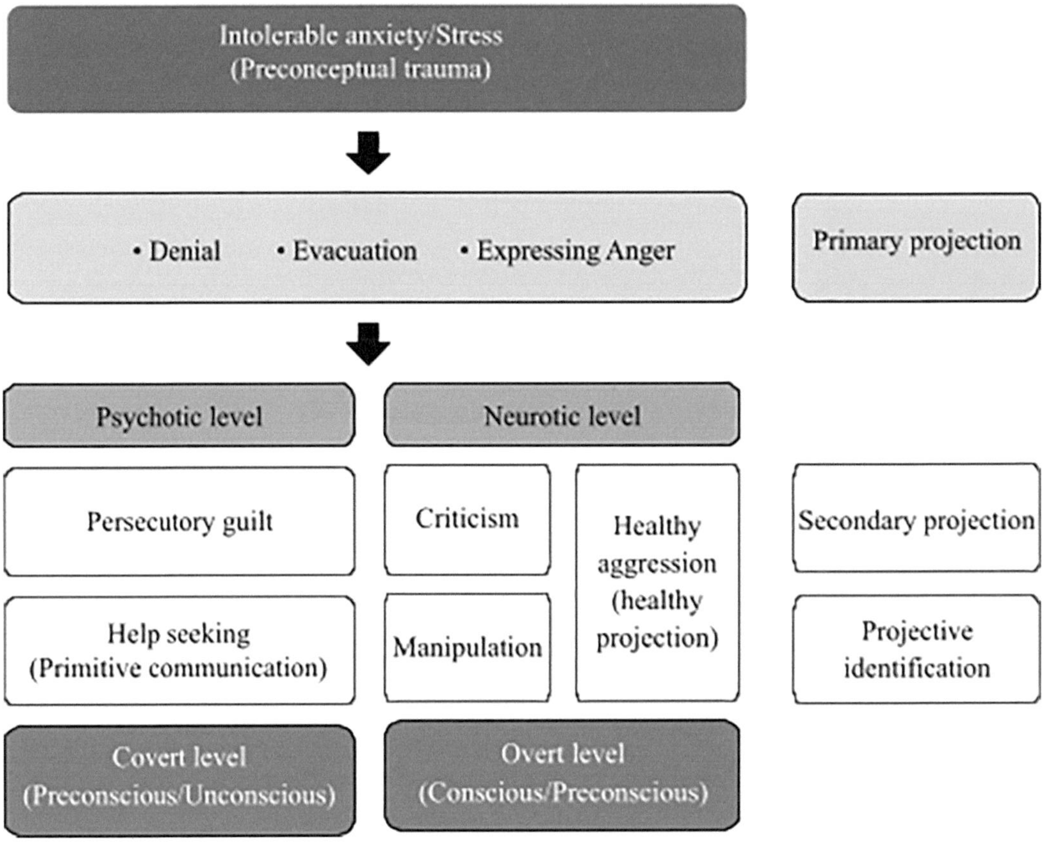

Fig. 18.2 Comparison of content according to type and level of projection

Diagnosis

A diagnosis of schizophrenia must meet all of the following criteria:

A. Two (or more) of the following symptoms must be present a significant portion of the time over a period of 1 month (or less if successfully treated), and at least one of them must be ①, ②, or ③.
   ① Delusions
   ② Hallucinations
   ③ Disorganized speech (e.g., frequent derailment or incoherence)
   ④ Grossly disorganized or catatonic behavior
   ⑤ Negative symptoms (e.g., diminished emotional expression or avolition)

B. For a significant period of time since the onset of the disorder, the patient's level of functioning in one or more major areas, such as work, interpersonal relationships, or self-care, has decreased significantly below the level achieved before the onset of the disorder. (or, if onset occurs in childhood or adolescence, failure to achieve expected levels of interpersonal, academic, or occupational functioning).

C. Persistent signs of disability continue for at least 6 months. This 6-month

(continued)

period must include at least 1 month (or less if successfully treated) of symptoms corresponding to Criterion A (e.g., active phase symptoms) and may include periods of prodromal or residual symptoms. During the prodromal or residual phase, signs of the disorder may be present only as negative symptoms or in a weakened form of two or more of the symptoms listed in Criterion A (e.g. odd beliefs, unusual perceptual experiences).

There are various levels of diagnosis for psychosis in addition to schizophrenia, and it is very complicated and difficult to differentiate and diagnose them in detail. From a psychotherapeutic perspective, it is more important to understand the recently proposed staging model than the diagnosis itself. The staging model for psychosis is divided into four stages, namely high-risk psychosis (stage 1), first-episode psychosis (stage 2), first-episode incomplete remission or relapse (stage 3), and severe, persistent or non-remission state (stage 4). While there may be several important psychosocial intervention goals at each stage, it is important to prevent psychosis in high-risk states, to prevent relapse and improve recovery in first-episode psychosis, to improve response and adaptation to symptoms in stage 3 or incomplete remission, and to manage and effectively manage and protect oneself in a case of severe stage 4. In particular, stages 2 and 3 require the most intensive psychosocial intervention, as this is when the most frequent relapses, highest suicide rates, brain changes, and continued functional decline occur. In other words, whether there will be improvement and recovery or a malignant course of gradual regression with frequent relapses is determined based on how optimal the treatment of the patient is during this period. Therefore, the period up to 5 years after the first psychotic symptom occurs, up to after treatment and recovery, is called the critical period.

Treatment

According to the UK's NICE guidelines (2014), cognitive behavioral therapy and family intervention are mentioned as important treatments that must be provided for psychosis/schizophrenia. Cognitive behavioral therapy (CBT) is a method of treatment where one monitors one's thoughts and emotions related to one's symptoms, recognizes the link between one's thoughts, emotions, and behaviors, reevaluates one's perceptions, beliefs, and inferences related to one's symptoms, and enhances new ways of coping with one's symptoms. CBT was found to reduce the length of hospitalization, readmission rates, and overall symptom severity, while also improving the patient's social function. Its effect on positive symptoms is limited, and while its effect on hallucinations was consistent, its effect on delusions showed mixed results. On the other hand, it was reported that there are no significant effects on improving drug compliance or insights into illness. Family mediation consists of supportive content, education about the disease, problem-solving, and crisis mediation. The guidelines state that at least ten sessions of family mediation should be provided, and research has analyzed it to be effective in reducing relapse and hospitalization rates. Finally, although psychoanalytic approaches do not have clear effects on symptoms, functioning, or quality of life, mental health professionals are recommended to consider them to understand their patients' experiences.

The American Psychiatric Association's guidelines (2004) mention Assertive Community Treatment (ACT), family mediation, and supportive employment as the main psychosocial interventions for psychosis/schizophrenia, with cognitive behavioral therapy listed as the fourth. CBT is effective in improving positive symptoms, but its effects do not extend to relapse, readmission, or social functioning. The Early Psychosis Asia network issued a declaration that CBT, which emphasizes Asian thinking such as awareness should be provided and that the hours of psychotherapy should be increased.

One of the important perspectives in psychotherapeutic approaches is the phase-specific approach. People who experience psychosis go through (1) an initial surviving stage where they must survive confusion, terror, and fear, (2) an existing stage where they have barely escaped from the swirling and overwhelming mental symptoms of the acute stage, have confirmed their existence or reality, and are just starting to live again, and (3) an active living stage where they deal with society and reality while rebuilding themselves. Pamella Fuller coined this the surviving-existing-living (SEL) model. In the surviving stage, it is appropriate to label and contain one's emotions, increase awareness of one's thoughts, normalize one's psychotic experiences, and participate in activity-oriented groups. During the existing stage, it is important to increase one's cognition and awareness, undergo cognitive behavioral therapy that includes regulating emotions, and receive counseling on one's job or career. At the living stage, it is important to undergo CBT or psychodynamic therapy that deals with the relationships between oneself and others, as well as receive vocational/academic support.

The Application of Meditation

Although there are quite a few studies on psychosis, here we will describe their results and implications, focusing on randomized controlled studies. The majority of treatment methods in the studies were various modified techniques based on mindfulness, as well as some studies of acceptance and commitment therapy, and one study on compassion meditation (Table 18.1). If we take a look at how effective the treatments were at addressing certain symptoms, they were as follows.

First, for positive symptoms, the effects were moderate to small in studies by Chien and Thompson (2014), Gaudiano and Herbert (2016), Chadwick et al. (2016), and no difference compared to controls in the studies by Langer et al. (2012), Lopez-Navarro et al. (2015), Moritz et al. (2015), Bach and Hayes (2002), Bach et al. (2012), White et al. (2011), and Shawyer et al. (2012). On the other hand, Braehler et al. (2013), Çetin and Aylaz (2018), and Davis et al. (2015) did not investigate the effect of meditation on positive symptoms because there were other primary outcome variables in their studies.

Second, for negative symptoms, studies by White et al. (2011) and Shawyer et al. (2012) showed positive results with effect sizes of 0.47 and 0.25, respectively. However, there was no difference compared to controls in the study by Lopez-Navaro et al. (2015).

Third, Moritz et al. (2015) reported significant changes in depressive symptoms, and White et al. (2011) reported an effect size of 0.43.

Fourth, in terms of the function of mindfulness, the effect size varied from 0.19 to 0.56.

Fifth, in terms of insight into the illness, although the effect sizes were small at 0.28, 0.29, and 0.39, the results were relatively consistent.

Sixth, in terms of the scale of mindfulness, the results of the studies showed strong effect sizes at 0.47, 0.50, 0.86, and 1.306 and were consistent.

In summary, there were a mix of small to medium effect sizes for positive symptoms, negative symptoms, and functioning. There was a moderate effect on depressive symptoms, but it was only a partial effect, which is not enough to draw conclusions. On the other hand, there was a small but consistent improvement for insight into the illness. The results of the scale of mindfulness consistently showed medium to very large effects. When analyzing its overall effect rather than on specific symptoms, the difference between pre- and post-treatment is a medium effect size. However, when compared to the control group, the effect size is small. Chien and Thompson's study had participants in their 20s, but all other studies were conducted with people in their 30s and older, and very few studies were conducted during the crucial period when patients need to receive intensive treatment. In particular, the attrition rate in these studies was less than 20%, which is lower than the results of other methods of psychotherapy. However, this is understood to be because the goal of the mindfulness approach is to change, accept, and positively adapt to rela-

Table 18.1 The contents and effectiveness of mindfulness-based interventions applied to psychosis

Type of intervention	Study	Subjects (n)	Treatment content	Dropout rate (%)	Primary results
Mindfulness MBCT	Langer et al. (2012)	SZ spectrum patients (23)	8 weeks of group therapy for 60 min/week	21.7	Improved response to stressful internal events compared to the control group.
MBPP	Chien and Thompson (2014)	SZ outpatients (107)	12 h, 2 h every other week	2.9 ~ 8.3	Improvement in psychiatric symptoms and psychosocial functioning, improved understanding of the disease/treatment, and improvement in readmission times over a two-year period.
MBPP	Çetin and Aylaz (2018)	SZ patients (55), C (80)	8 sessions (twice a week), 70 min per session, 10 min break, mental health education, counseling, and support	0	Effective for cognitive insight and adherence to medication.
MIRRORS	Davis et al. (2015)	SZ and SA outpatients (34)	8-week mindfulness-based stress reduction curriculum (with an added emphasis on self-compassion), 75-min group therapy twice a week	16.7	Showed a relationship between MIRRORs and high work performance and sustainability.
PBCT	Chadwick et al. (2009)	Outpatients with distressing voices (21)	Twice a week for 5 weeks (consisting of two 10-min sessions of meditation and a contemplative group discussion of 15–20 min)	22.7	No improvement in positive symptoms, but improvement in clinical function and mindfulness of painful thoughts and images.
PBCT	Chadwick et al. (2016)	SZ and SA patients hearing voices (54) C (54)	12 sessions at 90 min per session with 10 min of mindfulness practice	15	Helped with pain and perceived control of voice-related distress.
PBCT	Lopez-Navarro et al. (2015)	Patients with SMI (44)	26 sessions each 1 h, 15 min of guided meditation, frequent guidance, and 15 min of reflective group discussion	7	Improved psychological quality of life.
Internet-based	Moritz et al. (2015)	Patients with psychosis (90)	Mindfulness and Progressive Muscle Relaxation Manual (audio file with instructions provided)	29	No changes in paranoia over time or between groups.
Acceptance ACT	Bach and Hayes (2002) Bach et al. (2012)	Inpatients with positive psychotic Sx (80)	4 individual ACT and TAU treatments, 45–50 min per session	10	Over a four-month period, more symptoms were reported than in those who participated in TAU, lower belief in symptoms, and readmission rate was cut in half.

(continued)

Table 18.1 (continued)

Type of intervention	Study	Subjects (*n*)	Treatment content	Dropout rate (%)	Primary results
ACT	Gaudiano and Herbert (2006)	Inpatients with psychotic Sx (40)	3 individual ACT treatments of 1 h each	5	Overall improvement in emotional symptoms, social functioning impairment, and hallucination-related distress.
ACT	White et al. (2011)	Patients with psychotic disorders (27)	10 1-h one-on-one sessions	11.1	Improved mindfulness skills and reduced negative symptoms.
ABCBT	Shawyer et al. (2012)	Patients with psychosis with CHs (44)	12 sessions at 1-week intervals, 10 min of mindfulness training, ACT training and metaphors applied flexibility to promote detached acceptance of voices	9.1	No statistically significant difference between the two groups.
Compassion CFT	Braehler et al. (2013)	Psychotic patients (40)	16 sessions (2 h per session, once a week)	18	Clinical improvement and increased compassion

ABCBT acceptance-based cognitive behavioural therapy, *ACT* acceptance and commitment therapy, *C* controls, *CFT* compassion-focused therapy, *CHs* command hallucinations, *MBCT* mindfulness-based cognitive therapy, *MBPP* mindfulness-based psychoeducation programme, *MIRRORS* mindfulness intervention for rehabilitation and recovery in schizophrenia, *PBCT* person-based cognitive therapy, *TAU* treatment as usual, *Sx* Symptoms, *SZ* Schizophrenia, *SA* schizoaffective disorder, *SMI* severe mental illness

tionships rather than changing or correcting the contents of symptoms themselves. In addition, the number, intensity, and duration of mindfulness practice were appropriately modified so that participants could practice without difficulty.

Mindfulness's Mechanisms for Improving Symptoms

Here, we examine, "What are the underlying mechanisms of mindfulness-based interventions for improving symptoms?" The mechanisms for improving positive symptoms can be considered in the following three aspects.

The first is because mindfulness creates mental space. Because mindfulness itself maintains an attitude of observing without being attached to any object, thought, or emotion, it is a principle that creates a starting point to take a step back and look at things objectively rather than being preoccupied by idea of reference, persecutory delusions, or auditory hallucinations. This effect is expressed in various terms, such as distancing, decentering, strengthening the observing self, and increasing meta-awareness. One of the mechanisms that causes delusions to arise is feeling doubt or fear about the phenomena that arise in us, while saying, "Why did they say that to me? What is this?" and being lost deep in thought while trying to search for some kind of meaning. This phenomenon can be seen as the same as musing or ruminating, which involves repeatedly thinking about the cause or meaning of a negative event. In other words, by creating space in the mind, mindfulness-based intervention creates a starting point or opportunity to reduce the development or worsening of delusions that arise from ruminating on negative events. In addition, mindfulness-based intervention is also therapeutic in that if you have space in your mind, you have the flexibility to think more freely without being tied down to any one thought. However, it is difficult to sufficiently improve positive symptoms solely through methods of creating mental space such as distancing yourself from your thoughts. This is because a new corrective re-experience must occur through sufficient story sharing and reality testing to determine which parts of your thoughts are excessive and what the causes of these phenomena are. We can presume that the effect size of existing studies is small or medium and inconsistent because these details were not sufficiently integrated and implemented in existing research methods. Most people who suffer from psychosis have either had various traumatic experiences in childhood, or even if they haven't had one, they have negative emotions or schemas, such as low self-esteem or various complexes about themselves. Therefore, rather than just focusing on body scans or breathing, mindfulness-based intervention for psychosis requires training oneself to observe and accept one's negative emotions, thoughts, and complexes non-judgmentally and non-reactively. Through this, the patient experiences detachment and non-attachment along with a strengthening of their metacognition, and when sufficient story sharing and positive re-experiences follow, a re-perception of the symptoms a patient has experienced can occur at a sufficient level.

Second, there are the effects of acceptance itself. In the mind of a psychotic patient, they deny their situation and hate everything about it. And so they are angry externally and have a lot of feelings of hating and blaming others. However, rather than overtly showing it, the majority of psychotic patients project their anger subtly and covertly in a covert way, and are then afraid that others will find out or retaliate. Even though their level of anger and aggression is lower than that of patients with other diagnoses, acceptance refers to accepting (containing) the desire to be angry that secretly exists internally in order to soothe and endure it. This may block some of the mechanisms that form into delusions. In order for a patient to develop the strength to endure, the therapist and family must first tolerate the patient's long-lasting symptoms, slow recovery of function, and lack of courage (Bion 1962). The meaning of acceptance is not only related to the mechanism of positive symptoms, but can be very diverse and broad, including things such as receiving psychiatric treatment, taking medication, long-term monitoring of progress, having to endure the negative opinions and prejudices of those around you, having to handle things yourself, and acknowledging your own shortcomings. Therefore, the therapist must understand well that the patient has many burdens and difficulties they must bear and accept, and must encourage them.

Third is the effects of loving-kindness (Cí'ài, 慈愛 or Zì'ài, 自愛). In the West, there have been studies of treatments focused on compassion (Liánmǐn, 憐憫) or sympathy (Jīn xù, 矜恤). When we look at compassion or sympathy as feeling sorry for another person's pain or hardships, it is difficult to apply it directly to the patient's state of mind. Therefore, it appears that the choice of this word was incorrect as it caused confusion in the interpretation of the meaning of the word. If we look at a book on compassion-focused group therapy, you see that the contents of compassion include soothing oneself well, observing and looking at what one has experienced in a kinder and friendlier way. In addition, the book describes that the therapist's friendly and wholesome attitude towards the patient is conveyed nonverbally. If this is the case, the term loving-kindness meditation seems more appropriate than compassion. This is because, for loving-kindness meditation, you can start by soothing and loving yourself first if you have resistance towards or difficulty accepting the message to love others due to anger and resentment. It is known that psychotic patients feel strongly threatened and have negative views/schemas and emotions about themselves and others, and that these are associated with delusions. Therefore, appropriate levels of loving-kindness meditation appear to be effective in improving positive symptoms. Currently, there is only one randomized controlled study of loving-kindness meditation, and no detailed assessment of psychopathology has been made in this study. We hope that more active research in this field will be conducted in the future.

The Negative Side Effects of Meditation

The reason why there was a delay in applying mindfulness-based interventions to psychosis was due to concerns about possible negative side effects from meditation. The cases reported so far are summarized in Table 18.2. If we examine their main characteristics, there were more cases of psychiatric history than without, and the inten-

Table 18.2 Cases of mental symptoms related to mindfulness

Study	Target	Psychiatric history	Duration of meditation	Contents of meditation	Fasting?	Decreased sleep?	Symptoms	Diagnosis and treatment
Walsh and Roche (1979)	M (25)	Acute SZ episodes	1 week	Sitting & walking meditation, total silence	Yes	Yes (1 ~ 2 h)	Psychotic episodes	Thioridazine
	F (23)	Acute SZ episodes	2 weeks	18 h of practice a day	Yes	Yes	Acute SZ episodes	Thioridazine
	F (23)	SZ	Few days	Intensive meditation retreat	ND	ND	Suicidal ideation and acute SZ episodes	Chlorpromazine Hospitalization
Garcia-Trujilo et al. (1992)	M (20, 27)	Schizoid personality disorder	Few days	Intensive meditation practice	ND	ND	Acute psychotic episodes	Neuroleptics
Chan-Ob and Boonyanaruthee (1999)	F (25)	Depression	1 week	Temple meditation course, full attention on bodily movement	Yes (1 meal)	Yes (4 ~ 5 h)	Hallucinations, disorientation, labile affect, mild loosening of association, impaired insight	Brief psychotic disorder Haloperidol
	M (35)	ND	3 days	Rumination of thoughts on problems, walking meditation	Lost appetite	Yes	Hallucinations, delusions of grandeur, bizarre behavior, pressed language, loss of insight, flight of ideas	Acute psychosis, Bipolar Disorder Type 1 Haloperidol
	F (28)	Schizophrenic disorder	10 days	Temple meditation course	ND	ND	Persecutory hallucination, delusion, loosening of association	SZ Trifluoperazine
Yorston (2001)	F (25)	No	Few days (Yoga) and 2 years (Zen retreats)	Yoga course, encouraged psychological release, Zen Buddhist retreats	ND	ND	Delusions of grandeur, flight of ideas, increased talkativeness, over-activity, disinhibited behavior, labile affect	Manic episode Haloperidol
Sethi and Bhargava (2003)	M (20)	No	4 days	Total silence	Yes	Yes	Delusion of persecution, auditory hallucinations	SZ Olanzapine
	M (30)	Two Psychotic episodes (after meditation)	6 days	Intensive meditation	ND	Yes	Delusions, sleep disturbance	SZ Risperidone
Kuijpers et al. (2007)	M (24)	Hypomanic episode Mild depressive episodes	ND	Transcendental meditation, unguided and intense sessions	No	No	Visual impairment, hallucinations, ideas of reference and delusional convictions, pananxiety	Haloperidol, Risperidone
Sharma et al. (2016)	M (27)	No	1 year	Transcendental meditation, mantra chanting 2 ~ 3 h (daily) and 4 ~ 5 h (2 ~ 3 months before the onset of the symptoms)	ND	Yes	Hallucination, social withdrawal, decreased self-care	SZ Amisulpride

N/D no description, *SZ* schizophrenia

sity of meditation was much stronger (a very long period of practice, fasting, or reduced sleep), or had a mystical tone, such as transcendental meditation. The reason why these negative side effects occur is that in an analytical sense, meditation itself is like a "controlled regression," making it more likely that one will face repressed memories or traumas from the past. In addition, during meditation, various fantasies, imaginations or primitive thoughts may arise and one may feel a sense of unity with the universe. This is similar to the state that an infant feels when they coexist or are fused with their mother. In the section on diagnostic issues related to culture, the *Diagnostic and Statistical Manual of Mental Disorders: DSM-5* cautions that experiences of depersonalization or derealization that are internally caused when practicing meditation are common, but in these cases, they should not be diagnosed as a disorder. However, if the patient loses control over this as time goes by, it can become a problem. Therefore, when implementing mindfulness-based interventions for psychosis, the manual advises keeping the following points in mind. ① Practice meditation for a short period of time of no more than 10–15 min. ② Avoid long periods of silence. ③ For basic techniques for holding one's attention (body scan, focusing on breathing, etc.), provide additional guidance (every 30–60 s during meditation). The best group size is around 6 people. ④ Avoid analytical or insight-oriented meditation. ⑤ A person with at least 3 years of experience in mindfulness training and education should lead the treatment.

Conclusion

Up to this point, we have looked at the effects and side effects of mindfulness-based interventions for psychosis. Overall, small to medium effect sizes were shown for positive symptoms, negative symptoms, function, and illness, and on the mindfulness scale, there were medium to very large effect sizes. There were no side effects reported during the study and the dropout rate from the study was very low. This is due to the fact that the meditation techniques were appropriately modified and applied to suit the vulnerability of psychotic patients. Limitations of the studies include generally small effect sizes and lack of consistency in results. Mindfulness-based interventions have mostly been applied to patients in their 30s or older, and research on younger patients receiving them for the first time is very lacking. There has also been no research on the mechanisms by which the effects occurred. In particular, most of the contents of MBCT applied were mindfulness elements and did not integrate therapeutic elements of cognitive behavioral therapy. From a theoretical perspective, mindfulness-based interventions developed in the West have a fundamental limitation in that they do not encompass insightful elements such as impermanence and non-duality, which are core principles of Buddhism, nor do they implement a life of diligent practice based on the Noble Eightfold Path. However, despite these limitations, the results so far suggest that various mindfulness-based interventions can be safely applied to psychotic patients and that significant therapeutic effects can be obtained in various symptoms, functions, and illnesses. Currently in Korea, there are several studies reporting the effectiveness of cognitive behavioral therapy for psychotic patients. However, there is no research on mindfulness-based interventions yet. We hope that there will be much interest on the subject and more research will be conducted in this field in the future.

Bibliography

Korean Sources

Korean Schizophrenia Society Volume (대한정신분열병학회 편). Psychosocial interventions for patients with schizophrenia during the critical period (결정적 시기의 정신분열병 환자를 위한 정신사회적 중재). Seoul: Hakjisa; 2008.

Park J, Jeong Y-C, Ahn H-J. Medical care utilization status for patients with schizophrenia spectrum disorder at the time of first onset and for the following 2 years – current status of Korea as a whole and Gwangju Metropolitan City (조현병 스펙트럼 장애 환자의 첫 발병 시와 이후 2년간의 의료이용 현황 한국 전체 및 광주광역시 현황). 2015.

Young-Chul C. Understanding people with schizophrenia: when shared perception is linked to projection. Treatment and management (조현 장애인의 이해: 공유지각이 투사와 연결될 때. 치료 및 관리). 2018.

English Sources

American Psychiatric Association. Diagnostic and statistical manual of mental disorders. 4th ed. Washington, DC: American Psychiatric Association; 1994.

American Psychiatric Association. Practice Guideline for the Treatment of Patients with Schizophrenia. 2004.

Bach P, Hayes SC. The use of acceptance and commitment therapy to prevent the rehospitalization of psychotic patients: a randomized controlled trial. J Consult Clin Psychol. 2002;70:1129–39.

Bach P, Hayes SC, Gallop R. Long-term effects of brief acceptance and commitment therapy for psychosis. Behav Modif. 2012;36:165–81.

Bentall RP, Rowse G, Shryane N, Kinderman P, Howard R, Blackwood N, et al. The cognitive and affective structure of paranoid delusions: a transdiagnostic investigation of patients with schizophrenia spectrum disorders and depression. Arch Gen Psychiatry. 2009;66:236–47.

Bion WR. Attacks on linking. Int J Psychoanal. 1959;40:308–15.

Bion WR. Learning from experience. New York: Basic Books Publishing Company; 1962.

Birchwood M. Early intervention and sustaining the management of vulnerability. Aust N Z J Psychiatry. 2000;34(Suppl):S181–4.

Braehler C, Harper J, Gilbert P. Compassion focused group therapy for recovery after psychosis. In: Steel C, editor. Cognitive behaviour therapy for schizophrenia: evidence based interventions and future directions. Hoboken: John Wiley & Sons; 2013. p. 236–66.

Çetin N, Aylaz R. The effect of mindfulness-based psychoeducation on insight and medication adherence of schizophrenia patients. Arch Psychiatr Nurs. 2018;32:737–44.

Chadwick P, Hughes S, Russell D, Russell I, Dagnan D. Mindfulness groups for distressing voices and paranoia: a replication and randomized feasibility trial. Behav Cogn Psychother. 2009;37:403–12.

Chadwick P, Strauss C, Jones AM, Kingdon D, Ellett L, Dannahy L, et al. Group mindfulness-based intervention for distressing voices: a pragmatic randomised controlled trial. Schizophr Res. 2016;173:168–73.

Chan-Ob T, Boonyanaruthee V. Meditation in association with psychosis. J Med Assoc Thail. 1999;82:925–30.

Chien WT, Thompson DR. Effects of a mindfulness-based psychoeducation programme for Chinese patients with schizophrenia: 2-year follow-up. Br J Psychiatry. 2014;205:52–9.

Chung Y-C, Yoon K-S, Park T-W, Yang J-C, Oh K-Y. Group cognitive behavioral therapy for early psychosis. Cogn Ther Res. 2013;37:403–11.

Davis LW, Lysaker PH, Kristeller JL, Salyers MP, Kovach AC, Woller S. Effect of mindfulness on vocational rehabilitation outcomes in stable phase schizophrenia. Psychol Serv. 2015;12:303–12.

Dyga K, Stupak R. Meditation and psychosis: trigger or cure? Arch Psychiatry Psychother. 2015;17:48–58.

Freeman D. Suspicious minds: the psychology of persecutory delusions. Clin Psychol Rev. 2007;27:425–57.

Freeman D, Garety PA, Kuipers E, Fowler D, Bebbington PE. A cognitive model of persecutory delusions. Br J Clin Psychol. 2002;41:331–47.

Freeman D, Startup H, Dunn G, Cernis E, Wingham G, Pugh K, et al. The interaction of affective with psychotic processes: a test of the effects of worrying on working memory, jumping to conclusions, and anomalies of experience in patients with persecutory delusions. J Psychiatr Res. 2013;47:1837–42.

Fuller PR. Surviving, existing, or living: phase-specific therapy for severe psychosis. Hove, East Sussex: Routledge; 2014.

Gaudiano BA, Herbert JD. Acute treatment of inpatients with psychotic symptoms using Acceptance and Commitment Therapy: pilot results. Behav Res Ther. 2006;44:415–37.

Garcia-Trujillo R, Monterrey A, Gonzalezde JR. Meditation and psychosis. Psiquis Revista De Psiquiatria Psixologia Y Psicosomatica. 1992;13:39–43.

Jauhar S, McKenna PJ, Radua J, Fung E, Salvador R, Laws KR. Cognitivebehavioural therapy for the symptoms of schizophrenia: systematic review and meta-analysis with examination of potential bias. Br J Psychiatry. 2014;204:20–9.

Khoury B, Lecomte T, Gaudiano BA, Paquin K. Mindfulness interventions for psychosis: a meta-analysis. Schizophr Res. 2013;150:176–84.

Kim KR, Lee SY, Kang JI, Kim BR, Choi SH, Park JY, et al. Clinical efficacy of individual cognitive therapy in reducing psychiatric symptoms in people at ultra-high risk for psychosis. Early Interv Psychiatry. 2011;5:174–8.

Kim S-W, Jang J-E, Lee J-Y, Lee G-Y, Yu H-Y, Park C, et al. Effects of group cognitive-behavioral therapy in young patients in the early stage of psychosis. Psychiatry Investig. 2017;14:609.

Kirkbride J, Errazuriz A, Croudace T, Morgan C, Jackson D, McCrone P, et al. Systematic review of the incidence and prevalence of schizophrenia and other psychoses in England. PLoS ONE. 2012;7:1–21.

Kuijpers HJ, van der Heijden FM, Tuinier S, Verhoeven WM. Meditation-induced psychosis. Psychopathology. 2007;40:461–4.

Langer AI, Cangas AJ, Salcedo E, Fuentes B. Applying mindfulness therapy in a group of psychotic individuals: a controlled study. Behav Cogn Psychother. 2012;40:105–9.

Lopez-Navarro E, Del Canto C, Belber M, Mayol A, Fernandez-Alonso O, Lluis J, et al. Mindfulness improves psychological quality of life in community-based patients with severe mental health problems:

a pilot randomized clinical trial. Schizophr Res. 2015;168:530–6.

McGorry PD. The recognition and optimal management of early psychosis: an evidence-based reform. World Psychiatry. 2002;1:76–83.

McGorry PD, Nelson B, Goldstone S, Yung AR. Clinical staging: a heuristic and practical strategy for new research and better health and social outcomes for psychotic and related mood disorders. Can J Psychiatr. 2010;55:486–97.

Ministry of Health and Welfare (Korea). Seoul. The epidemiological survey of mental disorders in Korea. Seoul: Ministry of Health and Welfare; 2016.

Moritz S, Cludius B, Hottenrott B, Schneider BC, Saathoff K, Kuelz AK, et al. Mindfulness and relaxation treatment reduce depressive symptoms in individuals with psychosis. Eur Psychiatry. 2015;30:709–14.

Read J, Fosse R, Moskowitz A, Perry B. The traumagenic neurodevelopmental model of psychosis revisited. Neuropsychiatry. 2014;4(1):65–79.

Ripke S, Neale BM, Corvin A, Walters JT, Farh KH, Holmans PA, et al. Biological insights from 108 schizophrenia-associated genetic loci. Nature. 2014;511:421–7.

Sethi S, Bhargava SC. Relationship of meditation and psychosis: case studies. Aust N Z J Psychiatry. 2003;37:382.

Shapiro SL, Carlson LE, Astin JA, Freedman B. Mechanisms of mindfulness. J Clin Psychol. 2006;62:373–86.

Sharma P, Singh S, Gnanavel S, Kumar N. Meditation – a two edged sword for psychosis: a case report. Ir J Psychol Med. 2016;33:247–9.

Shawyer F, Farhall J, Mackinnon A, Trauer T, Sims E, Ratcliff K, et al. A randomised controlled trial of acceptance-based cognitive behavioural therapy for command hallucinations in psychotic disorders. Behav Res Ther. 2012;50:110–21.

Shonin E, Van Gordon W, Griffiths MD. Do mindfulness-based therapies have a role in the treatment of psychosis? Aust N Z J Psychiatry. 2014;48:124–7.

Trujillo RG, Monterrey A, de Rivera JG. Meditación y psicosis. Psiquis. 1992;13:75–9.

Varese F, Smeets F, Drukker M, Lieverse R, Lataster T, Viechtbauer W, et al. Childhood adversities increase the risk of psychosis: a meta-analysis of patient-control, prospective- and cross-sectional cohort studies. Schizophr Bull. 2012;38:661–71.

Walsh R, Roche L. Precipitation of acute psychotic episodes by intensive meditation in individuals with a history of schizophrenia. Am J Psychiatry. 1979;136:1085–6.

White R, Gumley A, McTaggart J, Rattrie L, McConville D, Cleare S, et al. A feasibility study of Acceptance and Commitment Therapy for emotional dysfunction following psychosis. Behav Res Ther. 2011;49:901–7.

Wong GHY. Early psychosis declaration for Asia by the Asian Network of Early Psychosis. East Asian Arch Psychiatr. 2012;22:90–3.

Yorston GA. Mania precipitated by meditation: a case report and literature review. Ment Health Relig Cult. 2001;4:209–13.

The Application of Meditation for Treating Physical Illnesses

19

Hoo Rim Song

Meditation is an important topic in psychosomatic medicine, which studies the correlation between mind and body. Research has continued to reveal that meditation, one of the most advanced techniques for dealing with the mind, can also be a means of controlling the body. From a medical perspective, it is reasonable to be interested in the efficacy of meditation for treating physical illnesses. Being one of the five areas of clinical focus according to the National Center for Complementary and Integrative Health (NCCIH) under the National Institute of Health (NIH) in the United States, meditation along with yoga has recently been used as an auxiliary treatment for mental or physical diseases by many medical institutions.

Strictly speaking, however, this can be likened to when Daofu (道副), the disciple of Master Bodhidharma (達磨大師), was not able to obtain the bone marrow of his master but rather only his skin. This is because the marrow of meditation is letting go of attachments and extinguishing defilements (Vipassanā) by observing the functions of the mind in a state of consciousness made clear through concentration (Samatha) to reach the ultimate state of peace (nirvana), and any medical efficacy of meditation would be merely incidental.

This perspective also reflects the differences between Eastern and Western views on meditation. Originally, meditation was developed primarily in Hinduism and Buddhism for the purpose of self-discipline or religious enlightenment. However, the method of meditation that is currently being widely applied is not its original form, but rather one that was transformed, accepted, and distributed from a pragmatic perspective in the West. Therefore, the religious aspects of meditation have been greatly reduced today, and there are many instances where it is accepted in a technical dimension, mainly focusing on its mental-physical effects. Conventionally, a practice with the following four basic elements is considered to be meditative today: (1) in a comfortable place with as few distractions as possible, (2) in a comfortable posture such as sitting, lying down, or walking, (3) focusing attention on a specific work, phrase, object, or the sensation of breathing, (4) observing and noticing phenomena non-judgmentally in the present moment.

Although the fundamental meaning of meditation was reduced and its goal was adjusted to become ordinary as a result, there are also advantages in that its accessibility improved and it has become possible to apply scientific methodology to the practice. In the United States, research has shown that the rate of experiencing meditation among the general public in 2017 was 14.2% for adults and 5.4% for children and adolescents.

H. R. Song (✉)
Forest of wisdom clinic, Goyang-si,
Gyeonggi-do, Korea

J.-H. Chae, H.-Y. Lee (eds.), *Meditation in Psychiatry and General Medicine*,
https://doi.org/10.1007/978-981-95-7147-5_19

Therefore, the application of meditation as a treatment for physical illnesses will continue to expand in modern society. In this chapter, we will describe how meditation is currently applied to physical illnesses, what its action mechanism is, things that should be considered in terms of its interpretation, and its future prospects.

Physical Illnesses Where Meditation Has Been Applied

From a psychosomatic medical perspective, meditation is applicable to most physical illnesses, and empirical effects of its application are expected. From an evidence-based medical perspective, however, there are four major physical illnesses for which data has been accumulated and which can be considered as therapeutic means, namely cardiovascular disease, pain, irritable bowel syndrome, and ulcerative colitis. Additionally, meditation is also applied to manage pain or stress caused by cancer, rather than the cancer itself. Furthermore, there are studies that have yielded positive results where meditation was applied to epilepsy, Human Immunodeficiency Virus (HIV) infections, asthma, premenstrual syndrome, and menopausal syndrome.

Cardiovascular Disease

It can be said that the application of meditation to high blood pressure and cardiovascular disease can be the very oldest yet still the most actively attempted field. Herbert Benson, a cardiologist at Harvard Medical School and director of the Mind-Body Medical Institute, found that practitioners of Transcendental Meditation (TM), a form of Samatha meditation where one concentrates on repeatedly reciting mantras that was popularized in the United States in the 1960s, lowered blood pressure, slowed heart rate, and reduced oxygen consumption while the practitioner was in a state of focus. He called this a wakeful hypometabolic state, in which physiological arousal is reduced, and he also found that this relaxation response can reduce cardiovascular strain and the effects of stress. In addition to TM, Benson and his colleagues developed several relaxation therapies that can induce a relaxation response, such as progressive muscular relaxation and relaxing imagery, and applied them to patients with cardiovascular diseases such as high blood pressure, arrhythmia, and coronary artery disease. Afterwards, Schneider et al. conducted a 3-month follow-up study in which 127 patients with mild hypertension were randomly assigned to three treatments: TM, progressive muscle relaxation, and lifestyle education. The results of the study showed that patients who practiced TM and progressive muscle relaxation had significantly lower blood pressure than patients who only received lifestyle education, and the degree to which blood pressure decreased was greater in the case of TM than in the case of progressive muscle relaxation. Actually, the relaxation response is only one of the biological reactions induced by meditation. Since the goal of meditation of achieving a clear consciousness was not intentionally pursued, it is possible that this difference influenced the results. There is still insufficient evidence that meditation is more effective than relaxation therapy for treating high blood pressure. In a meta-analysis on the effects of TM in lowering blood pressure, it was found that practicing transcendental meditation usually reduces systolic blood pressure to 4 mmHg and diastolic blood pressure to 2 mmHg. Regarding this, the American Heart Association (AHA) recognizes the effects of TM on treating high blood pressure, but expresses the opinion that it does not believe that the practice is superior to general improvements in lifestyle habits or exercise, nor that the effects can be solely attributed to TM compared to other meditation practices. In 2017 however, the AHA did review 57 meditation studies conducted without physical activity such as yoga and officially stated that meditation alone has the potential to lower the risk of cardiovascular disease. Of course, the AHA recommends using meditation as an adjunctive treatment for cardiovascular disease along with making general lifestyle improvements and exercising. Today, it is generally accepted that meditation can help improve high blood pressure, coronary artery disease, diabetes, hyperlipidemia, and hypercortisolemia.

Pain

After the 1990s, mindfulness meditation practices[1] such as Vipassanā received more attention than Samatha meditation. Among them, the Mindfulness-Based Stress Reduction (MBSR) program designed by Jon Kabat-Zinn of the Center for Mindfulness at the University of Massachusetts Medical School has been widely applied therapeutically. As an amalgamation of breathing meditation, sitting meditation, body scanning, Hatha yoga, awareness of stressful situations, eating meditation, and walking meditation, MBSR actually encompasses various techniques including Samatha meditation, relaxation therapy, and stretching rather than being limited to solely Vipassana meditation. It is also characterized as being relatively well structured and standardized compared to other therapeutic meditation methods. Typically, sessions of two and a half hours are held every week for 8 weeks, and short-term workshops of 2 days and 1 night or 1 day are held in parallel. Participants are asked to meditate at least five times a week for at least 45 min each day.

While existing pain treatment strategies seek to avoid pain or distract from it, meditation focuses attention on the specific sensory characteristics of pain and allows the patient to perceive it in a completely different way than before. Initially developed for patients suffering from chronic diseases related to pain, inflammation, and stress, MBSR has been reported to reduce overall symptoms in patients with cancer, rheumatoid arthritis, fibromyalgia, psoriasis, and multiple sclerosis, as well as reducing stress and mental problems. Afterwards, it was expanded to include treating cardiovascular diseases and gastrointestinal diseases, and then to treating patients suffering from mental symptoms such as anxiety and depression.

Therefore, MBSR is the main form of meditation that is practiced as a treatment for pain, and it is known to be able to reduce perception of pain, pain suppression behaviors, and the use of pain medication. However, despite the fact that various studies on MBSR have been attempted over a long period of time, it can be said that no study has yet provided conclusive evidence for its reputation. The most recent meta-analysis of 30 randomized controlled trials showed that MBSR had a mild effect in alleviating pain and depressive symptoms. However, due to qualitative issues in studies included in the meta-analysis, no definitive conclusions could be drawn.

The most cited study is one conducted with support from the NCCIH in 2016 that compared MBSR, Cognitive-Behavioral Therapy (CBT), and conventional treatment in patients aged 20–70 years with chronic low back pain. MBSR and CBT were provided on a schedule of 2 h per week for 8 weeks. The treatments had a higher effect on improving pain and function compared to conventional treatment, and this effect continued until the 26th and 52nd weeks after treatment was completed. There was no significant difference between MBSR and CBT. Considering this, meditation has the potential to alleviate pain through a cognitive shift toward pain. In other words, rather than being tied to or avoiding the pain itself, MBSR and CBT have been shown to have an effect on pain by moving to the position of the ego that observes and separates itself from the cognitive and emotional processes that respond to pain.

Meanwhile, another study conducted with support from NCCIH in 2016 found that meditation had an effect in reducing pain and unpleasant sensations similar to naloxone. This suggests the possibility that meditation can activate the brain's intrinsic opioid system. However, results from other studies show that meditation controls pain only at a cognitive level in higher brain centers without activating the intrinsic opioid system. Considering this, meditation itself appears to

[1]Mindfulness is a translation of the Pali word 'sati.' It means to 'carefully observe the mind's actions.' Today, mindfulness tends to be understood as a translation of Vipassanā meditation, but strictly speaking, 'sati' is a necessary element for both Samatha and Vipassanā mediation.

help improve pain in multiple ways, such as reducing pain receptors or inflammation, and at the same time changing the perception of pain.

Irritable Bowel Syndrome

Along with interest in the gut-brain axis, a small number of studies have been conducted to determine the effects of meditation on irritable bowel syndrome. In one representative study, 75 female patients with irritable bowel syndrome were randomly assigned to receive mindfulness training and support therapy on a half-day schedule once a week for 8 weeks. There was a significant difference in symptom relief rates after 8 weeks between the group that underwent mindfulness training at 26.4% vs the group that underwent supportive therapy at 6.2%. Even after 3 months, there was still a significant difference at 38.2% and 11.8%, respectively. In terms of the size of the effect, however, it was considered to have a potential therapeutic effect. In response, the American Gastroenterological Association (AGA) expected that mindfulness meditation may be effective for irritable bowel syndrome, but not in a significant way.

Ulcerative Colitis

MBSR treatment is consistently being attempted to treat inflammatory diseases. This is because mind-body medical approaches such as meditation have the mechanistic potential to improve the immune system. However, there are also no clinically definitive results for specific immune diseases. Among 55 patients with inactive ulcerative colitis in a preliminary study in 2014, the group that participated in MBSR for 8 weeks showed no differences in the progression of the disease, inflammatory markers, or psychological scale results compared to those who did not. However, the level of perceived stress during the disease activation period was low, which means that MBSR appears to potentially reduce the possibility of ulcerative colitis being activated due to stress.

Cancer

Meditation has the effect of reducing the emotional pain that comes with cancer. In particular, a lot of research has been done on breast cancer. In a representative study, prescribing 6 weeks of mindfulness meditation to young premenopausal breast cancer patients led to the finding that the level of perceived stress, inflammatory gene expression, and inflammatory signals were significantly reduced compared to those who did not. While existing research on meditation has focused on the patients' psychosocial adaptation to cancer while being reserved about its impact on the progression of cancer itself, interesting research results have recently been published showing that meditation can have effects at the cellular level. The telomere length in the chromatin of stage 1 and 2 breast cancer patients who practiced mindfulness meditation for 3 months was maintained throughout the entire period of the study. In contrast, patients who did not practice meditation had shorter telomeres over a three-month period. This suggests the possibility that meditation can reduce stress caused by cancer and at the same time have a direct effect on the progression of the cancer itself.

Things to Consider and Future Prospects

Today, meditation is widely welcomed by the public and has also become a medically important complementary therapy. However, in the current medical system, it is not being used as a priority treatment because, as seen above, no definitive results have been derived through studies such as RCT. There are a few things to consider here.

First of all, being an extremely subjective task, it is expected that there will be large differences between individuals who practice meditation and in terms of obtaining effects from it. Benson claimed that the simple meditation method he designed produced quick and satisfactory results even for beginners. However, since meditation generally presupposes one's ability to concentrate on paying attention, the results will vary depending on one's degree of concentration. Even if a structured group program like MBSR is implemented, each participant will have differences in how they learn meditation and the accompanying results will also vary. Because there are differences in the experience and capabilities of not only the patients themselves but also the program facilitators, limitations in achieving uniform results are to be expected. In other words, even if MBSR was implemented according to a manual in one study, there is no guarantee that the MBSR implemented in that study will be the same as the MBSR implemented in other studies. In addition, MBSR typically requires individual effort from participants during the course of the 8-week program and after the program ends. Thus, it is also highly likely that there will be varying efforts in the efforts that each participant puts in.

Additionally, MBSR is a comprehensive set of various techniques, and it is difficult to determine which elements among them have therapeutic effects. Even if one does not reach a state of clear consciousness, which is the primary goal of meditation, there may be effects that occur not necessarily through meditation alone, but through improving other secondary factors such as the one's relaxation response, emotional stability, or cognitive defusion. In cases such as yoga, it is difficult to distinguish between the benefits of meditation and the benefits of physical activity. In particular, because MBSR requires a lot of effort and time, there is a possibility that these factors may also have a therapeutic effect. The relatively small effect size of symptom relief from meditation may be because secondary factors indirectly intervened to produce improvement effects. In the 1970s, there was criticism that taking a hot spring bath and relaxing for the same amount of time as practicing meditation would both have a similar effect.

Although these criticisms were not raised through experiments, most studies on meditation are not double-blind, which modern medicine requires to eliminate bias, and either do not have a control group or have difficulty setting up a control group. In other words, setting up a control group is necessary to confirm the distinct effects of meditation, but because MBSR is an intervention with so many complex elements beyond just meditation, it is difficult to properly create a control group for it. To this, John Kabat-Zinn responded that the concept of meditation itself is inherently complex and that pure and independent meditation elements cannot be separated from the rest of MBSR, and that MBSR is an organic connection of various elements. Considering this, it can be said that MBSR focuses on the area of complementary and integrative medicine, which seeks to integrate elements and encompass them as a whole, as opposed to modern medicine, which seeks to separate, compare and analyze individual elements.

However, for evidence-based medicine, which is emphasized in modern medicine, just because there is a problem with the research methodology does not mean that the results should be excluded. Rather, evidence-based medicine sets the level of evidence differently depending on the methodology used. According to David Sackett, the founder of evidence-based medicine, evidence-based medicine does not simply rely on the results of clinical research, but is premised on recommending optimal treatment by aligning the doctor's experience and the patient's values. Therefore, it is not advisable to discount the many positive results and deny the clinical effects of meditation solely because of methodological issues. Although it lacks a high level of evidence, it is reasonable to consider mindfulness as a method of treatment to be applied to patients who need it.

Particularly in recent times, a lot of research is being done on how meditation affects brain function through cutting-edge brain imaging techniques. The advantage of brain imaging research is that objective indicators can be confirmed for those who are adept at meditation, allowing the effectiveness of meditation alone to be further verified. In the future, as studies combining clinical research and brain imaging research accumulate, it is expected that it will be possible to lay the foundation for a more scientific investigation of meditation.

Conclusion

In the process of practicing meditation, both physical and mental health improvements are attainable. There are a variety of practical meditation techniques that focus on acquiring these effects, such as relaxation techniques and MBSR. Many research results show that meditation helps relieve symptoms of chronic illnesses, and representative areas of its application include cardiovascular disease, pain, irritable bowel syndrome, ulcerative colitis, and cancer. Although it is difficult to clearly verify the effectiveness of meditation due to the structure of clinical trials, there is at least a considerable amount of evidence that secures meditation as an adjunctive treatment. We expect that meditation will continue to expand its scope of application to various illnesses in the future.

Bibliography

Bower JE, Crosswell AD, Stanton AL, et al. Mindfulness meditation for younger breast cancer survivors: a randomized controlled trial. Cancer. 2015;121(8):1231–40. https://doi.org/10.1002/cncr.29194.

Brook RD, Appel LJ, Rubenfire M, et al. Beyond medications and diet: alternative approaches to lowering blood pressure: a scientific statement from the American Heart Association. Hypertension. 2013;61(6):1360–83. https://doi.org/10.1161/HYP.0b013e318293645f.

Canter PH, Ernst E. Insufficient evidence to conclude whether or not Transcendental Meditation decreases blood pressure: results of a systematic review of randomized clinical trials. J Hypertens. 2004;22(11):2049–54.

Carlson LE, Beattie TL, Giese-Davis J, et al. Mindfulness-based cancer recovery and supportive-expressive therapy maintain telomere length relative to controls in distressed breast cancer survivors. Cancer. 2015;121(3):476–84. https://doi.org/10.1002/cncr.29063.

Casey A, Chang B-H, Huddleston J, Virani N, Benson H, Dusek JA. A model for integrating a mind/body approach to cardiac rehabilitation: outcomes and correlators. J Cardiopulm Rehabil Prev. 2009;29(4):230–8; quiz 239–240. https://doi.org/10.1097/HCR.0b013e3181a33352.

Cherkin DC, Sherman KJ, Balderson BH, et al. Effect of mindfulness-based stress reduction vs cognitive behavioral therapy or usual care on back pain and functional limitations in adults with chronic low back pain: a randomized clinical trial. JAMA. 2016;315(12):1240–9. https://doi.org/10.1001/jama.2016.2323.

Gaylord SA, Palsson OS, Garland EL, et al. Mindfulness training reduces the severity of irritable bowel syndrome in women: results of a randomized controlled trial. Am J Gastroenterol. 2011;106(9):1678–88. https://doi.org/10.1038/ajg.2011.184.

Hilton L, Hempel S, Ewing BA, et al. Mindfulness meditation for chronic pain: systematic review and meta-analysis. Ann Behav Med. 2017;51(2):199–213. https://doi.org/10.1007/s12160-016-9844-2.

Jedel S, Hoffman A, Merriman P, et al. A randomized controlled trial of mindfulness-based stress reduction to prevent flare-up in patients with inactive ulcerative colitis. Digestion. 2014;89(2):142–55. https://doi.org/10.1159/000356316.

Kabat-Zinn J. Bringing mindfulness to medicine. Interview by Karolyn A. Gazella. Altern Ther Health Med. 2005;11(3):56–64.

Kabat-Zinn J, Lipworth L, Burney R. The clinical use of mindfulness meditation for the self-regulation of chronic pain. J Behav Med. 1985;8(2):163–90.

Levine GN, Lange RA, Bairey-Merz CN, et al. Meditation and cardiovascular risk reduction: a scientific statement from the American Heart Association. J Am Heart Assoc. 2017;6(10). https://doi.org/10.1161/JAHA.117.002218.

Morgan N, Irwin MR, Chung M, Wang C. The effects of mind-body therapies on the immune system: meta-analysis. PLoS One. 2014;9(7):e100903. https://doi.org/10.1371/journal.pone.0100903.

Ooi SL, Giovino M, Pak SC. Transcendental meditation for lowering blood pressure: an overview of systematic reviews and meta-analyses. Complement Ther Med. 2017;34:26–34. https://doi.org/10.1016/j.ctim.2017.07.008.

Ray IB, Menezes AR, Malur P, Hiltbold AE, Reilly JP, Lavie CJ. Meditation and coronary heart disease: a review of the current clinical evidence. Ochsner J. 2014;14(4):696–703.

Richardson PEH. David Sackett and the birth of evidence based medicine: how to practice and teach EBM. BMJ. 2015;350:h3089. https://doi.org/10.1136/bmj.h3089.

Schneider RH, Alexander CN, Staggers F, et al. A randomized controlled trial of stress reduction in African Americans treated for hypertension for over one year. Am J Hypertens. 2005;18(1):88–98. https://doi.org/10.1016/j.amjhyper.2004.08.027.

Sharon H, Maron Katz A, Ben Simon E, et al. Mindfulness meditation modulates pain through endogenous opioids. Am J Med. 2016;129(7):755–8. https://doi.org/10.1016/j.amjmed.2016.03.002.

Wang C, Li K, Gaylord S. Prevalence, patterns, and predictors of meditation use among U.S. children: results from the National Health Interview Survey. Complement Ther Med. 2019;43:271–6. https://doi.org/10.1016/j.ctim.2019.02.004.

Zeidan F, Adler-Neal AL, Wells RE, et al. Mindfulness-meditation-based pain relief is not mediated by endogenous opioids. J Neurosci. 2016;36(11):3391–7. https://doi.org/10.1523/JNEUROSCI.4328-15.2016.

The Clinical Application of Meditation for Children and Adolescents

20

Young-Sook Kwack

Mental health problems in children and adolescents not only have a significant impact on learning and peer relationships, but if not treated early, often lead to mental health problems in adulthood. Mental health is therefore very important both from the perspective of an individual but also from a socioeconomic perspective. However, there is still a lack of understanding and interest in mental illness in Korea. In particular, not much is known about mental illness in children and adolescents, so it is rare for children to be admitted to the hospital before they show serious symptoms. Additionally, due to the nature of children at this stage of development, they are often reluctant to use psychotropic medication as they think that these drugs are intended to relieve symptoms rather than cure them. These children also often feel burdened by having to take medication for a long time and fear their side effects. Although in most cases this is the result of prejudice against drug treatment, there is still a lack of long-term research on the effects and side effects of medication on the development of children and adolescents. More research on this subject is therefore needed in the future. Additionally, in the case of mental illness during childhood and adolescence, patients often feel that psychological treatment is ineffective. In reality, psychotherapy alone has been shown to have limitations as there are many cases where its effects did not meet expectations.

It is desirable for consumers to have many different types of treatment to choose from. In addition to psychotherapy and drug treatment, mindfulness has been introduced as an alternative that is both effective and has no major side effects, and it has been applied as a therapy for various symptoms and illnesses. According to John Kabat-Zinn, the founder of MBSR, a representative program that clinically applies mindfulness, mindfulness is defined as 'consciously paying attention uncritically to the present moment.' Mindfulness is rooted in the tradition of meditation and can be considered to be one of several methods of meditation. This chapter investigates how mindfulness originated and evolved from meditation, what the differences are between meditation and mindfulness, the types of techniques of mindfulness-based programs, the evidence of their therapeutic effects and the application of mindfulness-based programs in various communities, including schools.

From Meditation to Mindfulness

As a method of practice that originated in the world of Buddhism in the East, meditation is aimed at 'obtaining one's true self without entan-

Y.-S. Kwack (✉)
National Center for Mental Health,
Seoul, Republic of Korea
e-mail: yskcpy@cheju.ac.kr

J.-H. Chae, H.-Y. Lee (eds.), *Meditation in Psychiatry and General Medicine*,
https://doi.org/10.1007/978-981-95-7147-5_20

glements or conflict in order to reach the state of Nirvana where there is no pain.' In the East, meditation has been a part of one's religious practice in order to reduce suffering and enhance positive qualities such as insight, wisdom, and equanimity. Focused attention and open monitoring, the representative forms of meditation, are rooted in the traditions of Zen, Vipassana, and Tibetan Buddhist meditation.

According to the literature, focused attention is also called concentrative meditation, and open monitoring is also called insight meditation. Meditation can be largely divided into focused attention, which involves paying close attention to a specific object, and insight meditation, which opens the mind to all objects and emphasizes 'awareness at this moment.' Among these, mindfulness can be seen as belonging to the latter. Other literature states that in traditional Vipassana meditation, concentration meditation is followed by mindfulness meditation, and both are used together to gain insight. As for meditation in Western culture, focused attention and open awareness have been mixed together into what is called mindfulness meditation. Mindfulness meditation has its origins in both Vipassana and Zen meditation traditions, but in Western cultures, Vipassana techniques are often chosen over Zen techniques. Eastern traditions require extensive training and include both focused attention and open awareness. Concentrative meditation can be considered as the primary basis for mindfulness-based interventions. Mindfulness-Based Stress Reduction (MBSR) is the only concentrative meditation technique with distinct roots in Buddhist philosophy, and it is based more deeply on Vipassana than Zen.

After Eastern meditation practice was introduced in this way to modern America, mindfulness meditation was developed within a scientific system so that it can be performed briefly and easily anywhere to suit the busy daily lives of modern people. In other words, mindfulness meditation can be seen as a Western style of meditation that is differentiated and developed from existing religious Eastern meditation methods. In the West, mindfulness meditation is a method of stress management, self-discipline, and psychotherapy.

Through mindfulness, participants attempt to accept unpleasant and painful experiences as they are, rather than trying to change them. However, because attempting to reduce one's suffering is an instinctive human response, many programs based on mindfulness focus on balancing the desire to change one's situation with an attitude of accepting reality. This is different from cognitive behavioral therapy (CBT), which focuses on changing one's perception and behavior. In other words, the goal of mindfulness is not to try changing one's thinking, but to change one's attitude towards thinking.

A Variety of Techniques

Five types of meditation practice were systematically investigated, targeting children and adolescents. They are (1) concentrative meditation, (2) insight meditation, (3) transcendental meditation, (4), the mind-body technique, and (5) the body-mind technique. The mind-body technique includes meditation and relaxation, and the body-mind technique includes yoga postures and tai chi movements.

The representative techniques for concentrative meditation as mindfulness-based interventions are Mindfulness-Based Stress Reduction (MBSR) and Mindfulness-Based Cognitive Therapy (MBCT).

MBSR is a 8- to 10-week program that trains patients in mindfulness to reduce stress by recognizing events and experiences from an objective perspective without being absorbed in their thoughts or emotions. When MBSR was first developed by John Kabat-Zinn at the University of Massachusetts Medical School in 1979, it was performed on patients with chronic pain and stress related illnesses. Now, the scope of its application has expanded and it has been proven to be a useful program for everyone, regardless of diagnosis or illness. MBSR is conducted as a group therapy once a week for two and a half hours for 8–10 weeks, and the program includes mindfulness meditation, self-awareness of the body, Hatha yoga, and defense using mindfulness in stressful situations.

MBCT was founded by J. D. Teasdale in 1991 and was originally developed to prevent recurrence in patients with a history of major depressive disorder. The program incorporates techniques such as mindfulness meditation into existing cognitive behavioral therapy, and aims to suppress the process in which stressful situations automatically lead to depressive episodes. Through MBCT, rather than just uncritically accepting negative stimuli and becoming immersed in those emotions, patients learn how to react less by stopping the natural flow of thoughts and looking at stimuli objectively. MBCT is conducted for 2 h once a week for 8 weeks, but a significant portion of the program is achieved through patients practicing mindfulness in their daily lives outside of class. During the 8-week MBCT program, participants learn to recognize that their thoughts and emotions do not accurately reflect reality, but are instead mental and internal events that occur within their own thoughts.

When MBCT is performed on children, they are encouraged to focus on memories of negative experiences, focus on the emotions that accompany those experiences, and become aware of physical sensations. After a few minutes, participants are asked to take a 3-min 'breathing space,' during which time they are asked to focus on their breathing and what is going on in their body and mind. Afterwards, in a relaxed state, participants tell themselves that they can now handle anything and resume focusing on their entire body. Participants are encouraged to use the 3-min breathing space they learned in their daily lives whenever they feel bad, helping them integrate formal training into their daily routines.

Both MBSR and MBCT emphasize one's attitude when meditating. Both emphasize a nonjudgmental, effortless, and relaxed approach. The more you practice, the deeper this attitude becomes, and you can move from concentration to a state of mental stability more easily since you are entering meditation without exerting much effort.

Research on insight meditation has been conducted targeting children and adolescents with ADHD. Insight meditation is usually practiced after the ability to concentrate and meditate is established. The goal of insight meditation is to just be in a state of observation. Rather than focus on any specific object, you focus moment to moment on anything that occurs in your experience. You observe every experience (thought, feeling, etc.) that occurs. Through a nonjudgmental process, one becomes detached from one's experience, is non-reactive, and gains insight and awareness. Types of insight meditation include Sahaja meditation, Sahaja Samandhi meditation, and Sahaja Yoga meditation. Among these, only Sahaja Yoga meditation was studied on children and adolescents.

Sahaja meditation is a 6-week insight meditation program that has been modified for children. Patients are expected to participate in meditation sessions at the clinical site twice a week and to meditate at home as well. Meditation sessions begin with guidance, sharing one's experience, and having shorter meditation sessions at home together with parents who have received meditation training.

Transcendental meditation is also called automatic self-transcendence, and here automatic means that the individual does not try to control their mental activity. Unlike in insight or concentration meditation, transcendental meditation neither focuses on controlling or even being aware of one's experience. Instead, it attempts to calm mental activity. During relaxation exercises, the practitioner repeats a mantra (a phrase spoken in silence) to block out distracting thoughts. Relaxation activities are used regularly to achieve a state of physical and mental calmness. This technique does not require concentration, reflection, or mental control. It reduces physiological arousal, but increases conscious arousal. This concept is somewhat difficult to understand for Westerners, so it may be difficult for children to understand as well.

The mind-body technique appears to link concentration meditation and insight meditation. In a sense, it even includes transcendental meditation through elements of relaxation. These include relaxation techniques such as MED-RELAX, progressive relaxation, or relaxation therapy. Deep breathing meditation is a mind-body technique used for testing anxiety. In addition, also included are techniques that combine posture, breathing, concentration, visualization, and electromyography biofeedback.

Meditation relaxation was used with Sri Lankan children traumatized by the 2004 Southeast Asia tsunami. According to its contents, the first hour includes psychological education, an evaluation of the child's problems, and then ends with a deep breathing exercise for at least 15 min. Each session begins and ends with 15 min of breathing exercises, where participants consciously focus on relaxing their mind as they inhale and exhale. The middle part consists of different meditations and relaxations, including inner peace meditation (25 min during the second meditation), uchchadana mantra chanting (25 min during the third session), progressive muscle relaxation (25 min during the fourth session), ice cream body relaxation (25 min during the fifth session), and inner light meditation (25 min during the sixth session). For each meditation and relaxation activity, the lead counselor reads content introduced in a manual in the same way.

For example, ice cream meditation is as follows: a bed sheet or mat is laid on the floor. The child is then asked to stand on it barefoot. Relaxation music is played and the background and the child are guided as follows: 'Stand up and put your hands up. Now imagine you are ice cream. This ice cream will gradually begin to melt in the air. Likewise, your body also gently relaxes (instructions are given very gradually and slowly while the music plays). The tension in your body decreases step by step and you melt a little more. The height of the ice cream decreases as it melts. Likewise, your height also slowly decreases. Slowly, little by little, and again, it melts. Now, it melts and spreads out on the floor (the sentence is repeated several times slowly until the child lies on the floor and relaxes).'

Participants are assigned homework to practice meditation techniques at home for 1 h every day. Progressive relaxation or relaxation therapy involves relaxing and tensing eight muscles, starting at the feet and ending at the head. Deep breathing meditation is a stress management strategy that involves focusing one's attention on breathing for a few minutes of quiet time. The practitioner sits in a comfortable position in a quiet environment and focuses their attention on breathing with an accepting attitude in order to develop their concentration. Fisher developed a focused meditation and insight meditation technique for children and adolescents in the latency period to help students become more receptive to learning in a classroom environment. Fisher provides four methods for use in a classroom environment: posture, breathing, concentration, and visualization. Posture techniques help with body control, breathing techniques help students prepare for brainstorming and free writing in a calm state, concentration helps memory, and visualization helps with imagination.

A posture technique for elementary school students is having them imagine themselves holding a needle. Middle and high school students make poses they have already learned with consent. Breathing involves alternating between slowly and quickly inhaling and exhaling. For training concentration, concentration games are suggested for children. Lastly, guided imagery is performed for visualization.

Neurophysiological Changes as Medical Evidence

Before examining whether meditation techniques actually have a therapeutic effect, it is necessary to first look at the medical evidence supporting neurophysiological changes. When Rubia compared the meditation states of experienced meditators and novice meditators (a control group), he reported that the parasympathetic nervous system, which is activated when resting, was more active in the experienced meditators. He also found that electroencephalography during meditation showed an increase in alpha waves, which are associated with anxiety reduction, and theta waves, which are important for emotional processing and maintaining attention, in the left frontal lobe. PET scans showed similar results, namely increased signals in the left frontal lobe, which is related to positive emotions, and in the limbic system, which is related to concentration of attention. In this way, the brain wave patterns observed during meditation and the specific brain regions activated can be viewed as objective evidence that signifies meaningful neurological changes through meditation, which supports the clinical application of meditation.

Research on the Therapeutic Effects of Mindfulness

Research on stress relief based on practicing mindfulness has mainly been conducted on adults, but research studies on school-age children and adolescents are being conducted little by little. Although there are limitations to these studies in that there are not many randomized control studies because most of them target small groups, the future of mindfulness-based treatment is bright when considering the results of the studies reported to date. According to Biegel et al., the advantages of MBSR for adolescents are as follows. First, it can be applied to various mental illnesses. Second, because it focuses on the present, it induces a more appropriate mental response to stress and related emotional and behavioral problems. Since much stress is caused by cognitive and emotional reactions to past or future events, MBSR helps people escape from cognitive and emotional events that cause stress and subsequent psychological problems through a calm and clear perception of the present. Third, the characteristics of MBSR, which emphasize paying attention to experiences, are considered to be well accepted by adolescents.

As a result of a randomized control study targeting 102 adolescents aged 14 to 18, children who completed the MBSR program reported in their self-evaluations that anxiety, depression, and stress were reduced, and their confidence and quality of sleep were improved compared to the control group. The rate of mood disorders was also significantly lower in the MBSR participant group. As the number of days practicing sitting meditation increased, the Global Assessment of Functioning score increased while the Mental Health Problem Scale (Symptom Checklist-90) score decreased, showing that MBSR influences changes in mental health. In the follow-up study, the overall functioning scale score was significantly higher in the MBSR participant group, showing a moderate effect size. Blind clinical measurements of mental health showed significant improvement in the treatment group, and significant improvement was also observed during a 3-month follow-up, showing that the changes were maintained. The evaluation conducted 3 months after the end of the program showed more improved results compared to the evaluation conducted immediately after and compared to the control group, suggesting that MBSR can be a good treatment and prevention method for adolescents' mental health.

Like MBSR, MBCT is also currently being applied to various diseases other than major depressive disorder (generalized anxiety disorder, cancer, suicidal thoughts, bipolar disorder, etc.), and research targeting children and adolescents is only just beginning. In a small-scale study targeting school-age and adolescent children, MBCT was found to be effective in improving internal problems such as anxiety and depression and externalizing problems such as ADHD, conduct disorder, and autism. Among these, the supplementation of mindfulness-based cognitive therapy in a study by Bögels et al. reduced behavioral problems in children with autistic disorder. However, the most impressive result of the study was the effect of continuously improving social skills in children with autism. The subjects were 14 adolescents with autism disorder, ADHD, oppositional disorder, conduct disorder, and externalizing symptoms, and mindfulness-based cognitive therapy was also administered to their parents at the same time. The study was conducted for 8 weeks and a follow-up survey was conducted 8 weeks later. As a supplementary method to control the impulsivity associated with ADHD, subjects were given half a cookie and instructed that if they did not eat it by the time they returned, they would be given the other half. In the meantime, they were instructed to focus on breathing to divert their attention from the desire to eat the cookie. Reinforcement was given for things such as doing homework and attending. After treatment, the child's social behavior questionnaire for parents showed a moderate or higher effect, and this effect was maintained during the follow-up. In the case of children with autism, they performed the best with regard to doing homework. Since the dropout rate was highest for oppositional disorder and behavioral disorder, it was suggested that individual training would be better for these patients. How to revise the technique according to the patient's diagnosis and age should be considered in the future.

In a study by Semple et al., Mindfulness-Based Cognitive Therapy for children was administered to a small group of children for 90 min per week for 12 weeks. The study assumed that anxiety interferes with concentration and emotional regulation. MBCT for children is a manualized group psychotherapy that was developed to increase the socio-emotional resilience (affective self-regulation) of urban children aged 9–13 from low-income families through improved mindfulness concentration. During the course of the study, behavioral problems were measured and assessed using the Child Behavior Checklist, State-Trait Anxiety Inventory for Children, and Multidimensional Anxiety Scale for Children. The results reported significant reductions in behavioral problems and moderate effect sizes. This suggests that MBCT for children is valuable as an additional intervention method for attentional and behavior problems and can reduce anxiety symptoms in children.

What is interesting about several studies related to mindfulness is that children often responded that there was no change after completing the program, but there were cases where parents and teachers evaluated that the children showed improvement. The studies mentioned several possibilities for this: first, there is the opinion that children may have had difficulty in evaluating themselves due to their immature ability to self-reflect compared to adults, whereas parents and teachers mainly evaluate children based on observing their behavior (especially for the reduction of ADHD symptoms such as inattention). On the other hand, there is an opinion that suggests a gap between the two may arise because children evaluate themselves based on their own subjective feelings. In other words, this suggests that MBSR can be more effectively applied to treat ADHD and behavioral problems. In fact, when Sahaja yoga meditation was used as an adjunctive therapy for 6 weeks in parallel with existing treatment for children with ADHD, it was confirmed that symptoms related to hyperactivity, impulsive behavior, and inattention were all improved, and the effect was maintained even when 50% of patients receiving treatment reduced the dosage or discontinued taking medication. However, rather than viewing meditation as a treatment that replaces medication, it would be more appropriate to view it as a method of treatment that can reduce the side effects of medication and maximize its effectiveness when combined with medication.

Even in Korea, more and more mindfulness research targeting adolescents is being conducted. A study was conducted on suicide, one of the serious problems of Korean youth, with the purpose of examining the effects of the Mindfulness-Based Teenager Suicide Prevention Program (MBTP) on suicidal thoughts, depression, and self-esteem. Program participants were measured on a suicidal ideation scale, a depression scale, a self-esteem scale, and a mindfulness scale. To prove the effectiveness of the program, a pre-post evaluation and a follow-up evaluation after 6 months were conducted to compare the experimental group with a control group that did not receive any treatment. The resulting data analysis showed that the suicidal thoughts and depression scores of the group that participated in MBTP were significantly reduced while self-esteem significantly increased. On the other hand, the control group showed no significant changes in relation to the scale. This suggests that MBTP is effective as a self-regulation program for suicidal thoughts and depression in adolescents. Additionally, the levels of self-esteem and mindfulness remained stable in the follow-up evaluation 6 months later, showing that the program has a lasting effect.

Another study sought to examine the effect of the MBCT program on the attention span of high school students. The results of a comparative analysis of the experimental group, the MBCT program group, and a control group showed that attention span and self-control significantly increased while anxiety and depression significantly decreased after students participated in the program compared to before. These results show that cognitive therapy based on mindfulness not only reduces negative emotions in high school students but also helps improve attention.

In a study targeting 42 fifth-grade elementary school students, a mind subtraction school-based meditation program was conducted four times a week for 8 weeks. The study then analyzed changes in depression, social anxiety, aggression, and salivary cortisol levels. The results showed a decrease in levels of all three. These results reveal that meditation can be effective in improving the psychosocial and behavioral aspects of elementary school students.

The Application of Mindfulness and Its Preventative Effect in Schools and Communities

Considering that meditation, the source of mindfulness, was originally a practice for the general public, mindfulness meditation can be implemented not only for the treatment of mental illnesses but also as a preventative measure to relieve stress and negative thinking in everyday life outside of hospitals, such as schools and community centers. In fact, the results of an 8-week randomized controlled study conducted on elementary school students aged 7 or 8 without mental illnesses showed an improvement in attention deficit and internal problems. In other studies, there was improvement shown in teachers' evaluation of their students in terms of attention, self-control, participation in school activities, and respect for peers. These results suggest that practicing mindfulness meditation regularly at school can help improve the overall mental health and academic achievements of students. In foreign countries, a range of mindfulness programs are being implemented in schools, including, for example, the University of Toronto's Mindfulness-Based Wellness Education (MBWE), the UK's Mindfulness in Schools Project (MISP), the US's Inner Kids Program, Cultivating Awareness and Resilience in Education (CARE), and Stress Management and Relaxation Techniques (SMART), as well as Spain's TREVA, Aulas Felices, and Meditación Fluir Programs.

What these programs have in common is the lack of randomized controlled studies. In some studies, the control group was a group of patients on the waitlist, rather than those of another mindfulness group or other curricular control group. There are also no studies on the long-term effects of these programs. Although the studies talk about positive effects, most of them target small sample groups, have weak research designs, and consist of subjective self-reports or observational evaluation data by participants or organizers. These materials are being used to promote these programs without any scientific procedures for reliability and validity.

Among these, the book *Mindful Games*, based on the Inner Kids Program in the United States, was recently translated and published as a meditation book for children in Korea. This book is a compilation of manuals for 10-plus years of nonreligious mindfulness professional training programs for children and families. The contents of the book are as follows:

The purpose of training is to develop life skills. Mindful play introduces six life skills, namely (1) focusing, (2) quieting, (3) seeing, (4) reframing, (5) caring, and (6) connecting. Of these, focusing is the central axis that supports the remaining five life skills.

The best way for parents or teachers to teach children to meditate is for them to meditate themselves. The specific methods will flow naturally from one's own actual meditation experience. Although meditation may seem like a passive action, it is a passive attitude as a strategy to finally recognize things that were not recognizable in an overly active state. Learning something new about something you did not know is one thing curious children love the most.

In addition, *Mindfulness Play* added more active and fun elements that took into consideration the child's developmental stage. The core training elements of sitting meditation, walking meditation, yoga, body exploration, and loving-kindness meditation were appropriately modified to suit the children's situation and level of understanding. The book also introduces 60 games using everyday tools such as breathing, our bodies, a pinwheel, a cup of water, wind, and stars. For example, breathing using a pinwheel allows the child to observe that the feeling in their body and mind changes depending on the way they breathe (fast and slow breathing, deep and shallow breathing, etc.). The book emphasizes that meditation experience from a teacher or parent must come first.

Recently, in Korea, a developmental and culturally sensitive Mindfulness-based Social-Emotional Growth (MSEG) Program was developed for children and adolescents. Kwack et al. (2024) emphasized this program's necessity to help students appreciate life, find personal meaning, build authentic relationships, and enhance resilience. By embedding mindfulness practices into the school curriculum, the authors expected schools to create an environment that supports mental wellness, reduces the incidence of mental health issues, and promotes overall well-being. Given the relative scarcity of mindfulness-related research in children and adolescents compared to adults, they are trying to get evidence of the effectiveness of their program by implementing it in schools.

Discussion

Through the various studies described above, it is known that mindfulness meditation can have positive effects in children and adolescents, such as improving attention, increasing the ability to cope with situations, relieving stress, and reducing anxiety and depression. However, cases that have been systematically proven through large-scale randomized control studies are rare, and most studies do not properly consider small sample sizes and control variables, resulting in large errors and failing to properly reflect the effects. Further research needs to be conducted through clinical studies with large samples and control variables to better understand the neurophysiological mechanisms and clinical effects of mindfulness meditation.

Additionally, since mindfulness meditation is a newly emerging method of treatment, we do not yet know what effects it will have on the brain or what its acute and long-term effects will be. Therefore, in order to overcome these problems, it is necessary to conduct research on any complications that may occur as a result of mindfulness meditation treatment before it is applied in a clinical setting. Like other treatments, mindfulness-based programs may have side effects. A multicenter study by Cebolla et al. (2017) showed 25.4% of attendees experienced an increase in mental suffering, as well as an increase in anxiety and feelings of confusion. Mindfulness meditation research done by Lustyk et al. (2009) reported participants with mental illness such as severe anxiety, depression, and psychosis had the most side effects. Specifically, guiding mindfulness without recognizing PTSD could result in re-experiencing trauma and even dissociation. In the case of psychosis, aggravations of hallucination and delusion were reported. More caution is needed in the case of children and adolescents because their ego strength and ability to self-control are not fully developed. Therefore, in the case of mental illness, mindfulness-based programs can be applied in a case-by-case situation along with evidence-based psychiatric treatments after a thorough psychiatric evaluation.

According to Sibinga et al., the biggest limitation for conducting an MBSR program was low participation and attendance rates. According to the study, 130 youths initially registered to participate in the sessions, but only 43 people actually attended, and only 35 of them attended more than 5 out of 9 sessions. Considering this, we can expect compliance levels for patients to be poor if this treatment were to actually be applied in clinical practice, and it is necessary to consider ways to improve compliance. The first measure to consider is increasing accessibility. Establishing a community-based program, such as the school-based MBSR program in the study mentioned above, can also be an alternative. Improving accessibility of treatment for patients so that they can easily learn and apply meditation techniques in their daily lives may help maintain compliance and long-term effectiveness.

Additionally, I believe that clinical experience and research on meditation therapy techniques that are appropriate for our culture are needed. Basically, I do not think that the basic philosophy or approach to meditation is very different between Westerners and Koreans. Buddhism and Zen (Korean: Seon) are widely and deeply rooted in Korean culture. They are thus cultural heritages that we are already very familiar with both consciously and unconsciously. However, if we try to apply a Western treatment that has been manualized as a specific treatment method to Korean people, we will need to take cultural differences into consideration. In particular, linguistic differences affect teaching, learning, and experience, so when revising the treatment to create a Korean version, we need to apply a detailed conversion to suit our language and reality, and we must also take into consideration differences in socio-cultural background as well as existing thoughts or attitudes towards meditation. In addition, we must find meditation training and guidance methods applicable in clinical settings through clinical experience and research on the Korean people. There are very few studies conducted on children and adolescents, both in Korea and abroad, when compared to adults, so more clinical experience and research are needed.

Conclusion

Meditation is commonly used for self-discipline and religious spiritual development. However, when we consider its effectiveness, it can also be used as a psychological treatment method in various fields including stress relief, and its scope of use is also expanding in psychiatric clinical trials. Additionally, mindfulness based on meditation can be seen as having a wide range of possibilities and applications as a way to reduce the limitations of existing treatment methods such as pharmacotherapy, and to maximize their effectiveness. In particular, mindfulness may be an option for children who are burdened by medication or are struggling with psychotherapy due to limitations with language. However, because there is still insufficient evidence for the effectiveness of mindfulness, it remains a supplementary treatment. In order for meditation to be widely used clinically as an evidence-based treatment, more high-quality research must be conducted in the future.

Bibliography

Ames CS, Richardson J, Payne S, Smith P, Leigh E. Innovations in practice: mindfulness-based cognitive therapy for depression in adolescents. Child Adolesc Ment Health. 2014;19:74–8.

Armon E, Kohls N, Giordano J. On the viability of neurotechnology and mind-body methods in pediatric mental health: perspectives on integrating new tools to complement old techniques. Eur J Integr Med. 2016;8(2):137–40.

Biegel GM, Brown KW, Shapiro SL, Schubert CM. Mindfulness-based stress reduction for the treatment of adolescent psychiatric outpatients: a randomized clinical trial. J Consult Clin Psychol. 2009;77(5):855–66.

Bögels S, Hoogstad B, van Dun L, de Schutter S, Restifo K. Mindfulness training for adolescents with externalizing disorders and their parents. Behav Cogn Psychother. 2008;36:193–209.

Catani C, Kohiladevy M, Ruf M, Schauer E, Elbert T, Neuner F. Treating children traumatized by war and tsunami: a comparison between exposure therapy and meditation-relaxation in North-East Sri Lanka. BMC Psychiatry. 2009;9:22. https://doi.org/10.1186/1471-244X-9-22.

Cebolla A, Demarzo M, Martins P, Soler J, Garcia-Campayo J. Unwanted effects: is there a negative side of meditation? A multicentre survey. PLoS One. 2017;12:e0183137.

Crescentini C, Capurso V, Furlan S, Fabbro F. Mindfulness-oriented meditation for primary school children: effects on attention and psychological well-being. Front Psychol. 2016. https://doi.org/10.3389/fpsyg.2016.00805.

Drigas A, Karyotaki M. Mindfulness skills training & assessment and intelligence. Int J Recent Contrib Eng Sci IT. 2018;6(3):70–85.

Eklund K, O'Malley M, Meyer L. Gauging mindfulness in children and youth: school-based applications. Psychol Sch. 2016;54(1):101–14.

Eom JW, Kim JM. The effects of the mindfulness-based cognitive therapy program on attention and reduction in depression and anxiety of high school student. Korean J Youth Stud. 2013;20(3):159–85.

Felder JN, Dimidjian S, Segal Z. Collaboration in mindfulness-based cognitive therapy. J Clin Psychol. 2012;68(2):179–86.

Fisher R. Still thinking: the case for meditation with children. Think Skill Creat. 2006;1(2):146–51.

Greenland SK. Mindful games: sharing mindfulness and meditation with children, teens and families. Boulder: Shambhahala Publications; 2016.

Grossman P, Niemann L, Schmidt S, Walach H. Mindfulness-based stress reduction and health benefits: a meta-analysis. J Psychosom Res. 2004;57(1):35–43.

Harrison LJ, Manocha R, Rubia K. Sahaja yoga meditation as a family treatment programme for children with attention deficit-hyperactivity disorder. Clin Child Psychol Psychiatry. 2004;9(4):479–97.

Haydicky J, Shecter C, Wiener J, Ducharme JM. Evaluation of MBCT for adolescents with ADHD and their parents: impact on individual and family functioning. J Child Fam Stud. 2015;24:76–94.

Kabat-Zinn J. An outpatient program in behavioral medicine for chronic pain patients based on the practice of mindfulness meditation: theoretical considerations and preliminary results. Gen Hosp Psychiatry. 1982;4(1):33–47.

Kabat-Zinn J. Wherever you Go, There you are. New York: Hyperion; 1994.

Kim CK, editor. Dictionary of counseling. Seoul: Hakjisa; 2016.

Kim DY, Son CN. The effects of a mindfulness based teenager suicide prevention program (MBTP) on suicidal ideation, depression and self-esteem. Korean J Health Psychol. 2012;17(2):323–39.

Kwack YS, Kang YH, Kim WD, Kim YH. The necessity of developing mindfulness based programs in school, SPECIAL ARTICLE Mindfulness based Social-Emotional Growth (MSEG) Program. Korean J Medit Med. 2024;4(1):1–6.

Lustyk MK, Chawla N, Nolan RS, Marlatt GA. Mindfulness meditation research; issues of participant screening, safety procedures, and researcher training. Adv Mind Body Med. 2009;24:20–30.

O'Brien KM, Larson CM, Murrell AR. Third-wave behavior therapies for children and adolescents: progress, challenges, and future directions. In: Greco LA, Hayes SC, editors. Acceptance and mindfulness treatments for children and adolescents: a practitioner's guide. Oakland: New Harbinger Publications; 2004. p. 15–35.

Perry-Parrish C, Copeland-Linde N, Webb L, Shields AH, Sibinga EM. Improving self-regulation in adolescents: current evidence for the role of mindfulness-based cognitive therapy. Adolesc Health Med Ther. 2016;7:101–8.

Rubia K. The neurobiology of meditation and its clinical effectiveness in psychiatric disorders. Biol Psychol. 2009;82(1):1–11.

Semple RJ, Lee J, Rosa D, Miller LF. A randomized trial of mindfulness-based cognitive therapy for children: promoting mindful attention to enhance social-emotional resiliency in children. J Child Fam Stud. 2010;19:218–29.

Sibinga E, Perry-Parrish C, Thorpe K, Mika M, Ellen J. A small mixed-method RCT of mindfulness instruction for urban youth. Explore. 2014;10(3):180–6.

Simkin DR, Black NB. Meditation and mindfulness in clinical practice. Child Adolesc Psychiatr Clin N Am. 2014;23(3):487–534. https://doi.org/10.1016/j.chc.2014.03.002.

Teasdale JD, Segal Z, Williams JG. How does cognitive therapy prevent depressive relapse and why should attentional control (mindfulness) training help? Behav Res Ther. 1995;33(1):25–39.

Travis F, Shear J. Focused attention, open monitoring and automatic self-transcending: categories to organize meditations from Vedic, Buddhist and Chinese traditions. Conscious Cogn. 2010;19(4):1110–8.

Walker L, Greene J, Garber J, Horndasch RL, Barnard J, Ghishan F. Psychosocial factors in pediatric abdominal pain: implications for assessment and treatment. Clin Psychol. 1993;26:206–13.

Yoo YG, Lee DJ, Lee IS, Shin N, Park JY, Yoon MR, Yu B. The effects of mind subtraction meditation on depression, social anxiety, aggression, and salivary cortisol levels of elementary school children in South Korea. J Pediatr Nurs. 2016;31(3):e185–97.

21 Meditation at the Workplace

Meerae Lim

Through modern times, the appearance of society changed from an agricultural society to an industrial society. The agricultural society was a society mainly composed of family and community, but as it moved to an industrial society, the role of family and community decreased and the workplace emerged as an important community. In fact, workers spend a significant part of their day at work. In other words, most people spend a certain part of their lives at work, whether that time is more or less.

Along with these changes in society, the concept of a healthy workplace has become increasingly important as the workplace receives attention in the field of health. In the early days, the concept of a healthy workplace was mainly focused on the physical working environment and the physical stability of workers during work. For example, the main concern was industrial accidents caused by health threats from harmful substances or physical risks in the workplace. However, this concept expanded its meaning with the expansion of the concept of health. In 1943, the World Health Organization (WHO) expanded its definition of health, defining "Health is a state of complete physical, mental and social well-being and not merely the absence of disease or infirmity." Since then, in 1998, it has been re-expanded and defined as a concept that includes spiritual parts, saying, "Health is a dynamic state of complete physical, mental, spiritual and social well-being and not merely the absence of disease or infirmity." The concept of a healthy workplace has also expanded from preventing physical risks to actively promoting physical and mental health. For example, in the past, to prevent industrial accidents, focus was placed on the physical elements of the environment related to safety and the work environment was created. Since then, it has recently been developed to make spatial elements, architectural details, and surrounding environmental elements in a way that can reduce workers' stress. Interest in mental stress has increased, and even the concept of interpersonal relationships in the workplace has been included as one of the important areas of health problems.

There are two main reasons why companies are interested in mental health. The first is the socially imposed obligation of employers. In recent years, cases of illness, suicide, depression, etc., caused by work-related stress being recognized as industrial accidents are increasing all over the world. If an employee's health is in danger of deteriorating due to overwork, the company should actively create a culture in which the employee can do the work at an appropriate level, as well as having the employee do less work. Second, it has been revealed that mental health problems affect the productivity of employees. The deterioration of mental

M. Lim (✉)
Pangyo Samsung Psychiatric Clinic,
Seongnam-si, Gyeonggi-do, Republic of South Korea

J.-H. Chae, H.-Y. Lee (eds.), *Meditation in Psychiatry and General Medicine*,
https://doi.org/10.1007/978-981-95-7147-5_21

health due to work stress can lead to frequent absenteeism and tardiness, which eventually leads to the resignation of skilled workers. It can also reduce the morale of the organization to which they belong and affect the relationships within the organization, thereby increasing the stress level of other people involved. Ultimately, deterioration of mental health can affect organizational productivity.

There are several differences between clinical practice and mental health interventions at the workplace. While clinical trials focus on the diagnosis and treatment of psychiatric diseases, efforts related to mental health at work focus on disease prevention and stress management. Psychiatric treatment in the clinical field is focused on the patient individual, but mental health management in the workplace is also important to the organization to which the individual belongs. In addition, it is important that mental health management in the workplace ultimately enhances individual work skills, enhances communication skills within the organization, and enhances productivity.

Reasons for the Introduction of Meditation

Workers are exposed to stress on a daily basis. According to studies on stress and work ability, it is known that when stress or appropriate pressure on work is applied to workers, their work ability improves in proportion. It can also be stressful if there is too little work pressure compared to the individual's ability. This is because it makes workers feel bored and adversely affects their identity as a worker. Therefore, as the pressure on work increases, the work ability may also improve. This is because the appropriate level of stress is given to work well by setting goals related to productivity. This appropriate stress can be called positive stress. However, work pressure above a certain level hinders work ability. Pressure that cannot be overcome by coping or adapting with one's own ability can be called negative stress. These negative stress results in depression and anxiety and reduces work ability.

Whether positive or negative stress, stress activates the sympathetic nervous system among the autonomic nervous system. Stress at work is often chronic. Pressure on work, conflicts in relationships with colleagues, and pressure on work performance are examples of chronic stress. Positive stress such as promotion also acts as chronic stress as the period of adaptation to new tasks or roles increases. Even constantly anticipating work difficulties becomes a chronic source of stress that activates the sympathetic nervous system.

Once the sympathetic nervous system is activated, adrenaline and noradrenaline are secreted, and blood pressure, pulse rate, and respiratory rate increase, triggering a "fight or flight" reaction. In the beginning, you are in a state where you can immerse yourself in a slightly tense state and perform your mission. However, if more than a certain amount of pressure is applied continuously, it causes negative consequences. Continuous hyperactivation of the sympathetic nervous system also causes inhibition of neural circuits that are not mobilized in that process. As a result, the learning ability to acquire new things decreases, anxiety and depression occur, and symptoms of overreacting to small stimuli appear. The hypothalamic-pituitary-adrenal axis is also involved, and adrenal hormones are secreted. As a result, immune function and nerve regeneration speed decrease, and nerve contraction occurs due to nerve overload. The sympathetic nervous system, which is chronically activated by stress, causes cognitive problems such as decreased attention, memory, and problem-solving ability, depression such as decreased energy and motivation, anxiety, fear, and sensitivity to surrounding stimuli. In this process, they gradually lose their resilience, cannot gradually do the things that usually restore themselves, and their human relationships gradually diminish and become alienated.

To reduce this response to stress, in 1979, Jon Kabat-Zinn's group developed the Mindfulness-Based Stress Reduction program (MBSR). Since then, several intervention programs based on mindfulness have emerged. With the introduction of these programs into the medical community, research related to meditation has also increased.

The results of the study on meditation summarized by Chaskalson and others are as follows.

1. People who are more mindful suffer less psychological distress such as depression and anxiety. A well-trained person is less neurotic, more outgoing, and reports more psychological well-being and satisfaction with life.
2. In the case of a well-trained person, he or she is more aware of his or her feelings, understands and accepts them, and can recover quickly when he or she feels hurt.
3. People who are more mindful have fewer negative thoughts, and even when negative thoughts occur, they can let them go easily.
4. People who are more mindful have stable and high self-esteem and are less shaken by external environmental factors.
5. People who are more mindful can enjoy more satisfying human relationships and communicate well with people. There is less discord in relationships with others, and there is less tendency to think negatively of the other person as a result of discord.
6. Mindfulness has a positive correlation with emotional intelligence, which is directly correlated with good sociality, the ability to cooperate, and the ability to see another person's perspective.
7. People who are more mindful are less likely to react defensively or aggressively when they feel threatened. Mindfulness increases self-awareness, and there is a positive correlation between mindfulness and vitality.
8. There is a correlation between good mindfulness and academic and personal achievement.
9. Meditation training increases concentration, occupational skills, productivity, and satisfaction with work, and builds better relationships with colleagues.
10. People who are more mindful control their behavior better, handle internal thoughts flexibly and control impulsive behavior well.
11. Meditation training increases blood flow, lowers blood pressure, and prevents the development of hypertension. This reduces the incidence and death of cardiovascular disease. In the case of cardiovascular disease, the severity of the disease can be reduced.
12. Meditating people are less hospitalized due to heart disease, cancer, and infectious diseases, and the number of outpatient visits is about half of those who do not meditate.
13. Mindfulness reduces addiction behavior and use of illegal drugs, prescribed medication, alcohol and caffeine.

Through non-judgmental perception training on thoughts, feelings, and senses, it is possible to clearly evaluate the perception of the current situation and the perception of one's ability to cope and prevent cognitive or emotional distortion of information processing. This reduces the responsiveness of the brain to negative emotional signals, which in turn reduces the stress response. These results related to the effects of meditation suggest that the use of meditation in the workplace can reduce workers' stress, increase efficiency, and increase creativity and productivity. In addition, meditation is shown to improve relationships with others, which is a very important virtue in the workplace that requires cooperation with colleagues. Therefore, programs targeting healthy office workers, not patients with diseases, are created and widely spread in the workplace, not in a medical environment.

An Example of Meditation at the Workplace

A Stress Reduction Program Based on Mindfulness

The Mindfulness-Based Stress Reduction (MBSR) program was created by John Cavatzin and has been implemented since 1979. The program runs over a total of 8 weeks. Mindfulness means intentionally paying attention nonjudgmentally to the here and now. Through this mindfulness, one trains to fully live here and now. This means not reacting automatically to stimuli, but living while actively making choices according to the situation.

MBSR consists largely of two forms of meditation. The first is official meditation, which is to stop what you are doing and perform it intentionally. These include breathing meditation, body scan, sitting meditation, and yoga. The second is informal meditation, which is a meditation that takes care of it while doing what is done in everyday life. These include eating, meditation, and mindful speaking and listening.

The program consists of nine sessions in 8 weeks. There are a total of 8 sessions held once a week for 2 h as a group, and on the 6th week weekend, there is a full day (6 h) meditation day for a total of 9 meetings. At times other than meetings, 45 min of individual meditation are given as homework every day.

Each session has its own theme. The first session is the introduction of participants and programs, and the second session connects to body scans with a topic of understanding the senses of the body. The third session is the time to learn and feel yoga. The fourth session is to recognize body reactions to stress, the fifth session is to recognize and accept stress as it is without responding to it in an autopilot state, and the sixth session is to overcome stress. The seventh session deals with the topics of eating and health, and the final eighth session concludes the entire session and concludes the program with plans for subsequent meditation.

Each session is designed to experience breathing meditation, sitting meditation, body scan, yoga, eating meditation, and walking according to the theme of the session, and as the session continues, the depth of meditation gradually increases. Until the sixth session, body scans or meditation is given as a task between sessions, but after the sixth session, after a full-day meditation training program, meditation should be trained more freely to suit each situation.

Low-dose MBSR is a simplified form of MBSR, which is modified for busy office workers. The session time has been reduced from 2 h to 1 h, the homework between sessions has been reduced to about 20 min, and meditation programs that work all day are omitted. Sharing sessions within the session mainly focus on discussing stress at work.

Google's Search Inside Yourself Program

The Search Inside Yourself (SIY) is a mindfulness-based emotional intelligence development program developed by Google's Chad-Meng Tan and launched in 2007. Emotional intelligence is the ability to monitor one's own and others' moods and emotions, discriminate against them, and use emotional information to think and act. This emotional intelligence allows you to have good work performance, excellent leadership, and the ability to create conditions for happiness. The fact that this emotional intelligence can be improved through training is also an important basis for this program.

This program has a clear scientific basis, is very practical, and is characterized by being written in a language that is easy for ordinary office workers to understand. The training period consists of a total of 20 h of courses for 7 weeks. Within that period, a total of three stages of training are conducted. The first step is attention training, which aims to bring participants into a calm and clear state of mind. The second stage is about self-understanding and self-control, which recognizes one's emotional flow in high resolution based on trained attention. The third step is to create useful mental habits, and it is about self-motivation, empathy, and leadership.

The Effects of Meditation on Office Workers

Research results of meditation programs for healthy workers are increasing. Here, we will briefly look at this.

First, programs based on mindfulness are effective in reducing stress and improving psychological ability when implemented for healthy workers.

It was found to reduce depression, anxiety, and tension and increase job satisfaction. Stress levels are lowered, and absences due to stress-related diseases are reduced. This is the same in the study comparing before and after participation in the program and in the study comparing the participating and non-participating groups.

Second, it was found that meditation programs based on mindfulness maintained good effects for a considerable period of time after the program. A study of the effects of MBSR on stress reduction among staff at a hospital showed that the effects of MBSR lasted throughout the year during the study period. In a study on the effectiveness of mindfulness-based programs in doctors, the stress of participants decreased after the program, and these results were found to last up to 15 months during the study period. In addition, after the program, participating doctors became more positive in their attitude toward patients, and the number of cases showing symptoms of burnout decreased further. This can be interpreted as the mindfulness-based program having a positive effect on their work.

Third, a short version of the meditation program tailored to the situation at work was also found to have a good effect. As a result of a meta-analysis of studies on the effect of performing the stress reduction program based on mindfulness as a whole and the effect of performing the short version, it was found that the effect of the two versions did not show a significant difference. This means that the length or method of the training program can be effectively adjusted according to the circumstances of the workplace, so that more people can receive meditation training and enjoy the positive effects of it.

Based on the results of research so far, mindfulness-based meditation programs do not seem to have a difference in stress relief from the effects of yoga or general relaxation programs. Body scan is a common factor of this intervention, and it may be because this common factor acts on the reduction of stress. In the future, further research is needed to find out the differences between each intervention.

Research so far has mainly focused on the stress reduction effect of meditation. In addition, many studies used the results of self-report tests on stress state and stress reduction. In future studies, it is necessary to develop indicators that can prove the effects of meditation more objectively. In addition, among the effects of meditation, research is needed on the effects of not only stress reduction but also improvement of personal ability, creativity in work, and relationship flexibility.

Conclusion

It was found that the introduction of the meditation program to the workplace restored the overall well-being and resilience of workers. In these workplaces, employees' stress levels are low, and absenteeism due to stress-related diseases is reduced. In addition, employees work more actively and productivity increases. Conflicts between employees will decrease and turnover will decrease. In addition, it can be expected that employee creativity and innovation will increase due to an increase in job satisfaction.

Bibliography

Carmody J, Baer RA. How long does a mindfulness-based stress reduction program need to be? A review of class contact hours and effect sizes for psychological distress. J Clin Psychol. 2009;65(6):627–38.

Chaskalson M. The mindful workplace, developing resilient individuals and resonant organizations with MBSR. Wiley-Blackwell; 2011.

Day A, Kelloway EK, Hurrel JJ. Workplace well-being: how to build psychologically healthy workplaces. John Wiley & Sons; 2018.

Geary C, Rosenthal SL. Sustained impact of MBSR on stress, well-being, and daily spiritual experiences for 1 year in academic health care employees. J Altern Complement Med. 2011;17(10):939–44.

Krasner MS, Epstein RM, Beckman H, et al. Association of an Educational Program in mindful communication

with burnout, empathy, and attitudes among primary care physicians. JAMA. 2009;302(12):1284–93.
Tan CM. Search inside yourself: Google's guide to enhancing productivity, creativity, and happiness. Emerald Publishing Limited; 2012.
Torbjörn J. The effects of a short-term mindfulness based intervention on self-reported mindfulness, decentering, executive attention, psychological health, and coping style: examining unique mindfulness effects and mediators. Mindfulness. 2012; 5(1):18–35.
Virgili M. Mindfulness-based interventions reduce psychological distress in working adults: a meta-analysis of intervention studies. Mindfulness. 2015;6:326–37.
Wolever RQ, Bobinet KJ, McCabe K, Mackenzie ER, Fekete E, Kusnick CA, et al. Effective and viable mind-body stress reduction in the workplace: a randomized controlled trial. J Occup Health Psychol. 2012;17(2):246–58.
Yarkes RM, Dodson JD. The relation of strength of stimulus to rapidity of habit- formation. J Comp Neurol Psychol. 1908;18:459–82.

Index

J.-H. Chae, H.-Y. Lee (eds.), *Meditation in Psychiatry and General Medicine*,
https://doi.org/10.1007/978-981-95-7147-5

MIX
Papier aus verantwortungsvollen Quellen
Paper from responsible sources
FSC® C105338

If you have any concerns about our products,
you can contact us on
ProductSafety@springernature.com

In case Publisher is established outside the EU,
the EU authorized representative is:
Springer Nature Customer Service Center GmbH
Europaplatz 3, 69115 Heidelberg, Germany

Printed by Libri Plureos GmbH
in Hamburg, Germany